The Treatment of Aphasia: From Theory to Practice

Edited by
Chris Code and Dave Müller

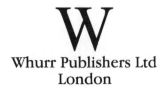

Whurr Publishers Ltd
London

British Library Cataloguing-in-Publication Data.
A catalogue record for this book is available from the
British Library.

ISBN 1-870332-33-4

Printed and bound in the UK by Athenaeum Press Ltd,
Gateshead, Tyne & Wear

Preface

There have been significant developments in the treatment of acquired language impairment over the last decade or so. We now have a well articulated theoretical framework for a variety of broad approaches and a research base to support the claim that aphasia therapy works.

In this book we have sought to bring together a comprehensive collection of chapters which will provide the reader with a survey of the current state of the art of aphasia therapy. We wanted to present theoretical reviews and the approaches which follow from theory. We hope we have done this. We wanted also to cover the manifestations of acquired language impairment in all modalities. This too we hope we have achieved. A further important aim for the book was to enlist an internationally representative group of authors. Our contributors are from Europe, America and Australia.

We believe this book will be accessible to students, clinicians, teachers and researchers in aphasia and related areas.

We have been aided in our efforts by our contributors who have worked hard to present scholarly but readable chapters that we hope have enabled us to achieve our aims. We are grateful to them for their patience with us and their response to our requests.

Chris Code and Dave Müller
(Sydney and Ipswich, 1955)

General preface

This series focuses upon disorders of speech language and communication, bringing together the techniques of analysis, assessment and treatment which are pertinent to the area. It aims to cover cognitive, linguistic, social and education aspects of language disability, and therefore has relevance within a number of disciplines. These include speech therapy, the education of children and adults with special needs, teachers of the deaf, teachers of English as a second language and of foreign languages, and educational and clinical psychology. The research and clinical findings from these various areas can usefully inform one another and, therefore, we hope one of the main functions of this series will be to put people within one profession in touch with developments in another. Thus, it is our editorial policy to ask authors to consider the implications of their findings for professions outside their own and for fields with which they have not been primarily concerned. We hope to engender an integrated approach to theory and practice and to produce a much-needed emphasis on the description and analysis of language as such, as well as on the provision of specific techniques of therapy, remediation and rehabilitation.

Whilst it has been our aim to restrict the series to the study of language disability, its scope goes considerably beyond this. Many previously neglected topics have been included where these seem to benefit from contemporary research in linguistics, psychology, medicine, sociology, education and English studies. Each volume puts its subject matter in perspective and provides an introductory slant to its presentation. In this way we hope to provide specialized studies which can be used as texts for components of teaching courses as undergraduate and postgraduate levels, as well as material directly applicable to the needs of professional workers.

David Crystal
Ruth Lesser
Margaret Snowling

Contributors

Evelyne Andreeswky
Institut National de la Sante et de la Recherche Mèdicale
INSERM-TLNP
Pavilion Claude Bernard
Hòpital de la Salpêtriere
47 Blvd de l'Hòpital
F-75634 Paris
CEDEX 13

Elizabeth M. Armstrong
Department of Speech Pathology
Royal Prince Alfred Hospital
Missenden Rd
Sydney, Australia

Shelagh Brumfitt
Department of Speech Science
University of Sheffield
Sheffield S10 2UR
England

Sally Byng
Department of Clinical Communication Studies
City University
Northampton Square
London EC1V 0HB
England

Sergio Carlomagno
Laboratorio di Neuropsicologica
Clinica e Neuroiabilitazione
Università degli Studi oli Napoli
11 Atenes
via Pansini 5,
Napoli
Italy

Françoise Cochu
Institut National de la Sante et de la Recherche Médicale
INSERM-TLNP
Pavillion Claude Bernard
Hòpital de la Salpâtriere
47 Blvd de l'Hópital
F-75634 Paris
CEDEX 13

Chris Code
School of Communication Disorders
University of Sydney
East St
Lidcombe
NSW 2141
Australia

M. Alison Crerar
Department of Computer Studies
Napier University
219 Colinton Rd
Edinburgh
Scotland

Anne Edmundson
The National Hospitals College of Speech Sciences
2 Wakefield St
London, WC1N 1PG
England

Susan Edwards
Department of Linguistic Science
University of Reading
Whiteknights
PO Box 218
Reading RG6 2AA
England

Andrew W. Ellis
Department of Psychology
University of York
Heslington
York YO1 5DD
England

Ralf Glindemann
Stattlich anerkannte Lehranstalt fur Logopaden
der Medizinischen Fakultat
der RWTH Aachen
Pauwelstrasse 30
D-5100 AACHEN
Germany

Allessandro Iavarone
Instituto di Scienze Neurologiche
Università Federica ll
Napals
Italy

Chris Marie Ireland
109 Burntwood Lane
London SW17 0AT
England

Richard C. Katz
Audiology & Speech Pathology
VA Medical Center
7th Street & Indian School Rd
Phoenix
Arizona 85012
USA

Ruth Lesser
Department of Speech
University of Newcastle
King George VI Building, Queen Victoria Road
Newcastle Upon Tyne NE1 7RU
England

Jaqueline McIntosh
The National Hospitals College of Speech Sciences
2 Wakefield St
London WC1N 1PG
England

Dave J. Müller
Suffolk College
Rope Walk
Ipswich IP4 1LT
Suffolk, England

Robert S. Pierce
School of Speech Pathology & Audiology
Kent State University
Kent
Ohio 44242
USA

Luise Springer
Stattlich anerkannte Lehranstalt fur Logopaden
der Medizinschen Fakultat
der RWTH Aachen
Pauwelstrasse 30
D-5100 AACHEN
Germany

Robert T. Wertz
VA Medical Center
Hearing & Speech Sciences
1310-24th Avenue
South Nashville
TN 37203
USA

Klaus Willmes
Neurologische Klinik
RWTH Aachen
Pauwelstrasse 30
D-52057 AACHEN
Germany

Linda Worrall
Department of Speech & Hearing
University of Queensland
Brisbane
Queensland 4072
Australia

Contents

Part I Treating the Individual

The first section in a book on the treatment of aphasia could address a wide range of topics. It would not be inappropriate to start with issues relating to diagnosis or indeed to overview a wide rang of theoretical perspectives relating to aphasia therapy. However, we have decided to include in our first section a set of linked papers which relate specifically to the requirement of all aphasiologists to address the individual needs of the aphasic person. This is, we believe, fundamental for those approaching the treatment of aphasia for the first time and to remind practising clinicians of the valuable role they play in helping the aphasic person regain his or her self respect in the context of the severe loss of language and related functions.

The importance of the individual in aphasia therapy is placed in a broad academic context in the challenging chapter by **Sally Byng**. She argues that our knowledge of aphasia therapy does not fully reflect the interaction between therapists and individuals with aphasia. She suggests that the relationship of treatment tends to be directed towards the language impairment or disability rather than focusing on the individual aphasic person. Instead, she suggests that therapy is an interactive process and that therapists and individuals with aphasia should be equal partners, hence emphasizing the role of the individual with aphasia in influencing and indeed determining the nature of the therapeutic process. She describes an interactional analysis which is an attempt to describe the process of therapy. This important chapter recognizes that at the heart of the process of therapy are those individuals with aphasia. It behoves all of us involved in the treatment of aphasia to regularly ask ourselves, 'What is aphasia therapy?' as a means of helping us monitor and reflect on our own practice.

The chapter which follows by **Shelagh Brumfitt** highlights the important contribution that psychotherapy can make in the treatment of aphasia. This chapter presents the case for aphasia therapists giving careful consideration to introducing and making available a wide range of psychotherapeutic techniques. It is recognized that not every aphasia

1

therapist is necessarily qualified to offer psychotherapy, but that those who do need to have a strong background in aphasia and indeed to have studied professionally in an appropriate and related field.

These suggestions are in line with the experiences documented by **Chris Ireland** in the following chapter and do highlight the need for developing approaches to the treatment of aphasia which explore eclectic approaches to supporting the individual. Her chapter is a very personal account of the impact of aphasia on one individual. Chris draws together her experiences and describes her own journey of self exploration in coming to understand from a personal perspective the impact of aphasia. This chapter is at the heart of coming to understand the needs of individuals with aphasia and is important to appreciate in the context of the development and evaluation of methods for treating each person with aphasia as an individual. This chapter makes a powerful and positive contribution to the literature.

Chapter 1
What is Aphasia Therapy?

SALLY BYNG

In a book on cognitive approaches to rehabilitation Basso (1989) makes the following pertinent observation about aphasia therapy:

> .. it is very difficult to know what aphasia therapy is... What occurs under the heading of aphasia rehabilitation in one place may have nothing in common with what occurs in a different place except for the fact that a speech therapist and a patient interact with each other. (p. 17, 23)

That this can be accurate reflection of the state of the art is concerning coming after several decades of published literature on aphasia therapy. The statement highlights a major problem: how can therapy be either developed, evaluated or communicated if we are not even clear what it is that we are considering?

In this chapter I shall suggest that the origin of these problems stems from the fact that currently our knowledge about therapy is *implicit*. As long as it remains implicit, therapy as a discipline in its own right will continue to be secondary to what seems to be considered the more theoretically robust, even respectable, field of diagnosis and will remain undervalued. I will reflect on why knowledge about therapy remains implicit, and explore ways in which we could be more explicit.

The Scope of Aphasia Therapy

In clarifying those aspects of the process of therapy for aphasia that are implicit, I am referring only to a part of the intervention that a therapist might undertake with a person with aphasia, that is the work that is carried out on the language impairment itself. The whole scope of a speech and language therapist's intervention with someone recovering from aphasia is, of course, much broader, as follows:

- a delineation of the uses of language made by the person with aphasia prior to becoming aphasic;

- facilitation of accomodation to changed communication skills;
- an investigation of the nature and effects of the language deficit with respect to the whole language system;
- an attempt to remediate the language deficit itself;
- an increase in the use of all other potential means of communication to support, facilitate and compensate for the impaired language;
- an enhancement of the use of the remaining language;
- an opportunity to use newly acquired and emerging language and communication skills, not just in a clinical environment, but in more familiar communicative situations;
- an attempt to change the communication skills of those around the person with aphasia to accomodate the aphasia. (Byng, 1993: 127–8)

This broad scope demonstrates the variety of skills with which a therapist needs to approach each person with aphasia. However, the kinds of therapeutic skills that I want to consider here are those that pertain, primarily, to the attempt to remediate the language problem itself. Methods of analysing the deficit have received a lot of attention, and although an accurate diagnosis of the deficit is an essential component of successful therapy, scant attention has been paid to analysing the process of therapy, so that the therapy itself has become the poor relation of the whole process or rehabilitation in aphasia.

The Implicit Nature of Knowledge about Therapy

Why has our knowledge of therapy become so implicit? Asking therapists to be explicit about exactly what they are doing in therapy is a hard task, not because therapists are unaware of what they are doing, but for two principle reasons. One is expressed by Howard and Hatfield (1987) as follows:

> Theoretically-motivated work from a variety of viewpoints has provided detailed analyses of the deficits underlying some aphasic patients' difficulties. Compared with these sophisticated analyses, many therapists' treatment techniques that are used in day-to-day practice appear too simple; they do not feel as if they do justice to the complexity of the problem. We suggest that this is because there is no explicit metatheory available that explicitly relates a deficit analysis to the process of treatment (p. 5).

The second reason is that what a therapist does becomes somehow intrinsic to his or her performance as a therapist. There seems to be an 'automatic pilot' that a good therapist develops and then switches on which suggests how to present a task, how and when to modulate it, how to respond to a specific response by the person with aphasia, and so on. Therapists make these decisions all the time, but on the basis of what criteria are these decisions made? How do we judge if we are right? How do we evaluate whether the therapy was appropriate and if it wasn't, what part of it to modify – the task, our interaction with the patient, the materials? Many therapists would call whatever process takes over *clinical intuition*, or the outcome of experience. The implication of these two responses is that there is nothing that can be done to make a good aphasia therapist, you either have to 'have it' or have to be told.

There will always be major aspects of the dynamic between the therapist and the person with whom he or she is working that cannot be captured by tangible means, but this does not mean that the whole process has to remain inaccessible to exploration, description and measurement. The process of therapy can be taken apart, to some extent, to explore how change through therapy is effected. Once a body of empirical data has been assembled the formulation of a theory of therapy can be attempted which would relate the analysis of the deficit to the process of therapy, as advocated by Howard and Hatfield.

What methods are available currently to make therapy explicit? In general the published literature provides the primary means of communicating therapy attempts between therapists. Howard and Hatfield (1987) approached their study of the field by describing eight different schools of aphasia therapy, such as the behaviourist school, the cognitive neuropsychological school, the pragmatic school and so on. They defined their delineation of the literature into these schools as 'Each of these is a group of therapists who hold certain common assumptions about the process of therapy and the nature of aphasia' (p.4).

This division of the literature into schools may, however, be misleading because it implies that the therapy process itself differs from one school to another, but it is not clear that such an assumption can be made. This is not to say that the therapy process would not be different from one approach to another, but rather that we do not know whether it is different, because the literature across all schools of aphasia therapy is not explicit in the details about the process of therapy, something generally referred to as a process about which we share a common understanding. I take Basso's observation, cited earlier, to mean that you cannot predict what kind of interchange is going to take place between patient and therapist, even if you know what sort of approach to therapy is being adopted. Yet is not the interaction between therapist and aphasic a primary point at which the therapy occurs?

The Literature on Aphasia Therapy: How is Therapy Reported?

In general, published therapy studies report very specific attempts at therapy, such as the outcome of one particular task or the effects of remediation of one particular aspect of the language deficit. Performance on a range of tasks or on a range of aspects of the language impairment is rarely systematically reported, in order to follow through all the stages of therapy. Longitudinal studies of remediation almost do not exist. The closest is the report that someone had *plateaued*, with the aphasia remaining stable for some time. Some reference might be made to the content of earlier therapy, but not in any detail. Most studies reported are of a relatively short duration – but the description of the therapy in those studies of long duration is not necessarily more involved and informative than the description of therapy given for a study of short duration.

The literature, therefore, does not reflect what happens in real clinical practice, when the therapist may see the person with aphasia up to several times a week for several months, working on a range of different aspects of the effects of the aphasia, constantly making decisions about what to do next. Any clinical aphasia therapist knows that to fill even one hourly session per week demands, if not a lot of materials, a lot of ideas and concepts about therapy tasks and ways of modifying the task and the materials as therapy is proceeding.

A major purpose of publishing studies describing therapy for aphasia must be to advance our knowledge about effective and relevant therapy procedures and develop our understanding about the process of therapy, so that other clinicians can read these studies and consider the methods described. However, Wertz (1984) suggests that in the literature concerning therapy for aphasia 'the tried is rarely tested', which suggests that the methods that have been described have not been very fully evaluated. Given the substantial literature on specific, successful therapies, it is surprising not to find more examples in the literature of these procedures being replicated. There are strikingly few studies which attempt faithfully to recreate a therapy previously described and to examine its effects further. If we look at other disciplines, such as experimental psychology, for example, we can see that work in that field has developed through different researchers replicating and extending the findings of other workers in the field, in order to refine the experimental effects and to examine crucial variables. We rarely see this kind of development in therapy. Some approaches might have been regularly applied, such as Schuell's stimulation approach, but because the level of detail about exactly what the therapy demanded is so general, it is hard to know how consistently the approach is being applied.

If we take the position of the clinician who might turn to the literature to discover what therapies might be appropriate, for whom, and how they should be applied, it soon becomes apparent that there are a number of basic assumptions underlying the way therapy has been described in the studies. I will go on to examine these in relation to some of the key elements involved in planning therapy that a clinician might be looking for. Although few specific studies will be cited, I would assert that there are general trends running throughout much (although not all) of the literature.

Determining the aim of therapy

There are a number of premises which might underlie the decision about the focus or aim of therapy, for example, the aim of therapy might be selected for its relevance to day to day language needs, or be based simply on an observed symptom or on a deficit highlighted in a standardized test (cf Byng and Lesser, 1993), amongst other things. In the majority of therapy studies, however, the aim for the selected focus of therapy is either not specified or seems to be based on the observation of a symptom. For example, the person with aphasia cannot name pictures so naming pictures is the aim of therapy. The functional utility of a therapy is often only sketchily specified, as is the relationship of the aspect of language being worked on to other aspects of the language deficit. Thus the relationship of the therapy to either the person's use of language, or to the overall language disorder is, in most cases, left unspecified. Perhaps some of the difficulty in demonstrating the effectiveness of therapy relates to this lack of specificity about the overall focus of therapy; if it is not clear what the focus for a therapy is within a person with aphasia's needs, it is hard to evaluate whether it has been successful.

Determining the rationale for therapy

The specification of the rationale for the therapy, that is, how the therapy is going to achieve the aims of the intervention, is a crucial aspect of the linking between the analysis of the deficit and the therapy procedure itself. A therapy procedure might be designed either to restore the functioning of an impaired aspect of language, eradicate a symptom, or establish a more efficient use of impaired language, for example. In the literature, however, the means by which the therapy is supposed to work is rarely specified in detail; there seems to be a general assumption that therapy will just modify the language in some unspecified way. This is not just an omission of theoretical interest, but one that has real implications for therapy. For example, what does the concept of restoration mean? Does it mean putting back something that is lost, and if so, how can that be achieved? Therapy might proceed differently depending on the hypothesis formulated.

Determining the strategies used in therapy

There is also lack of clarity about the strategies being used in therapy. The therapy could be intended to work on the function directly, or to establish an alternative means of carrying out that function or to bypass it altogether. If a decision is made to focus on gestural communication, then it is clear that the disordered function is being bypassed, but in cases other than these it is rare to find a specification that the therapy is requiring a function to be carried out using processes different from those with which it is normally carried out. Melodic Intonation Therapy (MIT) (Sparks, Helm and Albert, 1984) provides a good example of an attempt to specify the alternative mechanisms, that is right hemisphere involvement, but MIT could also be interpreted as the enhancement of a strategy used in normal language processing, of using information from prosodic contours. Thus even for relatively well-defined therapy procedures, the manner in which they may be working remains unclear.

Determining the tasks used in therapy

The tasks to be used in therapy are, in contrast, usually well described, especially those used in studies from a behavioural tradition and latterly the cognitive neuropsychological methodologies. Often the materials and the method of presentation are carefully described, but this level of details contrasts sharply with how the interactions in therapy are described.

Describing interactions in therapy

The interaction between the therapist and the person with aphasia is the point at which the therapy could be said to take place, and is therefore perhaps the most important part of the therapy process to describe. Yet it is the most difficult information to try to tease out of the literature. Again, studies with a behavioural orientation are often the clearest at describing what it is that the person with aphasia has to do, and these studies specify exactly how the therapist should respond. But there are two problems here – usually the range of permitted responses is extremely limited and has to be adhered to, and second, the manner of responding to the person does not generally appear to be dependent on any hypothesis about what the therapy is supposed to be doing for the person with aphasia. Thus the theoretical rationale for why the response made by the therapist should be effective in facilitating change to the language system is not made explicit.

Feedback is usually limited to correct or incorrect, but is rarely qualitative. Yet how many therapists in practice do not explain to someone with whom they are working why they had just done what they had done, or would not modify the task on the observation of patterns of performance. I am not suggesting that strictly behavioural studies, where procedures are adhered to and not modified, are necessarily inappropriate. What I am suggesting is that much therapy, in practice, does not proceed like that, in Britain at least. If we are to study how therapy proceeds, as practised by clinicians, we need to ensure that our studies reflect clinical practice (see Byng and Black, in press, for further discussion).

Additionally, in the vast majority of studies, a target response is demanded of the person with aphasia. Few published therapies allow the production of original language. There is rarely any flexibility described such as 'if the person does *a*, then the therapist does *x*, but if the person does *b* then the therapist does *y* and then goes on to *z*.' Admittedly this kind of therapy is harder to describe on paper and to transmit to other therapists, but we should not restrict the content and description of therapy interactions to those that can be explained easily.

Measurement of the effects of therapy

The effects of a therapy are often described in relatively limited terms. First, there is rarely an attempt to look at the effects of the treatment on an untreated but related function or an untreated, unrelated function. Equally, attempts to specify why there should be generalization to other items or functions are rare. However, the absence of any rationale for generalization does not stop researchers anticipating that generalization should take place. Using instruments for measurement of therapy effects, such as standardized tests, which assume that generalization, certainly across items if not across tasks, must take place, otherwise these methods of measurement would be seen to be inappropriate as barometers of change.

Assumptions underlying many approaches to therapy

A number of basic assumptions underlying many approaches to therapy are revealed as follows:

1. Practising a language task affects the language system and will thereby bring about some change in language processing. What this change might be and how the change is effected is not specified; there seems to be some implicit relationship between the task and the deficit that does not need to be spelled out.
2. The therapy is synonymous with the task. Therapy is described in terms of the tasks implemented, such as picture-sentence matching, repetition, picture pointing, and so on. A good example of this is PACE therapy (Davis and Wilcox, 1981; Glindeman and Springer, this volume) which is often described as an approach to therapy, whereas a more accurate description would be as a useful medium through which the therapy can take place. It does not describe the therapy itself, which would be the means by which the therapist conveys to the aphasic person how he or she can take advantage of all the means

of communication that they can utilize. Thus, in a description of therapy in which PACE has been used, a therapist would need to specify how, for example, a gestural or drawing technique was facilitated.

3. The parts of the therapy process which might have effected changes are not considered independently. Most therapies described do not represent a single therapeutic process, even if they involve only a single task. A single task might require a number of complex processes, but it may not be clear which of these processes was the most important for effecting change.

4. The person with aphasia often appears to be a passive recipient of therapy and has merely to practise, hence much of the existing literature could be thought of as describing *training* rather than therapy, which would involve an interactive process.

5. Therapeutic procedures, such as knowing when and how to modulate, modify and change the therapy are not accounted for, and thus may be undervalued.

6. The language to be used by the person with aphasia is very often specified in advance by the therapy task. Relatively few published therapy studies provide a chance for the person to use and modify his or her own language. Thus it is hard to see how this kind of therapy relates to the position that the person most often finds him- or herself in, of wanting to convey some entirely novel idea or piece of information.

7. Concepts of generalization are underdeveloped and based on unfounded assumptions, such as that practise on some items should affect similar untreated items and possibly bring about change in other aspects of language processing without a clear rationale for this taking place. Generalization is also often assumed to be the transfer of skills learnt in therapy to other situations, without specific planning for how this could be achieved.

The process of therapy

So far, although the process of therapy has been highlighted as a neglected entity, it has not been defined. By the *process of therapy* I am describing an essentially interactive process in which the therapist and the person with aphasia should be equal partners. Therapy can be conceptualized as comprising five main protagonists: the person with aphasia, the therapist, the language impairments and preservations, the focus of the therapy – either a specific aspect of the language impairment, a strategy to circumvent it or a preserved aspect to be emphasized – and the task and materials. As I have just suggested, the literature, in general, seems to take seriously only the role of the therapist and the task and materials; the aphasic person's part in the process is often neglected or is seen purely as the end point of what the therapist does with the materials. The impact of the aphasic person's response on what the therapist does is not generally considered.

But if we are considering therapy to be an interactive process, then the part of the person with aphasia has to be taken seriously. This shift of focus has implications for the way we are going to conceptualize, plan and implement therapy. These are not confined simply to such measures as including materials of interest to the patient or similar palliatives. Presumably any therapist is going to try to engage and empathize with the person with whom he or she is working. Rather I am trying to get at something more specific, which I will go on to describe.

First, the person with aphasia should, severity of communication disorder permitting, be involved actively in the decision about the focus of therapy, and insights offered should be interpreted and taken seriously. Keeping the five protagonists of therapy in mind, in the planning stages of therapy we need to consider the following:

1. How are the materials to be selected? What psycholinguistic and cognitive properties should they have and how do these relate to the nature of the impairment and the purpose of the therapy?
2. How are the materials to be used, i.e. what kind of tasks are we going to employ? This decision needs to be related explicitly to the hypothesis about what the focus of the therapy. The task and the materials are the *medium through which the therapy takes place*, rather than the focus of the therapy.

As an illustrative example I should like to contrast two therapy studies designed to remediate the same kind of language problem, but employing two very different tasks. Two therapy studies were carried out independently (Jones, 1986; Bying, 1988) with two people with agrammatic aphasia, whose spoken language was characterized by telegrammatic, single word or phrase utterances. Both therapies were based on the same hypothesis that the reason that these people could not produce structured utterances was because they had difficulty in co-ordinating aspects of the form of a sentence with its meaning and aimed to elucidate how these aspects are co-ordinated. However, the therapy proceeded in very different ways.

In Jones' study, BB was required to make judgements about sentences in response to questions about the role played by different constituents in the sentence. In the study I carried out, JG was required to order the written constituents of a sentence to match two pictures, to demonstrate what role a particular constituent played in the sentence meaning and how that role was represented in the structure of the sentence. In addition, having learnt some specific information about the structure of sentences in English through the task, JG was encouraged to use that knowledge to assist him in producing sentences. The results of the two different therapies were somewhat similar. Both people who had been aphasic for some years prior to the therapy made measurable gains in production of structured spoken language. In BB's case this was all the more remarkable because not only were the gains extensive but also he was not required to produce any language during the therapy.

The point of this illustration is to demonstrate that although the tasks were different, in one case a series of judgement tasks and in the other a sentence-ordering task and sentence-picture matching task, what was being conveyed *through* the tasks was the same or very similar. This highlights the need to recognize that the therapy is more than the task.

3. Central to this conceptualiztion of therapy is to anticipate a way of responding in qualitatively different ways to the person's responses. For example, what facilitators will be used, in the form of cues or different forms of feedback? Is the feedback intended merely to tell the person whether he or she is right or wrong? Or is it intended to inform the person about why a particular type of response or error was made, and how he or she might modify that response on the next occasion? Or, equally importantly, we might want to demonstrate how something that the person construes as an error is quite acceptable and communicative or a how a particular feature of the person's preserved communication skills can be developed further into an effective strategy. This is the point of interaction between the person with aphasia and the therapist that I am suggesting is crucial for an understanding of how the therapy process works and also possibly to the success of the therapy. I have already suggested that currently there exists no adequate methodology for describing this interaction.

4. I am making an assumption that the person with aphasia has to have some concept or understanding about the language impairment and how to modify it and work it before therapy can be meaningful. Only then can people with aphasia become active partners in therapy. Having a concept of the nature of the language impairment may not necessarily be at a conscious level, but may be tacitly or unconsciously comprehended. The person with aphasia does not, therefore, need to be especially motivated or insightful to be a real partner in therapy. Related to this point is that attempts to change language or communication processes have to relate to the person's *own* concept of what is wrong or he or she will not be in a position to be an active partner in therapy.

An analysis of interactions in therapy

One of the aspects of the process of therapy, therefore, that seems to almost entirely lacking from accounts of therapy is a description of the interactions between the therapist and the person with aphasia through which the therapy is conveyed. In order to provide an illustration of some aspects of the interaction that takes place between the aphasic person and the therapist, I shall present the results of a very preliminary attempt to capture the interactions in a particular therapy.

This interactional analysis, which is currently being developed more extensively (Byng and Jones 1993), is an experimental attempt to develop ways of describing the process of therapy. This analysis does not provide a model to be copied but rather a preliminary method of increasing awareness of the impact of each of the protagonists on the behaviour of the other. It may begin to alert us to a range of different dimensions when we are both planning and evaluating therapy.

The therapy that I shall describe represents three sessions taken out of weekly therapy that Dr Audrey Holland (AH) was carrying out with an aphasic man, LC. LC had good language comprehension skills, both for auditorily presented and written language. His spoken language was fairly fluent, but he had considerable word-finding problems, which responded to a variety of different cue types. His spoken language tended to sound empty and fragmentary because he had to leave an utterance incomplete when he got stuck for a specific word or a means of conveying his idea. Written naming was often easier than spoken naming. The therapy was intended to facilitate word retrieval, especially of verbs.

This study was carried out by videotaping these three therapy sessions, each of which involved a different task. Having transcribed these tapes, every interaction that took place was coded first by a single observer deriving the classification system from observation of the behaviours, and then by a group of speech and language pathologists viewing the tape together. The codes were analysed to look for patterns in the types of interaction that took place, that is, the aim of this procedure was to establish what LC said in response to AH and also to see what kind of responses AH made in reply to what kind of utterance made by LC.

As a result of the observational classification system, two main groups of interaction were observed for LC and four for AH. These were each subdivided into a number of different categories, but these will not be described further here. The two main groups for LC comprised *specific target responses* where he produced either a single word or a phrase or sentence in order to convey the information he wanted to get across. These responses could be either correct responses, related in form, or unrelated responses. The second group were termed *interactional responses* and these represented utterances which either developed a theme which he had already started, or which were comments made by LC on his own performance. They also included light conversational interchange.

The types of responses that AH made fell into four main groups. The first group consisted of *specific word information* cues, where some information about a specific lexical item that LC could not retrieve was provided. These cues could be phonological cues, orthographic cues, or simply a direct question which defines the area of search. A second category of cue type consisted of *supportive feedback strategies*, which included such parameters as elaboration or clarification of LC's utterances, positive feedback, requests for information etc.

A third category entitled *problem-solving feedback cues* represented a way of externalizing for LC for the word-finding process, and explaining the kinds of errors that he was making. In this way he was given information through which he could modify his own language and correct his own errors. These cues did not actually give LC direct information about the word for which he was searching, but helped him to retrieve information for himself. In this way these cues seem qualitatively different from the specific word information cues. The final category called *conceptual focus* cues represented a focus on a topic or theme by the therapist, or a refocusing by the therapist in response to a theme introduced by the LC.

Having coded every utterance made by AH and LC, the following features of their interactions were analysed: the most frequent response type for both therapist and aphasic; the type of interaction that most often resulted in LC producing a target response; the change in the proportion of response types in relation to the task; the pattern of response types made by LC in response to different cue types produced by AH; and the pattern of cue types made by AH in response to different response types produced by LC.

Some interesting aspects of the analysis which provide some qualitative information about how AH and LC interacted will be described briefly here. The number of responses classified as falling within each major category for both LC and AH remained fairly constant across the three sessions. LC produced on average twice as many specific target responses as interactional responses, although he did produce a good many of these, including being able to introduce a new topic or theme. AH also produced a similar pattern of cue types across the sessions, with the most frequently used cue being a specific word cue, closely followed by the supportive feedback strategies. Problem-solving feedback cues represented only a fairly small proportion of the total number of cues.

It is of particular interest to find out what kind of cues tended to precede LC's successful attempts to retrieve his target utterance. All cue categories preceded target responses, although at first glance it seemed that, in the cases where LC could not immediately retrieve the desired word or phrase, the largest number of targets were produced in response to a specific word cue or a supportive feedback strategy. We could suggest that these are the most effective cue types, however, when the total number of times a cue category was used is considered, it seems that problem-solving feedback cues were as good as specific word cures at eliciting targets. Thus all the strategies used to facilitate word retrieval were useful for LC.

In trying to determine what LC said in response to what kind of cue from AH, one or two features of the data will be picked out here. When AH used a specific word cue, on the majority of occasions LC replied with a specific target response of some kind. It is interesting to note that LC produced more target responses after the type of cue that represents a direct question than he did after being given some partial phonological information, although that was an effective cue type also. Maybe a direct question about a specific target focused retrieval more accurately and he could make use of this semantic information better than the phonological information.

Supportive feedback cues elicited both interactional responses and specific targets. There were no predominant patterns observable in the subcategories, however, there was one observation here of interest. AH often used positive feedback even when LC's response was not quite correct. The analysis showed that after such feedback LC often went on to produce the target correctly, even if he had been struggling severely. One feature of AH's therapy is to encourage the person with aphasia to accept a less than perfect piece of language if the communicative content has been conveyed, hence her use of this kind of cue. This piece of data suggests that this might indeed be an effective strategy – perhaps once the pressure was off, LC could more easily produce the target correctly.

The analysis also suggests what type of response from LC prompted which response from AH. Not surprisingly the conceptual focus cues nearly always followed a target response – AH moved on to another topic or point on LC's successful completion of a prior point. She produced more specific word responses than feedback strategies to specific targets responses from LC. There were some trends such as a tendency to use partial written cues after LC commented on his performance. These represented a comment from LC to indicate that he did not know a word, so AH gave him some of the letters to cue him. In addition AH often followed an elaboration of the topic by LC with a question to elicit a specific target. In this way she seemed to be picking up what LC wanted to express and getting him to be more specific.

AH used more supportive feedback strategies in response to interactional responses from LC, which presumably reflects normal communicative interaction. The strategy of using positive feedback in the presence of an error tended to be used specifically in response to a phonological approximation or an incorrect repetition. In these cases,

LC had struggled unsuccessfully for some time, and AH encouraged him to accept something less than the correct target. This seemed to be an effective strategy for LC. AH often used positive feedback after target responses, but a strategy of affirming and repeating back what LC had just said when he achieved a target was also evident. AH responded to LC's elaboration of a topic with an elaboration herself, again presumably a normal communicative interaction. The problem-solving feedback cues were used following a target response, as if to explain something about how LC got to, or had trouble getting to, the word he sought. They also followed a comment by LC on his performance.

There are a number of hypotheses that can be drawn from the data which can only be answered by further detailed study. For example, it would be interesting to know which of these response parameters AH would use when working with another aphasic person with word retrieval problems of a different origin, or which parameters are kept constant and which are more subject to change in line with change in the person. Keeping track of responsiveness to cues, for example, the ability to produce an interactional response to a feedback strategy, might be another way of monitoring progress in therapy. So often we are aware of change which is then hard to demonstrate in formal testing. It may be that what has changed is the ability of the person with aphasia to provide different kinds of responses to different kinds of input. Keeping track of the input and what it has elicited may provide useful data on progress to back up the therapist's observations.

This analysis is still at a developmental stage and, as yet, based on very little data, so these interpretations should be treated cautiously and with circumspection. A considerable amount of work remains to be done to develop this into a realistic tool for examining interactions in therapy (Byng and Jones, 1993). However, these preliminary data suggest that it may be possible to look in detail at patterns in the psycholinguistic dynamics between the therapist and the person with aphasia, if not the psychodynamics. With the kind of information gathered from this analysis, one could envisage passing on to another therapist or to a student some specific strategies or cues that could be adopted in a specific therapy for certain types of language impairment. A therapy could be planned round the categories of cue types to be used, that is, what kind of information or strategies will be conveyed and how, or what specific forms of feedback/information will be provided, in relation to the specific target of therapy. Information could be gathered for friends or family members about specific strategies to facilitate communication with the person who is aphasic.

Future research into therapy must reflect the clinical reality of therapy and not conform necessarily to received models about how to do experiments. Therapy is a discipline in its own right that demands the development of a methodology appropriate to its practice. Until we find some ways of examining the process of therapy itself we will not be able to relate the therapy to the disorder to generate theories of therapy. Making therapy explicit, and thereby recognizing the skills it requires, is not only vital for the development of our therapeutic skills, but also to realize the full potential of our service to people with aphasia.

Acknowledgements

This paper was first presented as the Seventh Annual Mary Law Lecture for Action for Dysphasic Adults, to whom I am most grateful for the opportunity to put together these ideas, which were formulated during the tenure of a Harkness Fellowship in the United States. I am indebted to Dr Rita Berndt, Maria Black, Dr Audrey Holland, Eirian Jones and Charlotte Mitchum for many illuminating discussions, which have contributed invaluably to the development of these ideas, and to AH and LC for allowing me to report on their therapy sessions which were coded collaboratively with Margie Forbes and Dr Davida Fromm.

References

Basso A (1989) Spontaneous recovery and language rehabilitation. In Seron X and Deloche G (Eds) Cognitive Approaches in Neuropsychological Rehabilitation. Hillsdale NJ: Lawrence Erlbaum Associates.

Byng S (1988) Sentence processing deficits: theory and therapy. Cognitive Neuropsychology 5(6): 629–76.

Byng S (1993) Hypothesis testing and aphasia therapy. In Holland A and Forbes M (Eds) Aphasia Treatment: World Perspectives San Diego, CA: Singular Publishing Group Inc.

Byng S, Black M (in press) What makes a therapy? Some parameters of therapeutic intervention in aphasia. European Journal of Disorders of Communication.

Byng S, Lesser R (1993) A review of therapy at the level of the sentence in aphasia. In Paradis M (Ed) Foundations of Aphasia Rehabilitation, Oxford: Pergamon.

Byng S, Jones EV (1993) Interactions in therapy. Paper presented at the British Aphasiology Society Conference, University of Warwick, UK.

Davis A, Wilcox J (1981) Incorporating parameters of natural conversation in aphasia treatment. In Chapey R. (Ed) Language intervention strategies in adult aphasia. 1st ed. Baltimore MD: Williams and Wilkins.

Howard D, Hatfield FM (1987) Aphasia Therapy: Historical and Contemporary Issues. Hove and London: Lawrence Erlbaum Associates.

Jones EV (1986) Building the foundations for sentence production in a non-fluent aphasic. British Journal of Disorders of Communication 21: 63–82.

Sparkes R, Helm N, Albert M (1974) Aphasia rehabilitation resulting from melodic intonation therapy. Cortex 10: 303–16.

Wertz RT (1984) Language disorders in adults. State of the clinical art. In Holland A, (Ed) Language Disorders in Adults. San Diego, CA: College-Hill. pp 1–77.

Chapter 2
Psychotherapy in Aphasia

SHELAGH BRUMFITT

Introduction

> If one uses the term Psychotherapy broadly, it is fair to say that all health professionals who interact with the patient have an opportunity, and perhaps ought to assume the responsibility, to incorporate psychotherapeutic principles in these interactions. This is probably true of the aphasia therapist and is undoubtedly widely practised by experienced speech pathologists (Sarno, 1981, p. 480).

Clinicians have long been aware of the distress experienced by aphasic patient, carer and family, but have been confused about the best way to respond to the problem. In Great Britain certainly, the psychotherapeutic approach is often controversial. Yet as Sarno (1981) indicates, the emotional needs of the aphasic patient have to be met in order to achieve the most satisfactory outcome in rehabilitation for both patient and relative.

Lewis and Rosenburg (1990) note that although there is literature on the use of psychotherapy with people who have congenital brain damage, or mild acquired neurological problems, there is very little on people with significant acquired damage. Yet it is these people with significant difficulties who have the major adjustment problems which may cause a poor outcome in rehabilitation. In addition, the specific needs of the aphasic patient are frequently overlooked in the literature which exists about generalized acquired brain damage.

An important distinction has been made about the process of psychotherapy with acquired brain damage. In general, psychotherapy is offered to people who are experiencing increased difficulty in coping with their lives. In contrast, the brain damaged person is forced to cope with a totally unpredicated event. Thus, although the concepts of psychotherapy are similar, the reason for it being offered are profoundly different.

The Application of Psychotherapy to Brain Damage

There are many features of psychotherapy with people who have general acquired brain damage which can be applied to aphasic people and their carers. For example, the head injured person is often offered psychotherapeutic help, and Rollin (1987) discusses the specific needs of this client group. Particular note is made of the effects on the family and the use of family caregiver support groups which aim to ameliorate some of the stress of living with a multihandicapped person. He suggests that family therapy be used to complement individual counselling.

Lewis and Rosenberg (1990) describe two main psychological disturbances which can be experienced by the acquired brain injured. These relate to anxiety, and problems with identity and self esteem. The anxiety appears to be frequently related to the increasing awareness of the deficit, but also to preexisting character traits and the point in the individual's life when the trauma took place. (For example, someone may experience a severe head injury when his or her life is in the midst of important other changes, such as, when leaving home and starting a family.)

Lewis and Rosenberg (1990) note how misleading it has been in past literature to view low self esteem experienced by these patients as entirely a neurological condition. Importantly, low self esteem and depression can result in poor motivation for rehabilitation. Indeed, patients can often be excluded from rehabilitation on the grounds of being poorly motivated. However, Lewis and Rosenberg (1990) stress the importance of working with these patients to help them understand what makes them depressed, and thus to help them work through their intense sadness. Mohl and Burstein (1982), quoted by Lewis and Rosenberg suggest that brain injury undermines the sense of self resulting in a 'disintegration of identity experienced as feelings of vulnerability, fragility and hopelessness' (1990, p.74).

The psychotherapy suggested by Lewis and Rosenberg 1990) focuses on helping the patient to express distress, eventually directing the patient's attention on to preserved abilities in order to make a connection with past and present self, also allowing time for the patient to mourn the lost self before a new self can emerge.

Pickett (1991) discusses the use of imagery psychotherapy in head injury rehabilitation. This approach is intended to help the patient work through the feelings of loss which have resulted from head injury and then to be able to adapt more creatively to the disability. Pickett views imagery as being particularly helpful in rehabilitation because using the imagination can be a relatively simple process which allows the individual a full sensory experience. This may aid memory ability in general and according to Pickett may be used to promote areas of the brain that have been unaffected by the trauma to assist the traumatized area. It is suggested that imagery helps the individual to understand more of a situation because the process uses all the senses (such as smell and taste) and that this increases the power of the image being developed. This may then help to reduce the confusion that occurs following brain damage. Although many of the statements by Pickett are based on clinical observation only and are very controversial, issues are addressed which need and deserve further exploration.

Other interesting approaches are described in the literature. Family therapy has been used to alleviate some of the adjustment difficulties experienced by patient and family. Soderstrom, et al. (1988) presented a model for crisis intervention and family therapy for head injured adults. Of particular interest is the fact that the patient is approached by a member of the psychotherapeutic team within ten days of admission to a neurosurgical ward. Although many patients may not be ready for psychotherapy, at least the principle is established of attempting to meet the emotional needs of the patient. When the patient is ready, crisis intervention procedures and family therapy are made available. Preliminary results suggested that patients who participated in the programme achieved an overall better adjustment to life as measured on the Psycho-Social Functioning questionnaire (developed by the research team).

Solomon and Scherzer (1991) offer some specific guidelines for family therapists working with the brain injured and their families. Their approach recommends a team consisting of a therapist specializing in family therapy and a therapist specializing in rehabilitation neuro-psychology. In a paper which presents a lot of practical detail, the reader is alerted to the roles the therapists need to take on in order to be effective. Note is made of the importance of sometimes being very direct with brain injured patients in order to increase their ability to organize and understand their lives. The therapist must provide the patient and family with information and feedback, but must be sensitive to manipulation by the patient or from the family members. This can affect the therapeutic relationship, but importantly it can undermine the strength of the family support unit if individuals feel they are being manipulated.

In addition to these approaches, there have been other attempts to help the acquired brain damaged person with the use of hypnosis (Crasilneck and Hall, 1970). In this approach hypnosis has been used to increase motivation towards recovery. Geva and Stern (1985) have reported a project which uses dreams as a way of enhancing the psychotherapeutic process. They argue that dream analysis does not require complex cognitive abilities and can counteract problems patients may have in using language and abstract concepts. Although patients are reported as initially having difficulty in remembering their dreams, persistence over time will achieve some success. The patients are first described as reporting short, simple dreams followed by dreams which are longer and more complicated and recounted more frequently. It is suggested that the use of these dreams in the therapeutic process is helpful in reintegrating the patient with the premorbid self.

The application of group psychotherapy to aphasic people

Blackman (1950) used group psychotherapy with aphasics injured mostly during the Second World War. The aim was to get the patient feeling better understood and more able to cope with rehabilitation. The group situation which Blackman described allowed the patients time to draw approval and support from other members. A particular note is made of the patient's renewed dependency on others. Often, the patient's dependency on spouse throws up feelings about parental relationships, 'a relationship from which he was emancipated at one time, but which has become again an actuality because of the head injury' (p. 156). Often these feelings would need to be drawn out in the therapy. The group also offered time for outpouring of hostility; this was seen as an important initial stage in the therapeutic process. Only when the anger and hostility about what had happened to them had been released, could the individuals move on to building a new identity. In later sessions one of the most positive remarks is recorded. 'In talking with the group and thinking about things important to us, makes me use more words. I also have a feeling that I stimulate and make some of the other members, who are not as verbal as I am, more talkative' (p. 158).

Blackman summarized the benefits as being about offering the aphasic an opportunity to express hostility and anger in a safe context. It also allowed the individual to develop a stronger sense of self, and by doing so, lessened the individual's need for dependency on parental figures.

Redinger, et al. (1971) reported on preliminary work which evaluated the effectiveness of group therapy with aphasic people. Of note, is the attempt to combine speech therapy with approaches generally used in psychiatry. At the beginning of the project, the group was set up for aphasic people only, but it immediately became clear that the aphasic people (who were significantly impaired) were very reliant on their spouses when attempting to communicate. Thus, spouses were included in the group. Six aphasic people attended regularly, with four accompanying spouses.

Three distinct stages were found to occur in the evolution of the group.

1. An initial period of anxiety, confusion and severe difficulty communicating with each other.
2. A period of complaints, misgivings and disappointments towards the home situation, the hospital environments and social circumstances.
3. A period of mutual understanding, friendliness and better adaptation to the home, the outside, and the hospital (p. 90).

The group was found to be helpful in many ways, particularly because it helped to break down some of the barriers which had built up since the aphasia had occurred and also because it allowed the exploration of conflicts (both intra and inter-personal) in a controlled setting with professionals available to give appropriate support. The authors noted the usefulness of being able to alternate between an intensely psychotherapeutic group and a social one. Often, the social compatibility enhanced the expression of topics which were painful. For example, the group often discussed food as a group of friends might. On one occasion, however, a member of the group revealed how painful it had been to find her friend expressing surprise that she could still cook even though she was now aphasic. The group member was able to talk about her loss of self respect and identity over this incident in the group context and gain support and understanding from the other members.

Group Psychotherapy for Spouses and Relatives of Aphasic People

The effect on the spouse and relatives of the aphasic person has been examined by many authors and summarized in Müller (1992). What is clear is that spouses and families experience many problems in adjusting to life with aphasic person and are frequently not given sufficient support. Williams and Freer (1986), for example, found that specific areas of concern for spouses of aphasic patients were the reduction in emotional support now available, and the changed life-style and sexual relationship with the partner.

Bardach (1969) has evaluated group therapy with wives of aphasic patients and concluded that these are an important adjunct to the total rehabilitation of the person. The wives were reported to have found that sharing the distress felt about their husbands' disability was a tremendous release which allowed them opportunities to express anger and frustration not revealed before. Derman and Manaster (1967) also reported the effectiveness of group therapy for spouses which appeared to improve aphasic and spouse relationships and clinician and patient relationships.

Währborg (1989) and Währborg and Borenstein (1989) have been influential in developing the concept of family therapy for aphasic people and their families. Their aims are to increase the family's sensitivity to the changes in the way the family unit functions and to allow them opportunity to express their distress at these changes which have been forced upon them. The therapist must emphasize the positive side of the family in the assumption that all members are aiming for an improvement in adjustment. Of interest is the focus on encouraging all family members to adjust their means of communicating with each other, rather than focusing solely on the aphasic person's way of communicating. Währborg and Borenstein (1990), in their evaluation of family therapy, concluded that most changes were observed in the aphasic person in terms of a reduction of depression and emotional and social isolation. As Währborg (1991) states. 'The aphasic state cannot be changed by family therapy but the quality of communication can' (p. 86).

Helping the individual aphasic person

There are many strands in the psychotherapeutic encounter which can be woven into the interaction in a speech and language therapy session (Brumfitt and Clarke, 1983; Ireland, this volume). Often, these facts of the interaction are implicit and not stated. If a therapist is able to be open enough to accept this sort of therapeutic relationship, the patient can start to attend to emotional needs as well as more straightforward remedial requirements. It may be that in the early stages of recovery, individual support and understanding is less threatening for the person than a group situation. What is certain, is that, as with the group therapy sessions, the aphasic person needs to feel understood in order to feel safe enough to express feelings. By allowing these feelings to be expressed, the person may be more open to rehabilitation and as Steward (1985) suggests 'Emotional healing must inevitably influence physical healing' (p. 81).

Brumfitt (1989) discusses the emotional responses of the aphasic person in relation to the features of bereavement described by Murray Parkes (1978). The process of realization which the newly bereaved person experiences is applied to the predicament of the aphasic person. It is noted that this process may take much longer in rehabilitation than is often acknowledged for the communication failure experienced by the aphasic person occurs only in a limited context in the hospital setting. When the aphasic person experiences the world outside, the full extent of the communication difficulties are then finally understood. Brumfitt (1989) emphasizes the importance of this in a rehabilitation setting. The response from the aphasic person may fluctuate depending on this or her experience outside. If the individual becomes acutely aware of failure he or she may be too immersed in distress to focus on rehabilitation.

Murray Parkes (1978) has also described the bereaved person's urge to search for the person who has been lost by death. Brumfitt (1989) draws parallels here with the aphasic predicament in that the person may be acutely aware of what life was like before. The sense of identity from the past may be a useful link in helping the person to establish a new identity. It is recommended that the aphasic person be allowed time to talk about the past self as a way of providing a more secure base from which to move forward. Being able to feel that part of him or herself is still intact can be very healing experience.

Rollin (1987) discusses some of the strategies that should be used when offering help. Of interest is his discussion on helping the person stop denying the disability. An example of this occurs when an aphasic person believes that one day recovery will spontaneously be complete, so that active involvement in rehabilitation is not necessary. A similar difficulty arises when an aphasic perceives the communication problem to be less than it really is. Rollin suggests that it is important to acknowledge this belief in the hope that this may stimulate discussion about the reality of the situation. Although denial has been rigorously discussed by Tanner and Gerstenberger (1988) and Gordon, Hibbard and Morgenstein (1988), my clinical experience suggests that there is at least a subgroup of aphasic people for whom denial is a means of avoiding psychological pain. These people need sensitive help if they are to come to terms with what has really happened to them. The duration of denial is certainly an important issue here. Denial in the short term may allow the person to buy time before facing the realities of the situation, whereas long term denial can only impede any sort of progress in rehabilitation.

Rollin also acknowledges the place of premorbid psychological problems and the difficulties faced by therapists who are trying to progress with rehabilitation. Trying to understand what has happened to the person before he or she became aphasic can often be productive and may often be the key to the person's behaviour now. Skenderian (1983) reports the man who suffered overwhelming feelings of imprisonment, degradation and isolation on becoming hemiplegic. In therapy the man revealed that he had been a prisoner in a concentration camp 40 years before and the present paralysis had brought to the surface many of the feelings he had experienced about imprisonment. Similarly, the balance of the relationship in a marriage may cause difficulties in the post-aphasic state. A clinical example of this occurred in a male aphasic and hemiplegic patient who refused to practise exercises for walking at home because in his words he 'had run about all his life for his wife and now it was time for her to do it all'.

Language Impairment and Psychotherapy

One of the assumptions made about psychotherapy is that the person can express feelings when given the opportunity to do so. Indeed, psychotherapy is often called the *talking cure*. Rollin (1987) describes the situation of professionals without training in speech and language therapy refusing to work with the aphasic person because he 'doesn't speak' (p. 64). There is no doubt that the aphasia is an added difficulty that may be overwhelming. Yet, the case for offering help is even stronger because the aphasic situation is so incongruous; the communication skills cause the emotional pain, yet the remaining communication skills have to be used to relieve distress. (Brumfitt, 1989).

It is well accepted that the non communication-impaired person will be less fluent when struggling to express emotion which is just coming to the surface. Being at a loss for words is well known to everyone. Thus the aphasic person's attempts at expressing emotion may need to be listened to with great care. Statements to check the person's feelings may need to be made more frequently than in a conventional psychotherapeutic situation. It may be necessary to be more directive than feels comfortable to help the aphasic clarify thoughts. Drawings and picture stimulus of different emotions may be necessary. Exploring the meaning of the loss of communication to the individual may be extremely difficult to do, but the application of the laddering technique as in Personal Construct Theory, can be productive (Fransella and Dalton, 1990). This can give a basis for moving forward and can be a useful task with some types of aphasic people.

With the severely impaired person such as in global aphasia, it may be unrealistic to think of psychotherapy as a long term process. Yet these people are frequently overlooked. What can be offered is an acknowledgement of the sadness and distress of the situation. The therapist may need to make statements about feelings for the individual. For example, 'I know you are feeling sad today.' This can be followed up with a drawing of a sad face and presented as a question, to explore how it really is. Although there is the obvious and ironic risk of putting words in the patient's mouth, it has to be appreciated that there is probably no-one else who is going to do this. The globally aphasic person may feel desperately trapped with unexpressed feelings and may be grateful for the therapist's attempt to unravel them. Brumfitt (unpublished case discussion, 1991) describes a severely impaired girl who was able to move through her emotional recovery by relying on the therapist to make statements about how she might be feeling, and then confirming or disconfirming those statements.

Future considerations

Although some doubt has been expressed about the lack of documentation of the neurological effects on emotion in aphasia, (Gordon, Hibbard and Morgenstein, 1988), it is clear that emotions are felt and expressed, and that therapists have to face these issues on an everyday basis. We clearly do need to find ways of assessing the feelings of aphasic people, particularly the severely impaired global aphasics who are frequently excluded from aphasia studies. The application of Personal Construct Theory (Kelly, 1955) has been partly explored (Brumfitt, 1985) to look at the aphasic person's self constructions in relation to other significant people. In this, the needs of the severely impaired individual are explored by developing picture stimulus as an aid to using a repertory grid. This work needs to be taken further. The Personal Relations Index developed by Mulhall (1977, 1978) looks at the interpersonal judgements of aphasic people and their families. Währborg (1991) however, comments on the lengthy time the administration of this procedure takes. The Code-Muller Protocols (Code and Müller, 1992) are now available for therapists to explore the aphasic perceptions of aphasic people, the significant others and therapists in their lives using a very simple procedure to aid counselling. Brumfitt and Sheeran (1995) are currently developing a visual measure of self perception.

Because so much of the literature applies the grief experience to the aphasic person's reaction (Tanner and Gerstenberger, 1988; Währborg, 1991; Brumfitt 1989), it is important for the phases of grieving to be studies more systematically. The relationship of the loss of language to emotional expression also needs to be explored. Part of the difficulty lies with the area of studies of emotion in general. Documenting an individual's emotional development is problematic if the individual is only expressing the emotion in a safe and valued therapeutic relationship. Finding an opportunity to record those emotions may seem contradictory to clinical work and it is understandable that this area is the least explored in aphasiology.

However, there are several forms of psychotherapy which could be explored further in relation to the aphasic's plight. For example, drama therapy may well have some potential. Art therapy, although not a pure form of psychotherapy, could also provide great opportunities, particularly for the severely impaired. As discussed earlier, the work by Pickett (1991) on imagery needs to be explored further, as does the work by Geva and Stern (1985) on the use of dreams. Little has been mentioned about the problems faced by aphasic people in resuming a sexual relationship, yet clinically it is known that physical difficulties may occur if there is a hemiplegia, and there may be specific difficulties associated with communicating sexual interest and needs. Wiig (1973) started the work on offering counselling in sexuality for the aphasic person, but this has not been further developed.

Whether or not psychotherapy becomes part of every therapist's clinical approach has yet to be determined, but as Währborg discusses, there have to be certain factors which are constant. The therapist has to be an aphasiologist in order to make full use of the aphasic patient's remaining abilities and in order to understand the range of problems which the patient might experience. The aphasic person must understand that psychotherapy is taking place and be willing for this to happen. Finally, Währborg emphasizes that the techniques which are used in psychotherapy need to accept communication attempts in any form (1991: p. 89).

There is a generally more accepting climate for expression of emotion than there was even 10 years ago. It is seen as much more acceptable for people to acknowledge feelings without seeming weak. Examples of this relate to many of the major disasters which have occurred during the last decade where group support and psychotherapeutic help is seen as an essential part of recovery. Although we are still exploring the efficacy of psychotherapy and counselling in aphasia, there is enough evidence to suggest that it is an important area for future development.

References

Bardach JL (1969) Group sessions with wives of aphasic patients. International Journal of Group Psychotherapy 19: 361–5.

Blackman N (1950) Group psychotherapy with aphasics. Journal of Nervous and Mental Disease 111: 154–63.

Brumfitt SM (1985) The use of repertory grids with aphasic people. In Beail N. (Ed) Repertory Grid Techique and Personal Constructs. London: Croom Helm 89–106.

Brumfitt SM (1989) A psychosocial case discussion. In proceedings of the summer conference of the British Aphasiology Society. Cambridge.

Brumfitt SM, Clarke PRF (1983) An application of psychotherapeutic techniques to the management of aphasia. In Code C, Müller D. Aphasia Therapy. London: Arnold.

Code C, Müller DH (1992) The Code-Müller Protocols. London: Whurr.

Crasilneck HB and Hall JA (1970) The use of hypnosis in the rehabilitation of complicated vascular and post-traumatic neurological patients. Journal of Clinical and Experimental Hypnosis 18(3); 145–59.

Derman S, Manaster A (1967) Family counselling with relatives of aphasic patients at Schwab Rehabilitation Hospital ASHA 9(5): 175–7.

Fransella F, Dalton P (1990) Personal Construct Counselling in Action. London: Sage Publications.

Geva N, Stern JM (1985) The use of dreams as a psychotherapeutic technique with brain injured patients. Scandinavian Journal of Rehabilitation Medicine-supplement 12: 47–9.

Gordon W, Hibbard M, Morgenstein S (1988) Response to Tanner and Gerstenberger Aphasiology 2 (1): 85–8.

Kelly GA (1955) The psychology of personal constructs. New York: Norton.

Lewis L, Rosenberg SJ (1990) Psychoanalytic psychotherapy with brain-injured adult psychiatric patients of Journal of Nervous and Mental disease 178 (2): 69–77.

Mohl PC, Burstein AG (1982) The application of Kohutian self psychology to consultation liaison psychiatry. General Hospital Psychiatry 4: 113–19. In Lewis L, Rosenberg S (1990) Psychoanalytic psychotherapy with brain injured adult psychiatric patients. Journal of Nervous and Mental Disease 178 (2): 69–77.

Mulhall DJ (1977) The representation of personal relationships: an automated system. International Journal of Man-Machine Studies 9: 315–35.

Mulhall, DJ. (1978) Dysphasic stroke and the influence of their relatives. British Journal of Disorders of Communication 13: 127–34.

Muller DJ (1992) Psychosocial aspects of aphasia. In Blanken et al. Linguistic Disorders and Pathologies: An International Handbook. Berlin and New York: Walter Degruyter.

Murray Parkes C (1978) Bereavement. Middlesex: Pelican

Pickett E (1991) Programme development: Imagery psychotherapy in head injury trauma rehabilitation. Brain Injury 5 (1): 33–41.

Redinger RA, Forster S, Dolphin MK, Godduhn J, Weisinger J (1971) Group therapy in the rehabilitation of the severely asphasic and hemiplegic in the late stages. Scandianvian Journal of Rehabilitation Medicine 3(1): 89–91.

Rollin WJ (1987) The Psychology of Communication Disorders in Individuals and their Families. Englewood Cliffs NJ: Prentice Hall.

Sarno J (1981) Emotional aspects of aphasia. In Sarno MT (Ed) Acquired Aphasia. New York: Academic Press.

Skenderian D (1983) Psychological aftermath of stroke: reflection of a personal construct psychologist. Paper presented at Fifth International Congress on personal construct psychology. Boston MA.

Soderstrom S, Fogelsjoo A, Fugi-Meyer KS, Stenson S (1988) A programme for crisis-intervention after traumatic brain injury. Scandinavian Journal of Rehabilitation Medicine–supplement 17: 47–9.

Solomon CR, Scherzer BP (1991) Some guidelines for family therapists working with the traumatically brain injured and their families. Brain Injury 5(3): 253–66.

Stewart W (1985) Counselling in rehabilitation. London: Croom Helm.

Tanner D, Gerstenberger D (1988) The grief response in neuropathologies of speech and language. Aphrasiology 2(1): 79–84.

Währborg P (1989) Aphasia and family therapy. Aphasiology 3: 479–82.

Währborg P (1991) Assessment and management of emotional and psychosocial reactions to brain damage and aphasia. Kibworth: Far communications.

Währborg P, Borenstein P (1987) Depression after stroke, some nosological considerations. Proceedings, First European Conference on Aphasiology. Vienna: Austrain Workers Compensation Board.

Währborg P (1989) Boreustein (1989) Aphasia and family therapy. Aphasiology 3: 479–82.

Wiig EH (1973). Counselling the adult aphasic for sexual readjustment. Rehabilitation Counselling Bulletin 17(2): 110–19.

Williams and Freer (1986) Archives of physical medicine. Rehabilitation 67: 250–2.

Chapter 3
100 Years on From Freud's *On Aphasia*: From Patient to Counsellor

CHRIS MARIE IRELAND

Introduction

For someone like me, who had a stroke nearly five years ago and lost her language completely (unable to talk, understand, read or write), to undertake the writing of this paper is a wonderful celebration of my battle for an active and involving life with others.

I am very grateful to have the opportunity to learn amongst so many people – my psychoanalyst, my speech therapist, friends and family, medical allies and new colleagues. I particularly appreciate my good friend, Jim Payne, who corrected my linguistic errors and typed the original draft, Roberta Green, who corrected my linguistic errors in the final chapter, Lyn Gregory, who typed it and Phil Sizer, who helped with the tables. Partnerships – good relationships – are the crux for human growth, particularly in the ability to depend on others when you have lost your previous capacity ('mature dependence', Fairbairn 1952). A psychotherapist once said that it is as important to learn to read people as it is to read books as the time we have is limited (Bion quoted 1990). Reading and writing are not easy skills now for me, but I keep on. I am a teacher and counsellor by profession and adapt my counselling skills to help others to face their loss, as I have.

To become less articulate, to lose one's fluency, to struggle with linguistic complexities, to face health problems and pain are very difficult tasks – but they can also give you a positive attitude. They keep you in touch with both basic and raw needs and enable you to see more of the caring issues in life. In this, the Kleinian approach is helpful for me – to see that every 'have' is balanced by a 'have not'; that there is no gain in life without a corresponding loss and that ambivalent feelings are inevitable within a complex life.

In this chapter I explore the losses with regards to language and the gains in adaptation to the disability. I draw some issues from the grieving models, examining the analytic process in the main, but also the humanistic and behavioural approaches when appropriate. I look at the effects of language disability on self-concept and personal relationships, and explore the partnerships between professionals and clients in the medical arena and within the therapeutic alliance.

There are also the issues around the non-disabled people's fears and defences regarding disability, particularly language problems. I contest that disability is a challenge which inevitably raises deep feelings within professionals. If this occurs they either need to attend to it by going through psychotherapy or counselling for themselves, or must at least be aware of their own limitations and refer on to trained counsellors (Jones and Byng 1989).

The Psycho-Analytic Process and Psychodynamic Counselling

I tried to read Freud's (1891) monograph *On Aphasia*. The paper was published 100 years ago, but, as a person with dysphasia, it is not accessible to me and probably only makes sense for those with neurological or linguistic training. Rizzuto (1990) indicated it was this monograph that laid the foundation of psychoanalysis, with the same concepts – object associations, representations, self-observations, spontaneous speech and transference. In seeking scientific validity for psychoanalysis and using a paternalistic style, I see the traditional Freudian approach as too detached and over-interpretative as in Freud's 1905 classical study of hysteria. But he was the pioneer of the psychodynamic approach as a rebelling child within his culture and time in the Victorian era; others have now introduced more humanity and spontaneity, to suit present times (e.g. Rycroft, 1985; Lomas, 1986; Miller, 1987a; 1987b 1990; 1991). Miller highlighted that child abuse was ignored by classical psycho-analysis.

Through the process of psychoanalysis, I own my growth – it belongs to me. My psychoanalyst needed to adapt to my needs and my language problems. At first, he needed to use helpful guessing to understand my communications (he was careful not to over-interpret and I showed my anger if I found him over the top). I had to write parts of words on a notebook as I was unable to say some words and worked sitting instead of lying on a couch. I needed visual cues. I transferred a lot of my anger onto him (some belonged to him and some to others. I remember I wrote down the words 'soul murder'. (I have recently come across the term in Rycroft's 1985 book.) I went, and am still going, through a cycle of very raw, basic emotions; hate, anger, sadness, depression, envy, greed, guilt, pain, vulnerability, and also understanding and growth of courage, love, adaptability, honesty and compassion.

I went back on the psychoanalyst's couch for a time. On one hand this is freeing, but I still have problems in building up trust because of the 'silent treatment'. At times, the therapist's silence can make you feel like being abandoned. As France put it; 'Total silence very rarely conveys warmth or friendliness' (1988). Sometimes silence can allow transference – uncomfortable early memories. At times it can be very painful and traumatic, particularly for a person with language impairment disability, to check out more than ordinary conversation – and analysis is not just an or ordinary conversation! Flexibility is needed: silence can allow you to explore the unconscious issues, free associations, dreams, etc. – raw data – but it can sometimes give a cold, uncaring message. But silence, as Luterman (1984) put it, is also a primary vehicle for promoting responsibility and it is vital...that we do not take that responsibility from the client.

Psychoanalysis is not easy. It is a demanding task which takes courage, energy, time and *money*! There are many difficulties. It is important to break down defences very slowly, at the pace of the patient, who is sometimes unable to cope well. There can also be unreality, or a distortion of reality, within the consulting room. But instead you have 'focus' giving time to reflect on the outside reality and the inner real feelings.

I am aware of these difficulties, so I work on them. I believe the art of the psychoanalytic process can allow people to get in touch with their basic needs and build up self-knowledge and self-belief – become more real 'through a personal act of understanding' to seek to find truth (Symington 1986). The process can allow individuals to tell their own story in their own words and in their choices of words even with their problems with language. This is a 'talk cure' and, given attentive listening, can go on to explore the inner world. I like the way Casement (1990) writes about the tension between 'wanting to create the atmosphere of a sandpit (playing with different shapes) rather than that of a court room' (p. 13).

Within the psychodynamic process applied in counselling there is the 'triangle of insight': 'Linking in the past will only produce relief and response, when it is relevant to a client's current experiences outside the counselling room, or present within it' (Jacobs, 1985: 11). The client, through transference, sees counselling as a mirroring of less-than-ideal parenting; the counsellor is not constantly available; acts like a controlling parent to set limits (time of session, rules – e.g., no acting out here – and payment) and is like an oedipal parent – not available as a partner for the client. The process is about re-experiencing, in order to grow within boundaries.

We are all affected by our past experiences. The only person I know who had a stroke died a few months later. I had bad experiences in staying in hospital as a child and as an adult. Losing language is losing a central part of the self. Past fears and anxieties (see Segal, 1985, both unconscious phantasies and couscious fantasies in everyday life). In the early days after a stroke, it is common to have fears of death and life feels out of control. Later there are fantasies, for instance, that sex might cause harm. The Kleinian (1940; 1956) element of the paranoid-schizoid was there – the 'why me?' feeling; the splitting of an idealized self before the stroke from a useless image after; the feeling of being robbed (raw feelings – fantasies of murderous/suicidal feelings) and of greed elements including the envy of others who seem to lead such enviable, independent, strong, active, social lives. There is also raw rage, if one allows oneself to express it.

The depressive position, which is adult depression, is a reactivation of infantile depression occurring in the actual mourning situation as an awareness of loss. This is a painful process. It helps people, through counselling/psychotherapy and transference, to go back to the source of their anxiety and, if someone else acknowledges their suffering, it can help them in the therapeutic processes of reconciliation and reparation. Transference allows negative and positive aspects of both hate and love and permits investigative meanings behind everyday issues. The basic fundamental task of transference 'is the road that will lead step by step to where the basic problem lies, in each individual case' (Herman, 1985).

To combat their problems in language people with dysphasia can explore alternative means of expressing themselves. There is an opportunity to tap inner resources and build up inner trust. I think many people cover their insecurity by too much talking with too little reflection. People with dysphasia can also develop their intuitive aspects to pick up hidden messages and body language. Other Jungian elements are also helpful – to explore *feeling* and *sensory*, and inner *thinking* through one-to-one reflective conversation for goals of self-understanding and self-realization (Jung, 1958). Music and other arts can also tap into spiritual and physical relaxation to build inner strength. Paining helps me to express deep feelings and communicate and explore in analysis – an adventure to the inner self as in Milner's work (1950). I am more aware of colour, shapes, images and body language since my stroke – like a visual compensation.

Losing language means that the person might need to face a *false self* (Winnicott 1986), built up from a lack of good enough parenting in childhood. Counselling can help a person to discover his or her *true self* – real need for love and care and the right to feel anger with others from the past.

Elements of Experience: Impairments and Disabilities in Dysphasia

I found the psychoanalytic approaches helpful to understand the complex process entailed in grieving, having myself had major losses (deaths, divorce, illness). Freud (1917) was the first to decide the process of grief work to help us to understand the term *object loss* (which is losing something or someone to whom one is attached). It is important that one of the goals of grief is to break the bond between the griever (the subject) and the deceased (the object).

In acquiring a disability, or losing an able self, adults may feel very distressed; it can help them understand that distress if they explore past experiences of loss or disablement, or childhood traumas or anxieties. People who have language problems frequently also experience the embarrassment of the inability of others to react constructively towards their difficulty in speaking. I have found some ignorance and embarrassment in public reaction. (This can be compared to the difficulty of reacting to the griever (Parkes, 1972).

I draw from other various psychoanalytic and psychotherapeutic studies to explain mourning through the losing of a *significant person* (of oneself – self-image before the stroke) and attachment, e.g. Bowlby, 1979; 1981; Erikson, 1965; Kast, 1990; Parkes, 1972; Leick and David-Nielsen, 1991; Miller 1987a; 1987b; 1990; 1991). The grief models are helpful but do not give a full picture. I prefer the term *elements* rather than the stages of grief models. With dysphasia there are no clear-cut stages. There is a constant struggle and people find themselves oscillating from one side to the other, particularly in new situations and in stress. I find it helpful to use the concept of *ongoing loss* (Leick and David-Nielsen, 1991).

Within my education and language experience, it is important to adapt theories/studies to each of our own life experiences thus becoming our own experts to debate and integrate inner knowledge. With chronic illness and language disability, the client can perceive him or herself both as a child and as an elderly person – with little or less energy – and feel more vulnerable and perhaps have other health problems, such as heart/blood problems; epilepsy. It is helpful for each person as a responsible adult to work on his or her own needs and processes and learn to taste life for qualitative rather than quantitative factors.

I have adapted various perspectives to my experience and to others (see Table 3.1). The table is an outline of the issues – dynamic, complex, unfolding and changeable:

There is debate between the *psychoanalytic approach* to language loss after having a stroke, which Tanner and Gerstenberger (1988) described as an emotional process characterized by language as a *symbol loss*, which can be followed by denial and depression, and eventually by acceptance and resignation, and the *medical model*, which views the patient's depression as one of the results of brain damage, not a psychological reaction (Gordon et al., 1988). As Tanner and Gerstenberger put it, 'A patient's psychological status cannot be separated from the neuropathology of speech and language' (1988:84). We must bear in mind that there could be the possibility of the presence of organic depression which may need treatment by medication. I see

Table 3.1 Exploring elements of the emotional issues of dysphasia after a stroke

A   Trauma - Confusion/shock

No or few words. Difficult to communicate and not to be understood.
Perhaps problems in use of one side of body.
(Elements of numbness, anxiety, very lonely, raw, fear, denial, dreamlike, etc.)

B   Anger - Chaotic emotions

(Elements of rage, why me?, raw feelings with the frustration with
problems in language and fighting for help, feeling the loss and abuse,
shame, pain, hate, splitting, greed, envy, fantasies/phantasies, etc.)

C   Mourning - Chaotic emotions

(Elements of grieving, the experience of loss, despair, depression, guilt,
sadness, 'alarm' (Parkes' term), 'stressed out' (Ireland's term), fears,
jealousy, vulnerability, powerless, loneliness, anxiety, etc.)

D   Searching, finding and separation

Searching	- Reflect on the past
	- Review the life-process
Finding	- Consent to the loss
	- Acquisition of skills
Separation	- Bargaining – give and take
	- Learning to process

E   Understanding, adaptation and acceptance

Gains and Losses	- Build confidence/courage/patience/care/sensitivity
	- More 'real' (Experimental)
	- Independence and Dependence
	- New creative/self expressive dimensions
Adjustment	- re language and physical disability (tiredness/travelling/pain/noise, etc.)
	- Working on 'pacing' and 'tactics'
Meaning of illness to each person	- Issue of understanding and acceptance but keeping on fighting and seeking if needed
	- Constant struggle: empowerment/ongoing loss, with others within social world

within the speech/language therapist's profession an entwining of the
competing approaches between the medical world and the emotional
processes which allow the patient to work on through the normal
process of grieving (as in Brumfitt, 1986 and Chapter 2, this volume).

I needed help from both my speech/language therapist to build my
linguistic skills, and from my psychoanalyst to face my losses and build
ego-strength to adapt and continue the emotional growth. I also

needed help from the medical personnel for my physical ailments. I think it is important to separate (and it is hard to do this) the physical problems, which need medical attention, and the psychosomatic symptoms, which rightly belong to the influence of 'avoided grief' as expressed by Leick and Davidsen-Nielsen (1991).

In summary, there are problems of delayed grief (which may come up later – perhaps by response to other unrelated, emotional triggers); avoided grief (psychosomatic illness/psychological – unreleased, repressed, pathological or disguised grief); and chronic grief (unable to grow through it).

Bowlby (1981) saw chronic mourning as a prolongation or extension of his first of four phases from numbing to extending 'to distorted versions of phrases of yearning and searching, disorganisation and despair' (p.138). People get trapped, with no opportunity to talk through their situation. As Parkes (1972) concluded in his studies, they need to be given 'the opportunity to talk freely about the disturbing problems and feelings that preoccupied them' (p.47). Counselling allows the client to give him or herself permission to grieve and to show that it is normal in spite of the intensity. One can also give support by identifying and discussing defences and coping styles which may lead to a denial of grieving.

Leick and Davidsen-Nielsen talk of grief work as *healing pain*. This is a demanding and tough process. The client will be very uncertain and vulnerable in trying to cope with the separation from the loss. The counsellor needs to be emotionally confrontational and in this psychotherapeutic experience can be very helpful. The counsellor also needs good skills in active listening, allowing the client to tell the stories in his or her own words and pace in confidence and building up trust.

The grieving model helps towards understanding of the emotional affects, which aspects of the disability of a stroke and language loss have had, but it is not necessarily in clear chronological steps or stages. I have accepted many of the limitations imposed by my impairments, but daily experiences provide challenges and give reminders that I need to confront the problem of how to learn again, to cope, and to keep on fighting against disability barriers (see Finkelstein and French, 1993). There is constant struggling; independence is crucial for self-respect and has to co-exist with the dependence of relying on others for help. It is an ambivalent process in Kleinian terms. The process is tiring and demanding and with physical problems and pain, it is natural to retreat. With help, one can come to terms with emotional pain, and this can give insights, but I do not see comparable benefits from the struggle against physical pain. The adult stripped of the skill of complex language, but still having intelligence, understanding and expertise developed through life, has to face the stripping of his or her defences, which are often based on language skills, after a stroke. The vulnerable feeling is similar to the insecurity of a child who is not understood by others, nor able to express complex meanings. The scale of vulnerability and difficulties are affected also by others' understanding and reactions and society's views of disability.

The adult's feeling of being striped bare and raw in counselling/psychotherapy can give him or her an opportunity to meet those feelings of loneliness isolation, anxiety and emptiness, felt as a child, in a context in which he or she feels understood and supported. To explore the early stages, as Erikson's Eight Ages of Man (1965) – particularly to build 'basic trust vs mistrust' and 'autonomy vs shame, doubt', can help the client in counselling to share the deep pain and may even help to repair damage from childhood. Luterman (1984) draws from the Erikson model, to give a developmental perspective to the counselling relationship for people with language disability. He also draws from existential psychotherapy (for example Yalom, 1981) – particularly when dealing with the notions of death, responsibility, loneliness and meaninglessness.

Miller (1980s and 1990s) sees the therapeutic process of helping clients to get to touch with their original, genuine feelings. Her approach is to work on the client's grief over the emotionally-deprived childhood. There is often a lengthy process of breaking down the idealizing of inaccessible parents before recognition of the painful reality of childhood can re-emerge. Counselling is giving understanding and empathy in taking on the client with conflicting emotions of pain, anger, guilt, shame, or jealousy and giving him or her a chance to repair part of the childhood trauma. Miller's work, particularly recently, is critical of classical psychoanalysis. She sees it ignoring injuries suffered in childhood and unable to find and face the truth.

The adult losses remind us of when we felt insecurity as a child – and can lead into the depressive position. But losses in life are inevitable, as Salzberger-Wittenberg put it, they are:

> part of our life experience and indeed necessary for the attainment of mature adulthood. For the work of mourning can lead to a greater integration, strengthening of character, the development of courage, and to deeper concern for others as we come to appreciate the preciseness of others and our own time of life (1970:112).

Exploring Relationships – Partnerships

Personal Relationships

The loss does not only affect the person who has had a stroke, but also the partners and children and those close. They might feel similar 'elements' – particularly shock and chaotic feelings. A crisis might bring an opportunity:

A crisis can lead to a new experience of identity. We can emerge from a crisis with new behaviour possibilities, new dimensions of self-expression, and new ways of experiencing the world, maybe with a new perception of meaning.

but

....even then the crisis may still overpower us. It may even lead to a breakdown (Kast 1990:3).

There is a test of the issue of dependancy/independency within the relationship and a test of the trust and love. There is also a test of the boundaries and separateness in an intimate relationship (Eichenbaum and Orbach, 1983). There are a lot or pressures and stresses – perhaps reversal of roles and the inevitable worry about money, loss of status and the occupational role.

There are also fears of death and increasing illness and sometimes worry about sex. There might be feelings of resentment, guilt and anger. The partner goes through a similar grieving process and this can bring unconscious repression. Earlier experience and unconscious expectations challenge the relationship with a severe crisis. I have seen some couples adapt well, but others get trapped in resentment, anger and guilt spirals.

Partnerships help in rehabilitation

There is some fear and ignorance of dysphasia within the medical community due to lack of training, stress, complexity of the issues and reduced resources. I think there is splitting off of the ill from the healthy – perhaps this is a defence mechanism to make it easier for medics to deny and avoid painful and deep feelings of their own disability and feelings of powerlessness. In the main I have received good medical help, but at times it has been less helpful. Within our culture, we project an ideal parent image onto doctors and nurses, giving them the remedies to our all illnesses. There seems to be a changing climate within medical treatment, with more professionals being eager 'to learn from the patient' (Casement, 1985).

Some medical treatments can be experienced by patients as 'torture' and 'abuse' with accompanying fear and anxiety (e.g. swallowing into a tube with a lot of noise (scan); 'rape' by pipe to check the heart (TOE Transoesophageal echo-cardiogram); electrocution by wiring electrodes on the head (EEC). Then after the tests the patient gets rat poison (Warfarin)!

Judd (1989) in her description of psychotherapeutic work with a dying child, shows her understanding of the child's experiences of fearful and agonizing treatments in a terminal illness. She works with him to allow him to share his feelings about illness and death. These are complex and agonizing questions for the medical profession and for all of our society.

Physiotherapy is very important in the early stages of rehabilitation of the physical problems that result from a stroke. I have found alternative therapies helpful – acupuncture, massage and yoga; transcutaneous electrical nerve stimulation (TENs) and painkillers can help to treat pain (See Sternbach 1987, Melzack and Wall, 1982). I feel it is important, as part of therapy, to try to be active and involved, with good rests when needed, and lots of treats!

My partnership with my speech/language therapist was central to my relearning. Our working partnership drew on her patience and expertise to work with clear steps and my previous knowledge of language. It was very hard and sometimes frustrating, but together we worked to break down my resistance to learn again. We liked and respected each other and built up our creative partnership with a lot of humour, honesty and inter-interested curiosity. She involved me and helped me to take on the responsibility to use my skills of counselling and training to run a support group and conduct sessions on assertiveness training.

Some speech/language therapists give so much of themselves that, like some other carers described by Bowlby (1979), they display 'a pattern of attachment behaviour' , which sometimes leads them into 'compulsive care-giving' (p.139). There is a challenge amongst the professional to fight more to build self-respect, gain better earnings and status within the health service, and to demand supervision to explore feelings about their work and clients. It is crucial that professionals, very much concerned with linguistic competence, also explore the emotions attached to the difficulty in talking, understanding, writing and reading.

Luterman (1984) explored the two theoretical counselling approaches within the speech/language therapy profession in the US – the humanistic (Rogers, Maslow) and the behaviourist (Skinner). The humanistic approach has the essential characteristics of unconditional positive regard, non-judgmental, accurate empathy and genuineness. Humanistic concepts are 'unclear and not readily amenable to scientific measurement; humanism requires a leap of faith, that given the time, the self-actualising drive will bubble through' (Luterman, 1984: 10) this gives 'an uncomfortable, unstructured framework' on listening, as opposed to action and prescribing through teaching skills. The behaviourist approach is not an equal relationship; the behaviour can be changed as a result of the systematic application of reinforcement.

There are also other partnerships to tap – volunteers (Stroke Association), particularly to sort out practical issues and offer friendship; disability groups to advise (if any are left after the current round of cuts!); and unions (mine is the National Union of Teachers, NUT) to help sort out complications with retirement. A newly disabled person particularly needs a lot of support, needs to learn the role of mature dependency and to build the spirit to learn to adapt. Belonging to a charity and campaign group, such as Action for Dysphasic Adults can help the spirit to fight and help with inter-support.

During a recession there are many pressures on the vulnerable individuals and on the charities serving them. Oliver's (1990) work shows that the issue of disability is a social rather than an individual problem. Jordan (1990; 1991) applies social policies to the speech/language profession. Disability groups are more organized and building a stronger voice, as shown by the BBC (1992) programmes: *Disabled Lives; Many Voices – One Message* (Morris 1992) and by publication of experiences of people with aphasia (Edelman and Greenwood, 1992; Ireland 1990; Ireland and Black, 1992). Lonsdale (1990) researched women's experience of physical disablement in a social and political context. Working with a team (see Gawlinski and Graesle, 1988) and campaigning enabled people with disabilities to feel less isolated and build up empowerment to fight for justice.

The Self-support Group

I have been involved with two groups since my stroke, but I was involved previously with self-support groups for women workers in education and a peer-supervision group for workers with adolescents. Group work, drawing from the Adlerian and Gestalt approaches (see Dryden, 1990), is about co-operative partnerships between equals, who work on goal changes to help to maintain relationships, encourage the dynamism, give insight and encourage new behaviour. The Feminist movement encourages women to share personal testimonies in groups and in publication (e.g. Virago; Women's Press). Ernst and Goodison (1981) give good guidelines in setting up self-help groups and addressing the issue of the politics of therapy. Whitaker (1985) examines how groups help people. In education and careers work, both use individual counselling and the group context to help with learning and give support (Ball, 1984; Egan, 1990). A group gives an opportunity to share experiences, anxieties and feelings of loss and loneliness and to explore, check out and build support for next steps. As Rogers puts it: 'In group therapy a person may achieve a mature balance between giving and receiving, between independence of self and a realistic and self-sustaining dependence on others' (1951: 293).

Assertiveness Training

Behaviourism and feminist counselling influence assertiveness training (see Smith 1975; Dickson 1982; Holland and Ward, 1990). I found role play helpful in my previous work, preparing young people to learn

how to handle anxieties about work/life experience and training teachers, youth and social workers, volunteers and women's groups. The
process to help change behaviour 'here and now' is goal-directed. I
work with a speech therapist helping groups of patients with cognitive
problems, helping them to practise facing difficulties with others – in
encounters with doctors, in personal relationships, in work and being a
consumer and claimant. There is one crucial issue – respect for oneself
and for others. There is a limitation on how much change can be
achieved, but it can help to reflect on how others see the person's
behaviour in building confidence.

Research Project: Counselling for People with Dysphasia

The practice of the concept of partnership is examined within a research
project in Counselling People with Dysphasia in Riverside Health
Authority, UK. The project has been set up with a grant from the
Department of Health via the charity, Action for Dysphasic Adults. I
have been a counsellor with a speech/language therapist for three
years, researching the issues of counselling adults with dysphasia.

There have been challenges to face within the working relationship.
We have regular supervision to help us to reflect on, and attend to the
emotional issues and counter transferences. The project is to explore
the emotional process undergone by those who have had a stroke,
resulting in language disability, within the therapeutic alliance.

I see the counselling process as reflecting on the past (recognition
of what has been lost, and the meaning attached to loss from the past
experience), the present (rebuilding with new experience everyday
life) and the future (new possibilities and new pathways). These are the
three phases: Beginning, Middle and Ending, described in Eichenbaum and Orbach (1983) and Jacobs (1988). Our project is a beginning
in counselling with those having dysphasia and also a research project
based on a qualitative approach. It will be an opportunity to explore
the emotional issues and what is helpful and what is not for the client.
We can learn from the client's views of counselling and in writing up
and disseminating their perceptions – this is part of the empowerment
process. Our project is small and not able to explore in detail the 'dis-
ablist society' ingrained in the 'individual conscious and institution-
alised practices' (Oliver 1992: 112). Both researchers are involved with
work on their own self-understanding and are continually learning
from the clients and offering thoughts for future services and more
development of 'emancipatory research' (Oliver 1992).

As for myself, I have found Brown and Pedder's (1979:95) outline of
the different levels of psychotherapy particularly helpful:

outer	(support and counselling)
intermediate	(clarification, confrontation and interpretation)
deeper	(exploration and analysis)

Support is a vital part of therapy at all levels. I see our project as drawing from the outer and intermediate levels in the building of trust and communicating and increasing understanding. Within a traumatic loss clients can feel deep disturbing emotions. The humanistic approach does not confront defences nor interpret unconscious processes such as transference. Some understanding of the intermediate level can allow the client to explore and have interpretations of unconscious motives, to explore early experiences (more aware of raw feelings), to transfer onto present experience and confront defences.

Rosen (1979) is helpful for our work on 'brief, focus psychotherapy' to draw from psychodynamic, cognitive, behavioural and client-centred approaches. We need to adopt 'a flexible, empirical approach to treatment' (p.57). We cannot offer a lot in short contracts. But in listening and giving a supportive, reflective time, we hope to enable the client to understand more of his or her needs. As counsellors we work with clients to reflect and to build more understanding on the trauma/chaos and grieving, to be held by boundaries and active listening, to explore dependency and independency and to face reality, the pain/creativity together.

Conclusion

This chapter has been an attempt to explore emotional issues and to adapt my counselling work to the needs of people with dysphasia. My self-exploration during psychoanalysis and my continued learning of the counselling process help to show what I can offer and also my limitations (see Asch and Russo, 1985). At the beginning of the chapter I wrote that this is a 'celebration of my battle for an active and involving life with others'. Another celebration is publication of a work in process with Maria Black to continue to explore living with aphasia. Since writing this chapter (between 1990 and 1993), the author continues to review and re-evaluate the above views with respect to aphasia and disability.

Acknowledgement

With thanks to Ray Wilson, Tutor Librarian at Suffolk College, for his help in chasing through some of the references.

References

Asch A, Rousso H (1985) Therapists with disabilities: theoretical and clinical issues. Psychiatry 48(1): 1–12.
Ball B (1984) Careers counselling in practice. London: The Falmer Press.

Bowlby J (1979) The Making and Breaking of Affectional Bonds. London: Tavistock/Routledge.

Bowlby J (1981) Loss, Sadness and Depression: Attachment and Loss. Harmondsworth: Penguin.

Brown D, Pedder J (1979) Introduction to Psychotherapy. London: Tavistock/Routledge.

Brumfitt SM (1986) Counselling. Bicester: Winslow Press.

Casement P (1985) On Learning from the Patient. London: Tavistock/Routledge.

Casement P (1990) Further Learning from the Patient. London: Tavistock/Routledge.

Dickson A (1982) A Woman in your Own Right. London: Quartet Books.

Dryden W (Ed) (1990) Individual Therapy: A Handbook. Milton Keynes: Open University Press.

Edelman G, Greenwood, R (Eds) (1992) Jumbly Words – The Experience of Aphasia from the Inside. Leicester: Far Communication Disorders.

Egan, G (1990) The Skilled Helper. Monterey, CA: Brookes/Coles.

Elchenbaum L, Orbach S (1983) Understanding Women. London: Pelican.

Erickson, E (1965) Childhood and Society. London: Penguin.

Ernst S, Goodison L (1981) In Our Own Hands. London: The Women's Press.

Fairbairn, WRD (1952) Psychoanalytic Studies of the Personality. London: Tavistock.

Finkelstein V, French S, (1993). Towards a Psychology of Disability in Disabling Barriers: Enabling Environments London: Sage.

France A (1988). Consuming Psychotherapy. London: Free Association Books.

Freud S (1891) On Aphasia - A Critical Study in Brain and Behaviour 4: Adaptation, In Pribram, KH (ED) (1969) London: Penguin.

Freud S (1891) Th Psychopathology of Everyday Life. London: Penguin.

Freud S (1905) Fragment of the Analysis of a Case of Hysteria In Freud S (1990) Case Histories, 1. London: Pengiun.

Freud S (1917) Mourning and Melancholia In Freud (1991) On Metapsychology - The Theory of Psychology. London: Penguin.

Gawlinski G, Graessle, L (1988) Planning Together. London: Bedford Square Press

Gordon W, Hibbard MR, Morganstein S (1988) Response to Tannes and Gerstenberger. Aphasiology 2: 85–8.

Herman N (1985) My Kleinian House. London: Quartet Books.

Herman N (1987) Why Psychotherapy? London: Free Association Books.

Holland S, Ward C (1990) Assertiveness – A Practical Approach. Bicester: Winslow Press.

Ireland, C (1990) I am not mad–I am angry. Nursing Times 45–7.

Ireland C, Black M (1992) Living with aphasia: The insight story In Working Papers in Linguistics 4 355–8.

Jacobs M (1985) The Presenting Past. Milton Keynes: Open University Press.

Jacobs M (1988) Psychodynamic Counselling in Action. London: Sage.

Jones E Byng, S (1989) The Practice of Aphasia Therapy: An Opinion Bulletin, College of Speech Therapists. Sept 2–4.

Jordan, L (1990) Social policy: What can it offer to speech therapists? College of Speech Therapists Bulletin.

Jordan L (1991) A profile of aphasia services in three health districts. British Journal of Disorders of Communication, 26: 293–315.

Judd D (1989) Give Sorrow Words: Working with a Dying Child. London: Free Association Books.

Jung C (1958) The Undiscovered Self. London: Routledge.

Kast, V (1990) The Creative Leap. Illinois: Chiron.

Klein M (1940) Mourning and the relation to manic-depressive states. In Mitchell J (Ed) (1986) The Selected Melanie Klein. Harmondsworth: Penguin.

Klein, M (1956) The study of envy and gratitude. In Mitchell J (Ed) (1986) The Selected Melanie Klein. Harmondsworth: Pengiun.

Leick N and Davidsen-Nielsen (1991) Healing Pain. London: Tavistock /Routledge.

Lomas P (1986) The Limits of Interpretation. Harmondsworth: Pelican

Lonsdale S (1990) Women and Disability. London: Macmillian.

Luterman D (1984) Counselling the Communicative Disorder and the Families. Boston MA: Little, Brown & Co.

Melzack R, Wall, P (1982) The Challenge of Pain. Harmondsworth: Pelican.

Miller A (1987) The Drama of being a Child. London: Virago.

Miller A (1987) For Your Own Good. London: Virago.

Miller A (1990) Thou Shalt not be Aware. London: Pluto Press.

Miller A (1991) Breaking Down the Wall of Silence. London. Virago.

Milner M (1950) On Not Being Able to Paint. London: HEB Paperbacks.

Morris J (1992) Disabled Lives. London: BBC Education.

Morris J (1989) Able Lives. London: The Women's Press.

Morris J (1989) Pride Against Prejudices. London: The Women's Press.

Nelson-Jones R (1988) The Theory and Practice of Counselling Psychology. London: Cassell.

Parkes CM (1972) Bereavement: Studies of Grief in Adult Life. London: Pelican.

Oliver M (1990) The Politics of Disablement. London: Macmillan.

Oliver M (1991) Social Work: Disabled People and Disabling Environments. London: Jessica Kingsley.

Oliver M (1992) Changing the social relations of research production. Disability, Handicaps and Society. 7(2):

Rizzuoto AM (1990) A Proto-dictionary of psycho-analysis. International Journal Psychoanalysis. (P2) 261–70 and 241–8.

Rogers C (1951) Client-Centred Therapy. London: Constable.

Rosen B (1979) Brief focus psychotherapy. In Block S (Ed) An Introduction to the Psychotherapies Oxford: Oxford Medical Publications.

Rycroft C (1985) The Psychoanalysis and Beyond. London: The Hogarth Press.

Salzberger-Wittenberg I (1970) The Psycho-analytic Insight and Relationship. London: Routledge.

Segal J (1985) Phantasy in Everyday Life. London: Penguin.

Segal H (1988) Introduction of the Work of Melanie Klein. London: Karnac.

Sternbach R (1987) Mastering Pain. London: Arlington Books.

Symington N (1987) The Analytic Experience. London: Free Association.

Tanner D, Gerstenberger, D (1988) The grief response in neuropathologies of speech and language. Aphasiology 2(1) 45–98.

Whitaker DS (1985) Using Groups to Help People. London: Tavistock/Routledge.

Winnicott DW (1971). Playing and Reality. London: Tavistock/Routledge.

Winnicott DW (1986) Homes is Where we Start From. London: Pelican.

Yalom ID (1981) Existential Psychotherapy. New York: Basic Books.

Part II: Pragmatic Linguistic and Functional Perspectives

The first chapter in this section by **Linda Worrall** leads on from the individual perspective presented in the first section of the book. The starting point for aphasia therapy is to find what the individual person with aphasia requires from therapy and to negotiate, such that treatment impacts upon his or her everyday life. This chapter sets aphasia therapy in the context of the World Health Organization's International Classification of Impairment, Disability and Handicap. In a broad ranging contribution it is suggested, and arguments presented to support, a top-down approach which encourages a broad view to be taken of the individual with aphasia in order that treatment relates to the individual's experience and hence has functional relevance.

Another contribution from Australia by **Elizabeth Armstrong** extends the functional perspective by overlaying a linguistic approach based on Systemic Functional Grammar. This emphasis, on the social rather than the cognitive role of language, is in line with the arguments put forward by Linda Worrall. The contribution of a functional linguistic analysis is proposed. This chapter offers a more detailed linguistic approach to the analysis of everyday communication whilst retaining the person-centred model supported by other contributors. It is argued that a grammar derived from the use of language helps support aphasiologists in analysing communication in everyday situations. These two contributions from Australia, although derived from different traditions, clearly overlap and present a persuasive argument for the functional analysis of communication.

The value of adopting a systematic and structured approach towards supporting the development of speech and language in everyday situations is emphasized by **Ralph Glindermann** and **Luise Springer** in the following chapter. This chapter presents in some detail how best to utilize PACE therapy which is shorthand for 'Promoting Aphasics' Communicative Effectiveness'. The advantages and disadvantages of this approach are reviewed and clear recommendations put in place derived from the experience both authors have had in implementing PACE therapy. The authors argue that PACE is particularly effective for certain deficits and disorders but cannot, and indeed should not, be used generically as a therapeutic tool for all individuals with aphasia.

The chapter by **Susan Edwards** which describes linguistic approaches to the assessment and treatment of aphasia, is set within the contemporary field of the study of aphasiology. The wide range of approaches adopted by aphasia therapists is recognized, but it is argued that there will always be a need to be able to describe in some detail the linguistic capacities and performance of individuals with aphasia. This, she argues, enables profiles to be established and base lines to be drawn to enable the effectiveness of intervention to be measured within the broader context of more expansive but less detailed pragmatic and communicative approaches. A major project to provide a descriptive framework for the analysis of spontaneous speech is presented and the value of this approach illustrated by reference to a brief case study. It remains important in trying to understand the needs of individuals requiring aphasia therapy to recognize the value of more traditional linguistic analysis alongside broader more holistic approaches to treatment. The major ability of the therapist involved in the treatment of aphasia is to be able to carefully select the most appropriate approach to help support those individuals with aphasia in achieving their goals.

Chapter 4
The Functional Communication Perspective

LINDA WORRALL

Of course, clinicians ask their patients what they want from therapy. Or do they? Of course, clinicians want their therapy to have an impact on their patient's everyday communication. But does it? These common-sense questions form the basis of the functional communication approach which has been seen as a non-theoretical, common-sense approach to the treatment of aphasia. The assumption that an aphasia therapist just needs to use common sense to apply the functional communication approach will be challenged in this chapter. The functional communication approach does use a lot of common sense but it needs to be applied systematically and rationally rather than in an *ad hoc* manner.

The first part of this chapter places the functional approach to communication into a theoretical framework. Ascribing to the belief that theory feeds practice and practice feeds theory, the second part outlines a practical approach to the assessment, treatment and management of aphasic clients using a functional communication approach.

There are two essential knowledge bases that a clinician must understand to apply the functional communication approach. The first is a clear understanding of the conceptual framework of the World Health Organization's classification of impairments, disabilities and handicaps (WHO, 1980). The second is an appreciation of the practical means by which functional goals of aphasia therapy can be accomplished. Hence, this chapter will explore both the theoretical and practical aspects of functional communication and will aim to encourage aphasia clinicians of all persuasions and experience to embrace this perspective.

Theoretical Framework

The most recognized framework for classifying the consequence of a disease such a stroke is the World Health Organization's International Classification of Impairment, Disability and Handicap (WHO, 1980).

47

This simple concept is described in terms of a continuum of Figure 4.1 and should help aphasia therapists understand the process of rehabilitation. It should help to set functional goals as well as inform them of all the aspects to be considered during rehabilitation. The broad concept of this classification system also allows aphasiologists to place various aphasia therapy perspectives within a continuum.

Impairment is defined as damage at the level of the organ. *Disability* is expressed in terms of the difficulty experienced performing everyday activities and *handicap* reflects the value that society attaches to the impairment or disability and the ability to earn a living, pursue leisure activities, etc. For example, a person who has a broken leg which is in a plaster cast has an impairment and a disability but no handicap. The impairment is the damage to the leg while the disability is the restriction to everyday activities such as bathing or walking outside the home. Society views a broken leg generally in a positive sense and a return to work and leisure activities is possible. However, if the broken leg left the patient with a permanent limp, then it is likely that there will be some handicap since society views people with limps in a negative way and it may not be possible for the person to return to work, leisure or sporting activities. A disability may remain as the person may be unable to perform some everyday activities but the impairment is likely to disappear.

Thus the terms impairment, disability and handicap can be viewed as points along a continuum. Applied to aphasiology, at one end of the continuum the impairment of aphasia is measured by brain imaging techniques and aphasia tests to determine the area of brain damage and extent of aphasia. Disability reflects the consequences of impairment in terms of everyday performance and activity; the traditional concept of functional communication falls into the continuum here. The traditional functional communication assessments such as the Communicative Abilities in Daily Living (Holland, 1980) or the Functional Communication Profile (Sarno, 1969) rate the performance of an individual on a core set of everyday communicative activities.

It could be argued that the goal of aphasia therapy should be to reduce the handicap resulting from aphasia. It is suggested therefore that the functional communication approach should aim to reduce the communicative handicap and therefore should be placed a little further along towards the handicap end of the continuum. The functional communication approach which takes the handicap of aphasia into account should place a lot of emphasis on the aphasic individual's view of his or her disability and impairment. This view of functional communication is a little different from the traditional view of functional communication since one aims to reflect the disability of aphasia and the other the handicap of aphasia.

To illustrate the difference, the concept of functional communication

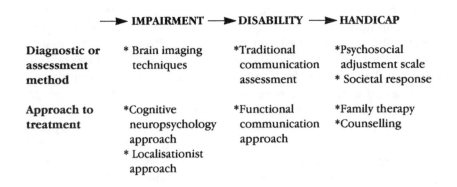

	IMPAIRMENT	DISABILITY	HANDICAP
Diagnostic or assessment method	* Brain imaging techniques	*Traditional communication assessment	*Psychosocial adjustment scale * Societal response
Approach to treatment	*Cognitive neuropsychology approach * Localisationist approach	*Functional communication approach	*Family therapy *Counselling

Figure 4.1 Assessment and treatment methods for the impairment, disability and handicap of aphasia.

as it is described in this chapter would accept that many patients are not concerned if they can't use the telephone or order a taxi. It may not be important to their perceived quality of life. Occasionally, a patient may not see his or her conversational difficulties as being particularly problematic. One particular retired male with a talkative wife found his aphasia a good excuse to spend a lot of time in his garden shed! The needs of aphasic clients and their significant others must be paramount and these should dictate the ultimate goals of aphasia rehabilitation. The traditional method of assessing the functional communication of these patients would have been to assess their performance in these tasks; perhaps the needs of the client may not have been taken into account.

At the far end of the continuum are approaches to treatment such as psychosocial adjustment and the needs of the family because they directly address the broader aspects of the handicap of aphasia. The value that society (including the patient and the family) attaches to the ability to communicate is an important aspect of these approaches.

In summary, the functional communication approach can be described as a top-down management approach focused towards the handicap end of the continuum, with the priority goal of aphasia rehabilitation being the reduction of the patient's handicap first and foremost, before considering the disability and impairment aspects.

The American Speech-Language-Hearing Association (ASHA) Advisory Panel (1990) on functional communication defines functional assessment of communication as follows:

Assesses the extent of ability to communicate with others in a variety of contexts, considering environmental modifications, adaptive equipment, time required to communicate, and the experience of the listener in the client's life. Special accommodations of the communicative partner to either receive or enhance reception of messages must be considered (ASHA, 1990:2).

This is an admirable attempt at a definition of the assessment of functional communication and it contains many important points for various communication disordered populations. However, there is little emphasis on the clients' stated needs or the variety of contexts in which the clients should be assessed. It cannot be assumed that there is a core set of everyday communicative activities in which all people engage. Smith (1985) found that individuals had a unique set of everyday communicative activities that were performed prior to their aphasia and also had a unique set of communication needs following their impairment. Thus, the following qualification could be added to the ASHA definition: assesses the ability of an individual to communicate in his or her *own everyday* environment.

The addition emphasizes the individual's *own* communicative environment, needs and activities. Finally, it is the *everyday* communicative environment in which the patients needs to be assessed. If the everyday communication of a patient includes the presence of a significant other upon whom the patient relies for help when a message is not understood, then the significant other should be included when assessment takes place.

In order to further clarify functional communication, some terminology must be discussed and the component parts must be related to each other. It is the purpose of the following sections to further describe communication and to state what it is not.

Functional Communication and Pragmatics

Many aphasiologists use the terms functional communication and pragmatics interchangeably. It is argued here that these terms refer to two related but different concepts. Functional communication has already been defined above and has essentially been coined from the clinical rehabilitation area. On the other hand, pragmatics is an area of linguistics that has been applied to disordered communication. Pragmatics has been defined as the study of the use of language in context (Bates, 1976) and because of the linguistic origins of pragmatics, it is mostly concerned with verbal language. Hence, functional communication incorporates pragmatics but it is not the same (see Chapter 5 for a fuller discussion of the role of pragmatics in aphasiology).

Functional Communication and Measuring Communicative Success

The terms used to measure the success of the communicative attempt in a functional sense are confusing and may include communicative competence, adequacy, appropriateness, effectiveness, or efficiency. However, these terms are not substitutes for the total concept of functional communication. The terms are used to rate the success of any communicative attempt on a scale ranging from successful to unsuccessful (see Figure 4.2). An important point on the rating scale is the point at which the message or the communicative attempt is adequate. Some clinicians use the term functional for this concept but it is suggested that the term communicative adequacy may be less confusing. It means that in a real life situation, the person would somehow be able to get the message across. The adequate message may be inaccurate with phonological, lexical or syntactical errors, inappropriate to the situation; or it may be very time consuming and inefficient. The sender of the message may be dependent on a relative or person nearby, but the essence of this adequacy level is that the message was successfully sent.

The goal of therapy with the more severely impaired aphasic person may be to achieve an adequate level of communicative effectiveness. That is, the goal is not to achieve accurate, efficient, independent or appropriate communicative attempts, the goal is simply to get the message across. For instance, an aphasic person may make many semantic and phonological errors when giving a phone message, but ultimately, the listener understands the message. The aphasic individual has therefore achieved an adequate level of performance for that task. However, some patients already have an adequate level of communicative effectiveness but require intervention to make them more efficient, more appropriate, more accurate phonologically, lexically or syntactically, or perhaps less reliant on other people. These may be the goals of intervention for those patients with milder language problems.

There is therefore a need to be able to judge a patient's communicative effectiveness as being somewhere along a scale ranging from totally inadequate with no attempt to communicate to completely and independently effective, with the point of adequate communication being

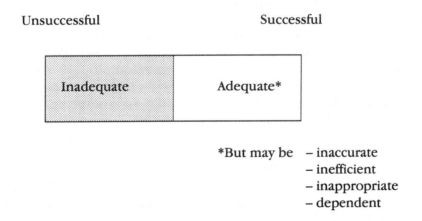

Figure 4.2 Terminology and conceputal framework for measuring communicative success.

an important initial priority for intervention for many patients. The clinician also needs to be able to qualitatively describe the ability of the patient in terms of level of independence from others, communicative efficiency, appropriateness to the situation, ability to repair conversational breakdowns, accuracy of message sending, and mode of delivery of the message. The qualitative description of the communicative attempt is important information necessary for planning appropriate intervention, while placing communicative units on a scale of effectiveness is a method for quantifying the overall functional communication status of the individual or to monitor progress.

Functional Communication and Outcome

The relationship between functional communication and outcome also requires clarification. The outcome of intervention with an aphasic client depends upon many factors, such as the general health of client or the severity of disorder, but in general, outcome is measured in rehabilitation facilities using simple rating scales of functional communication. Outcome measures purport to indicate the degree of benefit that the patient has obtained from intervention. They are being introduced alongside systems such as prospective payments and programme budgeting in order to contain health care costs and increase accountability (Frattali, 1992; Worrall, 1992a). While functional communication assessments are generally administered by a speech pathologist, outcome measure may be used by non-speech pathologists to rate functional communication on admission and discharge. It is therefore important for aphasiologists to be aware of how the outcome of aphasia therapy might be measured.

One such outcome measure, the Functional Independence Measure (FIM) (Hamilton et al., 1987) was designed for a range of rehabilitation patients including spinal, orthopaedic and amputee patients as well as neurological patients. The FIM covers six broad areas of patient functioning including self care, sphincter management, mobility, locomotion and social cognition as well as communication. It consists of a series of rating scales in each of the areas. The FIM rates communicative function on a comprehension and expression seven-point rating scale. However the validity of these scales must be questioned. For example, to achieve the highest rating of 7 in comprehension, the patient must be completely independent and be able to understand complex and abstract directions and conversations which are either spoken or written. Hence a patient who had poor literacy skills prior to the impairment would not rate as a 7 even though he or she can function well in his or her own environment. The use of a hearing aid automatically lowers the person's rating to a 6 even though comprehension may be excellent. The validity of equally weighting the components of communication (i.e., comprehension and expression) rather than the total communication attempt should also be questioned. This measure is conceptually far removed from the definitions of functional communication provided so far in this chapter. As Frattali (1992) argues, it is vital that the conceptual framework of functional communication be developed by aphasiologists so that outcome measures in rehabilitation incorporate valid measures of functional communication. Since future funding of speech pathology services may depend on accurate measures of functional communication, it would appear important that some time and effort be put into developing such a framework.

Accountability can also be measured in terms of consumer satisfaction. The functional communication approach outlined in this chapter goes some way to ensuring consumer satisfaction. There is also a trend toward consumer driven health services in some health organizations in Australia. The Australian Commonwealth Rehabilitation Service, for example, states that the client's needs are paramount and it is primarily the client's needs that form the basis of the amount and type of intervention. The consumer driven functional communication assessment process described in this chapter is therefore important in such a setting.

Practical Aspects

Functional Communication Assessment

Accurate and valid assessments are the key to successful aphasia rehabilitation. The process of assessment is a complex one which cannot be simplified into the single administration of a standardized aphasia test. An experienced clinician not only selects the tools that are appropriate to the situation but also needs to be a little creative to develop specific tools for unique situations. In addition, individual measures or probes need to be developed if the efficacy of therapy is to be monitored using a single subject experimental design.

The major functional communication assessments are the Functional Communication Profile (FCP) (Sarno, 1969), the Communicative Abilities of Daily Living (CADL) (Holland, 1980), and the Edinburgh Functional Communication Profile (EFCP) (Skinner et al., 1984). There are other lesser known assessments or research tools such as The Speech Questionnaire (Lincoln, 1982); the Communication Competence Instrument (CCEI) (Houghton et al., 1982) which have not gained wide acceptance. More recently, two functional assessments have been published which deserve some attention. These are the Communicative Effectiveness Index (CETI) (Lomas et al., 1989) and the Amsterdam-Nijmegan Everyday Language Test (ANELT) (Blomert et al., 1994).

The CADL and FCP are both well known and described in various other texts (see Simmons, 1986; Gerber and Gurland, 1989; Frattali,

1992) and will not be described here. The FCP was the first published assessment of its kind and the basic concept of the assessment has stood the test of time. The rating scale which judges the person's present status against his or her premorbid ability is an important principle which was not incorporated in subsequent assessments such as the CADL. For example, if an aphasic client did not have a telephone or refused to use a telephone prior to the stroke, then his or her subsequent inability to use a telephone should be rated considering the pre-morbid level. This assessment therefore takes into account the client's communicative needs. However, the FCP could now be revised and refined to include the knowledge of the last few decades. Aphasiology now requires a fuller assessment protocol to assess functional communication rather than one simple clinical profile. In addition, items like the 'ability to imitate oral movement' is surely not an everyday communicative activity!

The CADL introduced a radically different assessment procedure. Scoring a patient's ability in a real life or role play situation, such as going to the doctors, was a new concept and provided a more detailed method of examining functional communicative ability. The scoring system also introduced the concepts of adequacy of communication; the additional scoring system of Bartlett (1982) provided a method for assessing efficiency and method of communication. Unfortunately, the CADL did not translate well outside of North America because of cultural differences and it does not cater for aphasic clients who had no need for some of the communicative activities (institutionalized elderly people in general do not drive a car, shop for themselves, or visit a doctor).

The British assessment, the EFCP, does not appear to be well known in North America. For those who are unfamiliar with this assessment, it is an observational tool which allows the clinician to rate the success of communication in various speech acts such as greeting, acknowledging, responding, and requesting. Success is rated as non-communicating (no response, inappropriate, inadequate or stereotyped) or communicating (stereotyped, adequate, qualified or elaborated). In addition, a third dimension which categorizes the method of communication (speech, gesture, facial, vocal or written) is also entered onto the matrix. The EFCP has an extensive rating scale but the decision to assess at the level of the speech act aligned it with pragmatic profiles such as the ones proposed by Penn (1985) and Prutting and Kirschner (1983). It is therefore misnamed as a functional communication profile and the authors have not produced sufficient psychometric data to judge its reliability or validity.

The CETI is a more recent assessment procedure which is quite different from other assessments of functional communication. A set of everyday communicative situations was generated by groups of aphasic patients and their spouses. These were reduced to a core set of 16 situations which are rated on a simple scale by a significant other. Situations include 'Getting somebody's attention', 'Getting involved in group conversations that are about him or her', and 'Giving yes and no answers appropriately'. These are rated on a 10cm visual analogue scale with 'not at all able' at one end, and 'as able as before the stroke' at the other.

The Amsterdam-Nijmegan Everyday Language Test (ANELT) (Blomert et al., 1992) consists of scenarios of everyday life to which the patient is asked to respond. For example, 'You are now at the dry cleaners. You've come to pick this up and you get it back like this (hand patient shirt that is burnt at the front). What do you say?' The patient's response is rated on a scale of comprehensibility of the message and the intelligibility of the utterance.

While there are a range of assessments of functional communication available, it appears that few clinicians are using them. In an Australian audit of 68 aphasic stroke patient's clinical files in which 128 aphasia assessments were carried out, Worrall and Burtenshaw (1990) found that no published assessment of functional communication was used by any of the clinicians. The reasons that the clinicians gave for not using a published assessment included the inadequacy of existing published assessments, a preference for their own informal observational assessments, lack of access to the published assessments, unfamiliarity with the formal assessments, some patients not requiring a functional communication assessment because they were considered to be functioning normally or to be so severe as to not warrant a functional communication assessment. Some respondents considered it inappropriate to assess functional communication in the acute stage of recovery or in the institutionalized setting where a decreased level of communicative competence is required.

I will argue that functional communication should not be assessed using a single administration of a single test. The concept of functional communication is too complex for a single test administration. Instead a series of assessments using a variety of methods with which clinicians and patients feel comfortable would appear to have greater face validity at least. Such a serial assessment procedure, the Everyday Communicative Needs Assessment (ECNA) (Worrall, 1992b) is described next. The series begins with an interview to determine the communicative needs of the patient and a questionnaire to obtain information about the social networks of the patient, their preferences for conversational topics and an idea of their pre-morbid communicative style. The patient is then assessed in the real life situations that are important to them, their significant others and their lifestyle. The assessment situation is rated and the scores are then placed onto a profile form which provides a graphic representation of the patient's abilities.

Hence the ECNA aims to:

- be flexible enough for all aphasic clients (severe or mild, institution-alized or at home, acute or chronic);
- ensure that the activities that are relevant and important to the client are assessed:
- take into account pre-morbid personality, activities, and abilities;
- assess in detail, as well as provide a profile;
- be non-prescriptive so that clinicians can use professional judge-ment in its administration;
- be standardized so that the psychometric properties can be estab-lished.

Step 1: *Interview*

The patient and/or significant others are interviewed to determine the communicative needs of the patient. Table 4.1 shows a sample of the interview guide which lists everyday communicative activities. These may be used as prompts and/or as a record form.

Depending upon the stage of recovery of the patient, the four main questions concern whether the activity was performed prior to the stroke, whether the activity is performed now, whether the activity is missed if not carried out now, and then the perceived reasons for not performing the activity. Various prompts are used to determine the exact nature of the activity ('Do you need to be able to ring in case of an emergency?' 'Do you tend to telephone mainly friends or do you often have to look up numbers in the telephone book?'). The reasons for not being able to perform the activity now are coded as either a problem related to immobility, other stroke-related problem (e.g. mem-ory, perceptual difficulties, apraxia), aphasia or other reasons not relat-ed to the stroke.

Step 2: *Questionnaire*

The patient and/or significant others are asked to complete a question-naire. The questionnaire determines previous and present social con-tacts ('Who do you talk with on a daily basis?'); preferred conversational topics (e.g. family, hobbies, sport); and the pre-morbid communicative style of the patient (e.g. talkative, argumentative, reserved, got off the subject). It has been based on the social network interview schedule of Smith (1985), the communicative style adjectives of Green (1984) and Swindell et al. (1982), the communicative history form of Crystal et al. (1976) and numerous unpublished communica-tive history forms from a variety of speech pathology departments.

Step 3: *Prioritize problem list*

The clinician then prioritizes the needs of the client which will include the wishes of their significant other. Priority is given to communicative needs that are important for the patient's safety (e.g. obtaining help in

Table 4.1: Example of interview guide

Everyday Communicative Needs Assessment

1. Finances

- checking and paying bills
- writing cheques
- reading bank statement
- balancing accounts/budgeting
- organizing payment of rent/mortgage
- reading literature (Social Security/Veterans Affairs)
- filling in forms (Social Security, Veterans Affairs, Medicare)
- using an automatic teller machine

2. Using the Phone

- looking up numbers in phone book
- using Yellow Pages
- dialling emergency numbers
- writing down phone messages
- making appointment/business calls
- making social calls

3. Preparing food

- reading labels on food packets
- measuring ingredients
- reading sell by/use by dates and calculating food freshness
- following recipes
- making choices at mealtimes
- using the microwave and oven

4. General household activities

- following washing and ironing instructions on clothes
- following instruction leaflets for household appliances
- setting washing machine
- directing workmen (eg.plumber)
- dealing with people who come to door (eg. meter-reader)
- following written instruction re DIY jobs (eg shelves)
- writing note for milkman, home help, etc.
- caring for pets
- following instructions for use of gardening products
- gardening

Coding for reasons:
1. immobility
2. aphasia
3. other stroke related problems
4. other

an emergency) and have a high impact if met (e.g. if it allows the client to attend therapy by public transport).

Step 4: *Observe and rate performance*
The high priority needs of the client are assessed. Ideally, the clinician needs to observe the client performing the activity in real life. Holland (1983) argues that observation results in much better overall picture of the aphasic person and describes a case where an aphasic woman merely 'took up space' in one of their aphasic groups, but during a real life observation session coped far better than predicted as they went shopping, had lunch, and returned to explain their purchases to the patient's husband.

If the clinician has the flexibility of observing patients in the community or during home visits then this is ideal. Alternatively, communicative situations can be created quite realistically in the clinic so that natural behaviour can be observed. For example, if the client's need is to continue managing the family finances and one of the important and regular activities is withdrawing money from the bank using an automatic teller machine, then this can be created using information about the machines available from banks. Some will provide drawings or photographs of the machine upon request, while others even have life size models which can be used for demonstration purposes. The situation can be made more meaningful by having the client's own bank's automatic teller machine instructions. However, while roleplay can create opportunities for natural behaviour to observed, real life observation is potentially richer and is the observational setting of choice. While a client may be proficient at using the automatic teller machine in the clinic, a queue of impatient people may cause the patient to fail completely.

The Communicative Effectiveness Rating Scale (see Table 4.2) can be used to rate the success of each communicative attempt. This is a seven-point rating scale which essentially measures the effectiveness of a communicative attempt. The scale assumes that messages can be inaccurate (phonologically, semantically or syntactically), inefficient in terms of the content to time ratio, inappropriate to the situation, or even dependent on another person but still adequate for a real life communicative situation. Hence the scale is basically divided into 'adequate' and 'inadequate'. The ratings within each section are quantitative as well as descriptive, however, the scale is primarily ordinal. That is, more emphasis should be placed on whether the communicative attempt was a 5 or 4 rather than whether it fitted the description of the category perfectly. For example, if a patient has word retrieval problems when telephoning for a taxi and produces word approximations and many fillers such as 'um' and 'you know', but eventually the telephone operator for the taxi firm is able to send the taxi to the correct address, then this would be rated as 6. If the patient read from a card prepared especially for this purpose and became accurate and efficient in the process, then this would rate as a 7. A 5 rating is given when the aphasic person successfully enlists the help of another person but is accurate, efficient and appropriate. For example, some patients turn to their spouse in a conversation when they know they will have problems expressing themselves. A 4 rating would be given when help is enlisted only after some struggling communication attempts. Inadequate ratings are given to communicative attempts that have failed. An aphasic patient may hand over too much or not enough money when asked for the fare in a bus (3), or be unable to state his or her destination to the driver or any of the passengers (2) or simply refuse to attempt communication at all in a given situation (1).

Table 4.2 Communicative Effectiveness Rating Scale

Adequate	7	Independent, accurate, efficient, appropriate
	6	Independent but either inaccurate, inefficient or inappropriate
	5	Dependent but accurate, efficient and appropriate
	4	Dependent and either inaccurate, inefficient or inappropriate
Inadequate	3	Independent but either inaccurate, inefficient or inappropriate
	2	Dependent and either inaccurate, inefficient or inappropriate
	1	No attempt at communication.

Step 5: *Profile assessment*
A simple profile like the one in Table 4.3 is probably the most meaningful result of the ECNA. The mean and standard deviation of the ratings may also provide useful information. There can be no total score since the number of assessment tasks will vary. The reliability and validity of this method have yet to be examined.

Step 6: *Implement therapy and re-assess*
The ECNA is an intervention driven assessment process. When the patient's everyday communication problems have been identified, strategies can be implemented to either increase the independence of the patient or to increase the accuracy, efficiency or appropriateness. Re-assessment as a task will hopefully produce a higher rating on the Communicative Effectiveness Rating Scale.

Step 7: *Measure outcome*
A change in the mean rating of all everyday communicative activities can be used as a measure of outcome. It is possible to use the mean rating of everyday activities as an outcome measure in rehabilitation settings that are seeking to evaluate the effectiveness of the total rehabilitation process.

Table 4.3 Worked example of the profile of the Everyday Communicative Needs Assessment

Profile

Communicative activity		Rating	
		Adequate	Inadequate
		7 6 5 4	3 2 1
Phoning	– emergency		3
	– taxi		3
	– family/friends	6	
	– looking up directory		3
Shopping	– making a list, etc.	4	
	– asking for goods	6	
	–money handling	4	
Finances	– writing withdrawal slips	4	
	– balancing account	4	
Mean rating = 4.1			
S.D. = 1.2			

Functional Communication Therapy

Using the assessment process outlined above, the communicative needs of the patient are identified and the performance of the patient observed and rated. Functional communication therapy using strategies such as those listed in Appendix 1 are implemented to improve function as measured by the Communicative Effectiveness Rating Scale. Hence, the functional communication approach generally involves the use of compensatory strategies to circumvent the problems of language.

Functional communication strategies can exist at various levels. Using a top down process, at the top are rehabilitation strategies such as the use of a personal alarm system, installing a telephone with one-touch memory pads for frequently used or emergency numbers, using a telephone with a speaker and microphone so that another person can assist the aphasic person during a telephone conversation, carrying a card with the destination address written on it for taxi drivers, keeping a stock of pre-completed bank withdrawal slips which just require a signature, etc. Many of these strategies may not be suitable for elderly stroke patients who are not familiar with modern communication technology such as VCRs that 'talk' or word processors. However, younger aphasic patients may find these useful.

At the next level, strategies involve changing communicative behaviour. The aphasic person needs to learn to adapt his or her pattern of communication, as it may be that the aphasic person's message is often inadequate, inaccurate or inefficient. Some examples of these strategies include increasing the use of non-verbal behaviour so that the message is more accurate or more efficient. This can be done by either teaching a formal gestural system or by trying to augment any verbal skills with an increased amount of natural or spontaneous non-verbal behaviour such as facial expression, hand movement and head movement.

The patient could also be encouraged to use 'errors' to their advantage if it helps to maintain the conversational flow (using fillers such as 'um' or 'ah' or making mistakes and then correcting them) or to give a clue about the message by using circumlocutions or word approximations (Green, 1982). If word retrieval problems constantly interrupt the conversational flow, then strategies to trigger or cue the patient into the word can be used. Golper and Rau (1983) suggest that the clinician should first establish with the patient which cueing strategy is most successful. Bruce and Howard (1987) used computer-generated phonemic cues successfully with their patients. Another strategy is to encourage the patient to be more dependent if this ends up increasing the overall adequacy of communication. The patient could be encouraged to request repetitions if a message was not understood or to request that the listener guess what the speaker is trying to say, or to request help with the filling out of forms, etc. from clerks, shopkeepers, sales assistants, and so on.

Drawing has been used as a method by which aphasic patients with limited verbal skills can communicate part of their message (Lyon and Helm-Estabrooks, 1987). Bertoni et al, (1991) began their drawing therapy by using everyday pictographs to establish the functional relevance of pictorial representations. For those patients who perseverate and thereby reduce the efficiency of their communication, the Treatment of Aphasic Preservation or TAP Program (Helm-Estabrooks et al., 1987) utilizes strategies to reduce the effect of pereseveration. The communicative partners of the aphasic client (family, friends, staff and the community at large) can also be taught strategies to facilitate communication and these may include the use of comprehension checks, use of slower rate of speech and simpler syntax.

PACE therapy (see Chapter 6) is a useful method to accomplish many of the above aims. It can be used to increase non-verbal behaviour or generalize drawing therapy if the therapist models what is required. It can be used to increase the efficiency of message sending by timing messages sent. It can be used to encourage the patient to give the listener a clue by using the prompt system described by Davis (1980) or it can be used with spouses or family members to encourage more effective communication in the home (Newhoff, Bugbee, and Ferreira, 1981).

Some aphasic patients may not want to take a compensatory approach and may wish to remediate their language to a level that is as close to normal as possible. It is therefore necessary to use other approaches which aim to restore or substitute for lost linguistic functions with these patients. Hence the functional communication approach is not suitable for all goals of intervention or for all aphasic patients. However, many of the functional communication strategies can be used alongside other intervention to reduce the impact of the aphasia on the everyday life of the patient. In addition, functional communicative activities can be used to generalize new language skills.

Management Issues

As stated earlier, the functional communication approach dictates an overall client management plan that is practical in nature. Client management is the who, when and where of treatment (Wertz, 1983). That is, an aphasia therapist not only chooses what treatment to provide to the patient, but also who should give the treatment (aides, volunteers, family), when it will be given (intensive therapy, weekly, delayed) and where the treatment will take place (clinical facility, client's own home).

The first management issue concerns who should provide the intervention. Certainly some occupational therapists see their role as encompassing everything to do with function, therefore by implication, encompassing functional communication as well. This type of territorial dispute should not occur in a rehabilitation team which communicates well and ideally functional communication strategies can be implemented by all team members. However, if it does occur, it is suggested that speech pathologists should view the generalization of language into everyday life as part of their role as communication specialists.

In the broadest sense, the rehabilitation team should not only include the professionals, but also the family, friends, neighbours and carers of the patient. The speech pathologist has a major role in educating these members of the team. Those who are close to the aphasic patient may be better able to suggest strategies to assist the functional communication skills of the aphasic individual. The rehabilitation team may also include volunteers, whether they be part of a larger programme of trained volunteers or an individual with the skills and the time to participate in the rehabilitation of the aphasic person. The functional communication approach is particularly suited for use by non-professionals since, with professional guidance, it does not require too much knowledge of the complexities of aphasia and many tasks are readily understood by non-professionals. Since the functional communication approach is concerned with the practice of communicative strategies in everyday life, it would be most sensible to enlist the help of as many people from the patient's everyday environment as possible.

The next important management issue is when should intervention begin, for how long should it last and when should it be terminated. The functional communication approach should not only be used in the chronic stages when all else fails. It should be an integral part of therapy at all stages of recovery. If the functional communication approach is the top-down management approach described here, then it is simply a way of making sure that the client's wishes are taken into consideration and that intervention is as effective and efficient as possible. If the Everyday Communicative Needs Assessment reveals that the patient has adjusted well to the aphasia and would be content to have the communication skills required to drive his or her car, have a simple conversation with his or her spouse and weigh the biggest fishing catch, then the clinician should offer this service. If, however, the client needs to have high level communication skills to retain employment then this need can be met using the ECNA as a first step.

In the acute stage of recovery, there are many everyday communicative needs that confront the aphasic individual. It is important to assess how the patient is communicating in the hospital ward. While many of the needs of hospital and nursing home patients are anticipated by nursing care staff, many are not. The Everyday Communicative Needs Assessment can be based around some core activities of daily living such as going to the toilet, eating, drinking and taking medicine, transferring, walking, manipulating the physical environment, maintaining personal hygiene, and dressing and undressing. These activities are likely to be the focus of rehabilitation in the acute stage and it is important that the communicative needs that these activities require are considered by the clinician. Some of the everyday communicative problems of aphasic people in the hospital setting include understanding and being involved in the rehabilitation process, understanding the instructions of rehabilitation staff, ordering preferred food from the menu, being able to tell the time for appointments, reading and understanding written information about the cost of hospitalization or about how the bedside telephone or television works, using coins to purchase the daily newspaper delivered to the wards, reading about the outside world in the newspaper, or understanding the news or other items on the hospital radio. The other reason to start the Everyday Communicative Needs Assessment in the acute stage is to begin the preparation for discharge.

The current practice of speech pathologists in many Australian and British rehabilitation settings appears to be to argue the case for longer hospitalization for aphasic patients so that intensive aphasia treatment may continue. An alternative practice may be to use the time in hospital to prepare the patient for the communicative world outside. The aphasia therapist should be a vital part of the decision concerning where and when the patient is to be discharged. Many clinicians appear to rely on a judgement of the patient's abilities, based on a standard aphasia test. The relationship between an aphasia test and the ability to get help in an emergency or handle money is tenuous, yet the ability of the patient in such activities may be the difference between the patient returning to his or her own home or being admitted to a nursing home. It is therefore vital that a communicative needs assessment such as the ECNA be performed and the patient tested in situations that are as near to real life for the patient as possible. It is especially important to test the ability of the patient in matters of safety, particularly if the patient is to return home alone.

Illustrative Cases

The importance of assessing a patient's performance in everyday communicative activities is illustrated by the following two case studies. Both cases were elderly women who had been independently living at home alone prior to their stroke. One lady had a mild subcortical aphasia which was characterized by word retrieval difficulties. She was still working prior to her stroke and was living in a house owned by her son who lived in another state. Her husband had a history of alcoholism and was living in a nursing home. Despite her relatively mild aphasia, she was rated as 'inadequate' on many of the tasks that she and her son perceived to be necessary for her successful return to living at home alone. These included using the telephone in an emergency or phoning for a taxi to go shopping or visiting and handling money. After attempting these tasks, both the patient and her family decided that she could no longer live at home alone and took the option of moving into a hostel. The other lady had a severe aphasia, severe apraxia of speech and severe limb apraxia. Her verbal comprehension was very poor and verbal expression was limited to 'yes' and 'no' although she used facial expression to successfully convey her feelings. On the basis of these results, the decision may have been taken to admit her to a hostel or nursing home. However, she was adamant that she wanted to return home. An assessment of everyday communicative activities revealed that her communicative needs were confined to shopping, finances, seeking help in an emergency and answering the door. She was a virtual recluse except for the weekly visits of her son and his family. She was able to demonstrate how she would get help in an emergency by pressing the stored telephone number for her son's family and saying 'yes' and 'no' in her characteristic way. The family were prepared to take her shopping with them and take over her finances. She also demonstrated her abilities to deal with people who came to her door when the ambulance officers came to bring her into the hospital for speech therapy and 'told' them in no uncertain terms that she didn't want to go! While both cases had satisfactory conclusions, it may have been different if the discharge decisions have been based solely on standard aphasia test results.

The duration of intervention depends very much on the type of intervention decided upon and the response of the patient. Sometimes, patients are satisfied with a few quick and easy strategies which have had a high impact of their lives. For example, after several years of being dependent on her husband, a female aphasic patient became confident at using a taxi to come into the hospital for her outpatient appointments. A particular taxi firm had a system whereby the telephone operators have four set questions when a taxi is ordered: 'Your pick-up address? Going to? Passenger's name? Are you ready now?' The patient's oral reading was quite good so she had practised the responses from a written card. The number for the taxi was programmed into her telephone's memory and TAXI written on the button. She had her destination written on a card as well as a card explaining her speech problem if needed. She knew the approximate cost of the trip ($4.00) and gave the driver a $5.00 note each time and trusted the driver to give her the correct change. Her husband could have arranged for her to have an account with the firm but she preferred to pay cash. Following the success of a few trips she became more adventurous and her social life and feeling of independence increased to such an extent that she no longer wanted regular speech therapy.

Group therapy can encompass many of the aims of functional communication therapy. While the definition of group therapy for aphasia remains a contentious issue (Aten, 1991; Fawcus, 1991; 1992; Loverso, 1991; Pachalska, 1991a; 1991b; Repo, 1991; Springer, 1991), most authors agree that communicative strategies can be practised in such a setting. Indeed, Aten et al. (1982) found that group therapy using a functional communication approach produced significant functional gains as measured by the CADL.

An experienced therapist who uses a top-down management

approach will often challenge the system of service delivery in their rehabilitation facility. Using the functional communication approach, the therapist would argue for inclusion in the home visiting team of aphasic individuals and may ask to provide a domiciliary service rather than treat out-patients in hospital. Permission to take the patient on trips to the bank, shops or on public transport are requested and the family are positively encouraged to initiate strategies to overcome particular problems.

The clinician who uses the functional communication approach also develops a habit of collecting real life assessment and therapy material. Menus from pizza restaurants, cafes, coffee shops, take away outlets and expensive a la carte restaurants are useful, as are bank forms from all banks, instructions sheets for automatic teller machines, promotional material for various products, recipe books, newspapers, highway code book, bus timetables, social security forms, tax forms etc.

Conclusion

The functional communication approach begins with a top-down assessment in which the broadest view of the patient functioning in his or her environment determines the type of intervention required. Functional communication therapy uses various forms of compensatory strategies to reduce the handicap resulting form aphasia. This chapter has emphaized the need for a thorough and real life assessment of the patient's needs and abilities. An assessment process is proposed that ensures that the client's communicative needs are paramount.

In an effort to stimulate further debate about what aphasia therapy hopes to achieve, a theoretical framework was proposed and the terminology of functional communication defined. Finally, the relevance of the functional communication to outcome measures and the future funding of speech pathology services was noted.

It is important to note that the functional communication approach is complementary to other approaches such as the cognitive neuropsychology approach. The philosophy of top-down management, however, dictates that the needs of the client are paramount and that gains are ultimately measured in terms of reducing the patient's handicap.

Appendix 1

Strategies for Everyday Communicative Activities

Finances

* Arrange for a standing order to pay bills, mortgage or rent.
* Keep a stock of pre-completed cheques, withdrawal or deposit slips that just require a signature.

- Use Fast Cash or similar method of withdrawing money from an Automatic Teller Machine that requires limited reading ability.
- Enlist help from a family member to check bank statements with an aphasic nursing home resident.
- Enlist help of a family member to set aside coins for purchase of newspaper or phone use while in hospital.

Phone

- Make a personalized phone book with photos of family and friends next to their numbers and group names and numbers according to family or some other meaningful way rather than alphabetically.
- Install a phone with several one-touch key pads for often used or emergency numbers.
- Use a personal alarm or security phone which doesn't require communication to get help.
- Install an answering machine so that the spouse or carer can leave the aphasic person at home and not be concerned that he or she cannot answer the phone.

Household Activities

- If answering the door is a safety problem, fix a safety catch.

Travel

- Have a card with the destination written on it.
- Have a regular booking made with a taxi service for a nursing home resident to visit a friend.
- Always carry a card which explains the person's communication problem with his or her name and a contact phone number of close relative or friend.
- Pay by credit card.
- Have an account with a taxi service.

Shopping

- Purchase generic shopping lists so that the shopper merely has to tick a box or place a small peg next to the item required.
- Pay by credit card or by electronic funds transfer which directly debits the money from the purchaser's account.

Leisure

- Utilize talking books from the public library.
- Change newspaper/television news channel to one that is more pictorial.
- Change to a VCR that is programmed using bar codes or that instructs the user verbally.

- Try word processing letters so that errors can easily be erased and a spell check can be made.
- Use printed Christmas cards.
- Ask family/friends to telephone or fax a booking for the theatre or a concert and pay by credit card so that the aphasic person doesn't have to pay by cash.

References

American Speech-Language-Hearing Association (1990) Functional Communication Measures Project: Advisory Report. Rockville, MD: ASHA.

Aten JL (1991) Group therapy for aphasic patients: let's show it work. Aphasiology 5(6), 559–61.

Aten JL, Caligiuri MP, Holland AL (1982) The efficacy of functional communication therapy for chronic aphasia patients. Journal of Speech and Hearing Disorders 47: 93–96.

Bartlett CL (1982) A modified scoring technique for communicative abilities in daily living. In Brookshire RH (Ed) Clinical Aphasiology Conference Proceedings. Minneapolis, MN: BRK Publishers.

Bates E (1976) Language and Context. New York: Academic Press.

Bertoni B, Stoffel A-M, Weniger D (1991) Communicating with pictographs: a graphic approach to the improvement of communicative interactions. Aphasiology 5 (4 and 5), 341–53.

Bruce C, Howard D (1987) Computer-generated phonemic cues: an effective aid for naming in aphasia. British Journal of Disorders of Communication 22: 191–201.

Crystal D, Fletcher P, Garman M (1976) The Grammatical Analysis of Language Disability, London: Edward Arnold.

Davis GA (1980) A critical look at PACE therapy. In Brookshire RH (Ed) Clinical Aphasiology Conference Proceedings. Minneapolis, MN: BRK Publishers.

Fawcus M (1991) Managing group therapy: further considerations. Aphasiology 5(6), 555–7.

Fawcus M (1992) Group work with the aphasic adult. In Group Encounters Speech and Language. London: Whurr.

Frattali CM (1992) Functional assessment of communication: merging public policy with clinical views Aphasiology 6 (1): 63–83

Gerber S, Gurland GB (1989) Applied pragmatics in the assessment of aphasia. Seminars in Speech and Language 10 (4): 263–81

Golpher LAC and Rau MT (1983) Systematic analysis of cuing strategies in aphasia: taking your 'cue' from the patient. In Brookshire RH (Ed) Clinical Aphasiology Conference Proceedings. Minneapolis, MN: BRK Publishers.

Green G (1982) Assessment and treatment of the adult with severe aphasia: aiming for functional generalisation. Australian Journal of Human Communication Disorders 10 (1): 11–23.

Green G (1984) Communication in aphasia therapy: some of the procedures and issues involved. British Journal of Disorders of Communication 19: 35–46.

Hamilton BB, Granger CV, Sherwin FS, Zielezny M, Tashman JS (1987) A uniform national data system for medical rehabilitation. In Fuhrer MJ (Ed) Rehabilitation Outcomes: Analysis and Measurement. Baltimore, MD: Paul H. Brookes.

Helm-Estabrooks N, Emery P, and Albert ML (1987) Treatment of aphasic preservation (TAP) program. Archives of Neurology 44 1253–5.

Holland AL (1980) Communicative Abilities in Daily Living. Baltimore, MD: University Park Press:

Holland AL (1983) Remarks on observing aphasia people. Brookshire RH (Ed) Clinical Aphasiology Conference Proceedings. Minneapolis, MN: BRK Publishers:

Houghton RM, Pettit JM, Towey MP (1982) Measuring communicative competence in global aphasia. In Brookshire RH (Ed) Clinical Aphasiology Conference Proceedings. Minneapolis, MN: BRK Publishers.

Lincoln NB (1982) The speech questionnaire: an assessment of functional language ability. International Rehabilitation Medicine 4: 114–17.

Lomas J, Pickard L, Bester S, Elbard H, Finlayson A, and Zoghaib C (1989) The communicative effectiveness index: development and psychometic evaluation of a functional communication measure for adult aphasia. Journal of Speech and Hearing Disorders, 54: 113–224.

Loverso FL (1991) Aphasia group treatment, a commentary. Aphasiology 5(6), 567–9.

Lyon JG, Helm-Estabrooks N (1987) Drawings: its communicative significance for expressively restricted aphasic adults. Topics in Language Disorders 8: 61–71.

Newhoff M, Bugbee JK, Ferreira A (1981) A change of PACE: spouses as treatment targets. In Brookshire RH (Ed) Clinical Aphasiology Conference Proceedings. Minneapolis, MN: BRK Publishers.

Pachalska M (1991a) Group therapy for aphasia patients. Aphasiology 5(6), 541–54.

Pachalska M (1991b) Group therapy: a way of reintegrating patients with aphasia. Aphasiology 5(6), 573–7.

Penn C (1985) The profile of communicative appropriateness: a clinical tool for the assessment of pragmatics. The South African Journal of Communication Disorders, 32: 18–23.

Prutting C, and Kirschner D (1983) Applied pragmatics. In Gallagher T Prutting C (Eds) Pragmatic Assessment and Intervention Issues in Language. San Diego, CA: College Hill Press.

Repo M (1991) The holistic approach to rehabilitation: a commentary. Aphasiology 5(6), 571–2.

Sarno MT (1969) The Functional Communication Profile: Manual of Direction. New York: University Medical Center, Institute of Rehabilitation Medicine:

Simmons NN (1986) Beyond standardised measures: special tests, language in context, and discourse analysis in aphasia. Seminars in Speech and Language 7, (2): 181–205.

Skinner C Wirz S, Thompson I, Davidson J (1984) The Edinburgh Functional communication Profile. Winslow, England: Winslow Press Agency.

Smith L (1985) Communicative activities of dysphasic adults: a survey. British Journal of Disorders of Communication 20: 31–44.

Springer L (1991) Facilitating group rehabilitation. Aphasiology 5,(6): 563–5.

Swindell CS, Pashek GV Holland Al (1982) A questionnaire for surveying personal and communicative style. In Brookshire RH (Ed) Clinical Aphasiology Conference Proceedings. Minneapolis, MN: BRK Publishers.

Wertz RT (1983) Language intervention context and setting for the aphasic adult: when? In Miller J D, Yoder D., Schiefelbusch R (Eds) Contemporary Issues in Language Intervention. Rockville, MD: American Speech-Language-Hearing Association.

Worrall L, Burtenshaw EJ (1990) Frequency of use and utility of aphasia tests. Australian Journal of Human Communication Disorders. 18, (2): 53–67.

Worrall L (1992) Functional communication assessment: an Australian perspective. Aphasiology 6 (1) 105–10.

Worrall L (1992) Everyday Communicative Needs Assessment. Available from the Queensland 4072, Australia: Department of Speech and Hearing, The University of Queensland.

World Health Organization (1980) International Classification of Impairments, *Disabilities, and Handicaps.* Geneva-Switzerland: World Health Organization.

Chapter 5
A Linguistic Approach to the Functional Skills of Aphasic Speakers

ELIZABETH M. ARMSTRONG

The question of how to facilitate improvement in an aphasic person's ability to communicate is the ultimate concern of the clinical aphasiologist. In other words, the clinician is concerned with improving the speaker's ability to convey meanings to a listener – to ask and respond to questions, to make statements, to recount events, to give directions, to explain why something has happened or why something should happen. The clinician's job is to explore the linguistic resources available to the speaker to fulfil these functions, to find ways of maximizing the use of retained resources and increasing the range of meanings he or she can convey, (see also Chapter 7).

In recent years there has been a growing interest in examining the aphasic speaker's abilities in connected speech and everyday communication situations in an attempt to directly address the issue of how an aphasic speaker communicates (Wagenaar et al., 1975; Yorkston and Beukelman, 1980; Holland, 1980; Ulatowska et al., 1981; 1983; 1989; 1990; Davis and Wilcox, 1985; Shewan, 1988; Saffran et al., 1989; Vermeulen et al., 1989; Ferguson, 1993; Edwards et al., 1993). Rather than extrapolating potential for communication from test results which examine communication subskills (such as naming) in decontextualized tasks, analysis of texts or discourse enables the clinician to look directly at the communication skills of the individual and the kinds of meanings he or she is able to create.

To date, the main grammatical approaches to text analysis in aphasiology have come from two main perspectives. One has been involved in applying structural grammars to discourse analysis (see Crystal, Fletcher and Garman, 1976 (the LARSP); Wagenaar et al., 1975); Saffran et al., 1989. Such analyses are actually mainly concerned with sentence-level phenomena, with a text characterized largely in structural terms by what happens in its constituent sentences. The second perspective has again utilized structural grammar principles to analyse sentences and has called sentence phenomena part of the microstructure of a text (see Ulatowska et al., 1981; 1983; Glosser and Deser,

1990). However, this perspective has also included a view of the overall macrostructure of the text and has utilized principles taken from the work of linguists/psychologists such as Van Dijk (1977); Kintsch (1977); Van Dijk and Kintsch (1978); Longacre (1976); and Rumelhart (1975). Analyses coming from this perspective provide information on a text's structure in terms of constituents such as setting, complicating action and resolution, as identified in a narrative text.

The framework used to describe discourse in this chapter – systemic functional grammar – is that proposed by Michael Halliday whose functional approach to language is concerned with the uses to which language is put as well as its internal form. Systemic functional theory is one of the few grammatical theories which sees text as its basic unit of analysis and relates all grammatical ranks – morpheme, word, group and clause to overall discourse meaning. Hence, the notion of separating microstructure and macrostructure is not so relevant, as one is seen as intricately related to the other. Microstructure in particular is analysed in relation to the role it plays in building up the macrostructure of the text. As the theory also relates wording and meaning to extralinguistic context, it has great relevance to the analysis of functional communication. Indeed, that is its central concern. Cohesion analysis is the main part of Halliday's theory to have been utilized in aphasiology to date (Piehler and Holland, 1984; Lemme et al., 1984; Bottenberg et al., 1985; Armstrong; 1987; 1988; 1991; Coehlo et al., 1992) but it has been discussed in terms rather isolated from the total theory. Hence, its relationship to meaning and context *per se* has not been fully explored.

It is the intention of this chapter to look at some of the ways in which aphasic speakers express their meaning, utilizing Halliday's systemic functional grammar as the basis of analysis, and to propose ways of facilitating the communication of aphasic speakers, again using this framework. Within the confines of the chapter it seemed most feasible to present basic principles and broad-based approaches to treatment rather than detailed linguistic analyses. For greater detail of the analyses themselves, the reader to referred to Halliday (1985a; 1985b); Mattiesson (in press); Hasan (1985); Martin (1992); Armstrong (1988; 1992; 1993).

What Do We Mean by Meaning?

First, it is important to examine the notion of meaning. Halliday discusses three types of meanings – ideational, interpersonal and textual. Ideational meanings are concerned with the interpretation and representation of experience. Referential meaning (e.g. naming), is one aspect of this, as are relations between entities and attributes, an action and its goal, an actor and an action as well as logical connections between messages and propositions. Interpersonal meanings are concerned with the interaction between speaker and listener and are reflected in such aspects of language as tense and modality – conveying when something happened in reference to the current situation, degrees of definiteness of the information presented. In addition, the nature of the interaction, be it a request or ordering, etc., is of interpersonal significance. Textual meanings are concerned with the way in which the other two types of meanings are presented as information developed in context. Cohesion is involved in this aspect, as is the organization of given or new information and thematization of certain aspects of the text, all contributing to the continuity and coherence within the text.

Halliday thus proposes that meanings are more than simply a representation of a set of facts related to the real world. When speakers communicate, they do more than simply state facts. And even the representation of a fact depends on the speaker's perspective, with representational meanings realized accordingly – through choices of particular lexical items, patterning of clauses, use of modality and in the thematizing of particular aspects of events. Hence, meaning is multifaceted, each of the above types of meanings contributing to the ultimate language production.

In addition, a text is not simply a matter of the cumulative effect of the meanings of individual words or sentences contained therein. If a clause is taken out of a text, it may not always make sense standing alone, for example, *he saw it in the distance*. There is clearly some dependency on the pronominals *he* and *it* which are identified explicitly elsewhere in the text. The distance is also made clear elsewhere. Texts or discourses have their own meanings which are not simply the sum of their component parts. Similarly, in a narrative discourse, temporal or causal connections may be made between clauses which are essential to the text's continuity and coherence. In these cases, the ordering of the clauses and/or the conjunctive relationships between them are as important as the content of the individual clauses.

To date, meanings conveyed during aphasic discourse have been investigated largely from a macrostructural perspective, although cohesion has certainly a focus as well. The work of Ulatowska and colleagues and that of Glosser and Deser (1990) have demonstrated relative intactness of text macrostructure in mildly and moderately aphasic speakers, reflecting the speakers' ability to convey the gist of a story, while still having difficulty at the sentence level in terms of providing details due to word-finding problems. In terms of cohesion, numerous authors (Ulatowska et al., 1981; 1983; Dressler and Pleh, 1988; Glosser and Deser, 1990; Armstrong, 1991) have reported the difficulty aphasic speakers have in maintaining clear co-reference throughout a text – using pronominals and demonstratives in particular without ultimate explicit referents.

Systemic-functional grammar examines the so-called microstructure of a text and in essence relates it to the macrostructure. Unlike other grammars in which the sentence is usually the upper limit of syntactic analysis, systemic-functional grammar regards the text as the basic unit analysis. While the same ranks (with the exception of the clause complex) are analysed in other grammars (the phrase or the clause), what happens at these ranks is related to what happens in the text overall. In addition, discourse is seen as a semantic notion rather than a syntactic one. Hence, it is not merely another level beyond the clause, and its analysis has immediate semantic ramifications. The analysis of the microstructure is not unrelated to the meanings contained in the macrostructure – it helps to explain the macrostructure. Indeed, one cannot properly be looked at without reference to the other.

I will now return to the notion of the different types of meanings conveyed and outline the ways in which they are realized in the wording of a language. Because of space limitations and because of their obvious applicability to the deficits already identified in aphasia, I will focus on ideational and textual meanings only in this discussion. For discussion of interpersonal meanings in aphasic discourse, the reader is referred to Ferguson (1993).

Ideational meanings

The category of ideational meanings is divided into two sub-categories – experiential and logical. Experiential meanings concern 'the expression of some kind of process, some event, action, state or other phenomenal aspect of the real world' (Halliday, 1985a; 18). Hence, the experiential metafunction is one aspect of representing what is going on in the discourse. At the rank of clause, its output is the grammar of transitivity – the configuration of a process, its participants and circumstances. Transitivity analysis is similar to the grammar of predicate argument structure and thematic roles discussed by Jackendoff (1987). An example of such a clause is depicted in Figure 5.1:

The other car	pushed	me	off the road
Actor	Process	Goal	Circumstance

Figure 5.1: Transitivity analysis of a clause

When one is looking at experiential meanings, one is really concerned with something happening – an event – and the participants or circumstances associated with that event. Halliday sees the process as central to the meaning – what is happening. He proposes four main types of processes (realized by verbs) which encapsulate these meanings – material, relational, mental and verbal processes.

Material processes are processes of doing. They 'express the notion that some entity "does" something – which may be done "to" some other entity' (Halliday, 1985a; 103) and they involve an obligatory Actor and optionally a Goal. Examples include *walk, hit, eat, drive, catch* and include the process in the above example. Relational processes are processes of being, having and being at. They relate an entity either to another entity, an attribute of some kind or a circumstance, as in Figures 5.2-3.

the dog	was	white
Carrier	Process: relational	Attribute

Figure 5.2: Transitivity analysis of a clause involving a relational process of 'being'

the boy	had	a new toy
Carrier: possessor	Process: relational	Attribute: possessed

Figure 5.3: Transitivity analysis of a clause involving a relational process of 'having'

Mental processes are processes of sensing and hence involve feeling, thinking or perceiving. Consider the following examples:

I	loved	the play
Senser	Process: mental	Phenomenon

Figure 5.4: Transitivity analysis of a clause involving a mental process of feeling

I	heard	a good joke
Senser	Process: mental	Phenomenon

Figure 5.5: Transitivity analysis of a clause involving a mental process of perceiving

Verbal processes are processes of saying. Verbal clauses 'represent symbolizations involving a symbolic source, the Sayer' (Matthiesson: 232). Consider Figure 5.6:

She	said	he came over yesterday
Sayer	Process: verbal	verbiage

Figure 5.6: Transitivity of a clause complex involving verbal projection

A text can be characterized in one regard by the types of processes used within it. For example, Martin and Rothery (1981) outline the typical process patterns in different genres. In what they call the narrative strand, they identify four different genres – the observation/comment, in which mental and relational processes predominate, recounts, in which material and mental processes predominate, narratives, in which material processes predominate, and thematic narratives, in which material processes again predominate. The types of processes can be related to the types of meanings these sorts of texts convey. For example, recounts contain a predominance of material processes as they are about what happened at a particular time, whereas commentaries (observations/comments) are more concerned with personal interpretations and attitudes to events and thus contain more relational and mental processes. In the expository strand, reports are characterized by relational and behaviour processes, where exposition is dominated by relational process. Differences here can be explained again in terms of meaning – reports are decidedly more abstract than recounts, for example. As Martin and Rothery say:

> Reports are not principally concerned with reconstructing or imagining experience. Rather they interpret experience: they describe, classify and attribute habitual behaviours to their subject matter (Martin and Rothery, 1981: 30).

It is of interest to examine the process usage of aphasic clients to see just how they are utilizing this resource for meaning. Do they have a good variety of process types or do they use predominantly one or two? Do they use processes appropriately to the context or genre? Are they able to use mental and verbal processes to report ideas and conversations? And are they able to utilize a range of processes successfully in the one text? Given the genre characterizations just discussed, it is important that client language samples should be obtained in as many different contexts as possible, certainly using different genres, such as narratives, explanations, discussions, casual conversation and even different topics. One should not expect a speaker to use all process types equally in all texts. In fact, this would be quite inappropriate. However, one can still look for variety of process types within the one text. Consider the following example taken from an aphasic speaker, RD, in which he was recounting a holiday taken at the Gold Coast in Queensland with his family. The prompt was, 'Tell me about a good holiday you've had – I think you've been to the Gold Coast haven't you?' The following was the aphasic speaker's recount:

1. That — up the Gold Coast...good one yeah
2. Pick on that one
3. What we did with the kids?
4. Mum did
5. We went
6. And Played
7. We did things
8. Uh...went...to pool
9. Went swimming

10. And walks
11. Get into things
12. We'd get
13. I'd like the kids out
14. And make 'em like kelevans
15. Kids on kids
16. And they like to get out
17. And make junks
18. Make things
19. Make a giant (—)
20. Gotta get out
21. And do it
22. Kids (—) we get away by ourselves
23. Go out and uh...
24. Play silly buggers
25. And play around a lot
26. We have some fun that way

In this text, one sees almost total usage of material processes. Now the predominance of material processes demonstrates the speaker's retained awareness of appropriate process usage for this particular genre. However, the fact that materials were used almost exclusively is somewhat less appropriate. If such a pattern was found across numerous texts, indicating limited resource usage on the part of the speaker, one could walk on introducing other aspects to the text in the form of other processes to add some variety of meaning, such as adding relational processes and even some verbal processes. The clinician could facilitate these by asking questions such as, *What was the motel like? How big was it? What was the weather like?* These questions could stimulate relational processes, with responses such as, *It was fine, It was wet, The motel was big, The motel was new*, etc. Questions such as, *How did you enjoy it? What did the children think of it?* could elicit clauses or clause complexes containing mental processes such as, *We loved it there. They thought it was great.* A variety of cueing techniques including modelling (verbally and/or visually) and/or sentence completion tasks could be used to elicit such responses from more severely impaired clients who could not simply be asked questions and reply.

The above text was taken from an aphasic speaker at one month post onset of his stroke. As part of a recovery study underway, another version of the same recount was obtained from the speaker at six month post onset. The later version contained a greater variety of processes as is evidenced in an extract from this text below (processes were not worked on in the speech therapy received by this speaker in the intervening period):

Cl: Last time you were telling me about the Gold Coast

1. The Gold Coast... oh we went up there with the kids the last time

Cl: Yes tell me about that

2. Uh that was the two boys over here
3. They were what fourteen and fifteen...fifteen sixteen something like that...And Mum and meself
4. Uh...we went up there
5. We only had a week day seven days uh...ten days altogether
6. Cos we went up there for a couple of days seven days actually at the Gold Coast
7. And uh...oh we had fun with the kids
8. (–) Gold...Seaworld with the girls
9. Uh they could spend a full day couple of days there
10 ....not trouble to get it all
11. And we went all places round [they went]
12. Then we just had our days at the um...motel [where we stayed]
13. We were right at the pool
14. And they had it all worked out
15. ...twelve...looks...twelve...uh to get to 'em...just to get from out of her place into the pool
16. (–) and you're in
17. And for the kids that was good
18. And we'd go down to the pool
19. Um...we did our time up there
20. Oh they thought
21. It was good
22. They could have anything [they wanted]
23. They thought
24. We were queens
25. I said
26. I'm not a queen
27. That was a big thing at the time
28. And uh...they thought
29. It was beautiful

In this version, one can see more use of relational processes, (they were fourteen, we were right at the pool, it was good) so that the speaker was able to add different types of descriptive information and some evaluations. In addition, mental processes were also used, reflecting what the children thought of the holiday. Hence, rather than simply reporting what they did, other aspects of the holiday were included. This text confirmed the initial impression that material processes dominated somewhat abnormally at one month post onset and that greater variety of meanings would be appropriately conveyed if a greater variety of process types were used. Hence, the process itself can be a focus of treatment.

However, as well documented in aphasia, there are numerous other aspects of disruption occurring at clause level. These are associated with both word-finding difficulties and syntactic problems. For example, a speaker may produce clauses such as the following:

> The woman ate...
> The boy chased...

In certain contexts, goals might be required in these clauses to complete the meaning, while in the following examples, circumstances could have been supplied:

> The man went...
> The woman walked...

If an aphasic speaker was to make such omissions in a text, where such constructions did function as incomplete clauses, work at the clause level would be very important, focusing on those aspects which were problematic. However, seeing such omissions as part of a difficulty with creation of a clausal process rather than a difficulty in retrieving isolated words is central to this approach. While the word-finding difficulty is acknowledged as such, the function of the word is examined within the clause. Actor, Goal, Circumstance are treated in a clause and discourse context, rather than according to its class membership alone, as in a noun. This approach is similar to the approach employed by Byng (1988) in her 'mapping therapy' applications – the main difference, however, is that using a systemic-functional approach, one would treat within the context of discourse rather than isolated sentences. Using a systemic-functional approach, a genre could be chosen as the focus of treatment (recount, expository or procedural). A topic could then be decided upon, with relevant processes chosen and meaningful sentences associated with that topic constructed. The amount to which the client is involved with the construction of the sentences themselves obviously depends on severity. The milder ones could construct their own with simple cueing procedures – sentence completion techniques – while the more severely impaired could simply be required to repeat relevant sentences, could copy them in writing, or even just have them supplied by the clinician. The clinician can then prompt increased awareness and production of the problematic functions.

An example of the sort of stimuli is a set of pictures depicting the following story:

> A man is walking in a park on a windy day. His hat is lifted off by
> the wind and blown into a tree. The man tries to get his hat with

his walking stick but is unable to do so, finally giving up and walking away. Two birds come along and make a nest out of the hat.

Following presentation of the story, the clinician can elicit the particular focused on functions by asking such questions as, 'Who lost his hat?' 'What did he lose?' 'Where did he lose it?' – again with varying degrees of cueing needed to elicit a response depending on severity.

The other important perspective when analysing texts for experiential meaning is that referred to above when discussing processes used. It is not only a matter of looking at what is problematic or erroneous in the person's discourse – but also what is missing. What resources are not being used at all? For example, at the rank of clause, is the speaker never supplying circumstances? Is he or she never producing clauses involving recipients? And at the phrase/group rank, is he or she always only supplying simply noun phrases? Can the person's language not only be corrected but also enhanced through extending resource usage?

Logical Meanings

In terms of logical meanings, the output is the system for combining clauses, or, as Halliday terms it – the creation of clause complexes. While a detailed discussion of this is available in Halliday (1985a, 1985b), suffice to say the system encompasses a variety of ways in which clauses can relate logically to each other. Halliday recognizes two sorts of relationship – the structural one, closest to the traditional notions of co-ordination and subordination, and the logico-semantic one – consisting of the sub-categories of projection and expansion.

Projection involves one clause projecting another clause. These are associated with mental and verbal types of meanings, where a speaker reports ideas or verbal interactions:

I said
I would go

He thought
He wanted an apple

He said
Don't go to the theatre

Expansion is the means by which one clause expands on another in some way. It is divided into a further three sub-categories – those of elaboration, extension and enhancement. *Elaboration* does not involve the secondary clause providing any new information, but rather re-stating, clarifying, exemplifying or refining what is already stated in the primary clause. Consider the following examples:

The road was not wonderful
It had a lot of broken bitumen on the left hand side

We went into a most terrific skid
Doing a figure eight around the road

In the first example, the second clause elaborates on why the road was not considered to be wonderful, as suggested in the initial clause. The second example involves the second clause elaborating on the nature of the skid referred to in the first clause.

Extension involves the addition of some new information by either simple addition, by replacement or by provision of an alternative. For example:

So the local quack came round
And took one look at me

And we went into a most terrific skid
Grounding two tyres off

Enhancement involves the qualification of one clause by the other – by reference to time, place, manner, cause or condition. Consider the following examples:

We had absolutely no money at all
So we borrowed a car

Before I realized
I was in the ambulance

In aphasic discourse, one finds both errors in the ways in which clauses are combined – often signalled by an error in conjunction usage, and predominance of certain patterns at the expense of others (Armstrong, 1992)). For example, in the following aphasic version of the Windy Day text described above, there is a predominance of extension relations. This can be contrasted with a normal speaker's version of the same story in which there is a greater variety of relationships present, reflecting a much more intricately structured text containing significantly more variety in meaning – both in terms of time and circumstances:

Aphasic speaker FP's text:

1. The gentleman's walking along this wind...wind driven street
2. And...his hat is...taken off
3. And thrown up into the tree
4. And he tries to get it
5. And he couldn't get it with his hanger...with his walking... water... his walkstick

6. And he gives it away
7. And a bird comes around
8. And spots [this hat sitting in the bough of the tree]
9. And sits there
10. And drinks
11. Has a...has...
12. And she takes part in it

Normal text:

1. Well in this story a gentleman's walking through...a parkland on a very windy day
2. Looks like a wintery day
3. Because he's wearing a coat and a hat
4. And the wind is blowing a lot of leaves around
5. And unfortunately it blows his hat off
6. And his hat sailed through the air
7. Landed in the fork of a tree
8. And when it landed
9. It was upside down
10. So that the concave part of the hat was facing upwards
11. And he tried to reach it with his walking stick
12. But couldn't do so
13. And while he's attempting to do this
14. Some birds came along
15. And found
16. It was a very convenient place to build their nest
17. So they hopped inside the hat

Again, there is no right or wrong way of using logical relations. However, when looking at language as resource for meaning, one can see the richness of the second version as compare to the first.

In addition, the clinician has to focus on the meaning need of the client or perhaps even the best types of meanings to compensate for his deficits. For example, elaboration may sound tangential and repetitive for one speaker, but be used quite successfully to clarify problematic information by another. For example, if a speaker is doing the latter, then perhaps increasing this strategy may be of value and add to his meaning potential. Consider the following re-statements, clarifications produced by an aphasic speaker discussing his hospitalization following his stroke:

> And I just lay there
> And said very little to anybody
> And didn't food me
> They more or less...give me...food no food

In this example, he realize his 'error' in the third clause and corrected this in the following clause. In the following example, he tries to be more specific in his information through elaboration:

> Friday Saturday Sunday Monday I didn't have any food or...
> I apparently was intervened

In the next example, in which the speaker was discussing setting off on a holiday, a word-finding difficulty is compensated for in a clarification attempt:

> Saturday night we stayed at a your air...
> Anyway you would stay overnight

Again working within the context of a particular genre and topic, the clinician and client can go about constructing a text related to that topic, focusing on one or two sorts of relations felt to be the most pertinent. For example, if the client was being encouraged to use elaboration, the clinician could encourage a re-stating of certain clauses in different ways – with the purpose of clarification. The client could be asked to discuss a happy event in his or her life. From clinical experience, weddings have proved to be a good topic for discussion. In order to focus on elaboration, one could encourage starting the text with a short discussion about the size of the gathering. The clinician could facilitate this by asking about this and encourage elaboration in the following way:

Cl: *So tell me about the size of the wedding*

Pt: It was quite a big wedding

Cl: *Were there many people there?*

Pt: Oh about a hundred

Cl: *So you had lots of people – all relatives?*

Pt: No – about half relatives and half friends

From the information, the text could then be gone over again – this time with the client doing most of the talking. The clinician and client would first go over the information provided, perhaps write it down (either completely or using key words as cues) and then the client would restate the information in the following way:

> We had a big wedding
> There were about a hundred people there
> About half were relatives
> And half were friends

It is also important to remember when structuring texts for clients in this way that their participation in the planning of stimuli is important. For example, if the client preferred to make *wedding* thematic in the first clause and not *we* (i.e. focus on the wedding rather than the participants as the starting point to the clause), this is quite a viable option and the clauses may follow another route:

> The wedding was big
> A hundred people were there
> Both relatives and friends were there

While clinicians often make the comment that such activities may only be of value to the more mildly affected clients, it should be pointed out that the goal in such activities is meaning, not perfect structure. Hence, any combination of clauses including the key points would be acceptable depending on the abilities of the speaker. For example, a more severely impaired speaker may produce the following version:

> Big wedding
> hundred
> relatives...friends

When working from a meaning perspective, there is less focus on structure, although structure must obviously be incorporated into the planning of the treatment. However, if one is focusing on elaboration, for example, the meanings involved are the focus of treatment rather than the form they take. So rather than focusing on one kind of syntactic structure, the clinician focuses on a kind of meaning and may encourage a variety of syntactic structures to facilitate such meaning.

Taking this perspective, even severely affected clients could benefit from at least the notion of clause complexing. Of course, we are not talking of globally aphasic individuals here. However, even speakers restricted to the single word level may benefit from having the notion of continuity of ideas reinforced at some level. Consider the following extract from a text in which an aphasic speaker SE was describing the lead-up to the rupture of her cerebral aneurysm – related at first to some difficulty at work:

1. Jump from truck um...um...boss from uh from...oh...
2. Cos um stroke...

Cl: See if you can tell me about that

3. I was um...stroke um...or...

Cl: Who had the stroke?

4. Me

Cl: Right. When you had your stroke. Right. What was it to do with your boss and the truck? What was that?

5. Boss um...headache um...used to...uh five months or so before that
6. And um um...went to doctor from...uh...Glenfield
7. Was um...
8. She...she told me...
9. It was um never...stroke..me um for...um...two months or go
10. That uh...when um...I go doctor from Ingleburn
11. He uh oh um scan
12. She um...and..andurim

Cl: Aneurysm

13. Yeah
14. Um...um...one day um...and uh...specialist called...Smith
15. Easy...uh...uh...doctor was uh...operation

Cl: But what were you telling me about a truck? Or about your boss?

16. We had a...um...accident at uh work
17. And we had um...um...cos uh he had uh...(—)

Cl: So who had the accident

18. Me

Cl: And it was something to do with your aneursym?

19. Yeah

Cl: What sort of accident?

20. It had...falling from a up the truck for um...three fall

Cl: You fell out of a truck at work

21. Yeah

This text was largely dialogic as the client did not offer many speech attempts without prompting. And yet in clauses 5–12 it is clear that she was capable of developed speech to some extent. While analysis of this text and this client's language skills in general remain beyond the scope of this chapter, suffice to say that she was capable of some clause complex formation and that this was encouraged in treatment, even though her skills at the clause level were far from intact. It is of significance that most aphasic speakers (except for very severely or globally impaired individuals) still manage to express their meaning at least to some extent, even given their limited or compromised linguistic resources. Hence, it is very important to consider how this occurs as well as considering the limitations encountered. Much has been written on the need for a strength-based approach to aphasia therapy as well as a weakness-based one (Holland, 1991). In exploring both perspectives, the clinician has a fuller appreciation of the possibilities for improvement in the aphasic speakers ability to express their meaning.

As can be seen, this approach thus goes against the more traditional constituency-based approach to treatment – working at the single word level first, then the clause level, then text level. It is more a top-down approach to language treatment. As text is seen as a semantic unit in systemic-functional grammar, rather than a syntactic one, it always forms the basis for any treatment paradigm, as facilitating meaning is the aim of that paradigm. While one might be restricted to single word production in treatment, those single words can be treated in the context of a text (language in use) and can be taught or elicited in such a way that they perform some function. They may function as a single statement or command or may form the basis of a more extended attempt at communication, in which a number of connected ideas are conveyed and the sorts of semantic relations just described are involved.

Textual Meanings

In terms of the textual metafunction, cohesion is one of the outputs. The main aspect of cohesion discussed in the aphasiology literature to date is the difficulty aphasic speakers have with co-reference. However, other aspects of cohesion (as discussed by Halliday and Hasan, 1976) are worth reiterating here and expanding upon – in particular, aspects of lexical cohesion.

For a text to be coherent, numerous criteria must be met. However, lexical cohesion is one way of drawing the text together. When a speaker is speaking, the context largely determines what will be said. If, for example, one is discussing the weather, words from a fairly finite range will almost surely occur during the discourse – fine, wet, hot, sunny, cold, humid, rain, sleet, snow, temperature, etc. The fact that these words are related to each other in some way in a text means that the text is then lexically cohesive. They are related to each other through one of the following sense relations – repetition, synonymy, antonymy, hyponymy, meronymy or collocation. Repetition obviously involves reference to the same person, place, thing, quality via the same lexical item throughout a text. Synonymy involves a relationship of similar meaning between words, whereas antonymy involves opposite meanings. Hyponymy involves a category/member relationship, for example, furniture/chair, and meronymy involves a part-whole relationship, for example, nose/face. Collocation is one of the most general types of relationships through which certain words will co-occur in a text by virtue of the topic. The list of words related to the weather example above is an example of words which are collocationally related – although some, of course, also fall into the other categories.

When one examines lexical cohesion in aphasic discourse, one sees the limited variety of sense relations used. This is not surprising given the lexical difficulties aphasic speakers have. The following cohesive chain analysis of aphasic speaker FP's Windy Day text quoted on pp. 80–1 demonstrates the relative lack of lexical cohesion. And what lexical cohesion exists is mainly achieved through the device of repetition, with some of synonymy. The predominant form of cohesion in this text is grammatical – with the use of co-reference (through pronominalization) and ellipsis. Ellipted words are signalled by (E) and in this text, these are credited with forming the cohesive chain referring to the bird in the story:

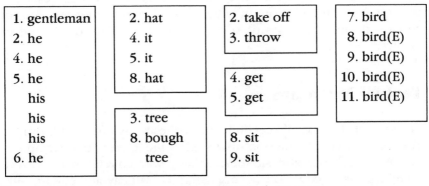

Figure 5.7: Cohesive chains Formed From FP's Windy Day text

In such a text, an increase in variety of lexical cohesive devices could be considered as an aim in increasing its cohesion.

To work on lexical cohesion would again involve deciding on a topic to be discussed so that the resultant language would be in some context. The clinician and client could then develop a list of words relevant to that topic – again with appropriate degrees of cueing involved depending on severity. Facilitation techniques could include the client having to choose appropriate words from a larger selection of words, some of which are not related to the topic, semantic cueing by the clinician involving talking 'around' a target word, for example, what is happening when you have an umbrella up to stop you getting wet, you usually stay indoors, etc., and simple synonym/antonym tasks, done in the context of the topic at hand. For collocational words, the client can be assisted by discussing participants, processes and circumstances associated with the topic as described in the section above related to transitivity at the clause level.

After a word list is generated, the clinician can assist the client in building a text using these words. The text can be written down, or taped and the client can then rehearse in order to ultimately produce the text independently. Involvement of spouses, friends and others is important as the text then has some function in communicating information to other people, rather than being clinically produced for artificial purposes only. Topics used can relate to current affairs, personal events, sport, etc. – the clinician must negotiate these with both the clients and their families to ensure maximum relevance. Different genres such as recounts, reports, procedural discourse, expository discourse, casual conversation can all be attempted in order to make the treatment tasks as natural as possible and as functional as possible.

Conclusion

The application of systemic-functional grammar to the treatment of aphasia offers a framework in which the discourse of speakers can be analysed in terms of both specific and overall meanings. Words at the phrase, clause and clause complex ranks are related to their function in the text and the meanings to which they contribute, rather than being seen in isolation or in a sentence context only. In viewing language in this way, meaning becomes a focus of analysis and treatment. Therapy is geared towards capitalizing on skills retained to some extent by the aphasic speaker, increasing use of resources to expand varieties of meanings expressed and correcting ambiguous or confusing aspects of language usage. While structure is less of a focus than meaning, the two are intricately tied together in this grammar. Therapy is encouraged to take place in a context-driven framework, while maintaining a grammatically-based approach. Hence, the notion of functional therapy is broadened somewhat to include not only the context/meaning based 'language in use' notions previously employed, but also more ideas on the specific sorts of language actually used to accomplish everyday communication.

References

Armstrong EM (1987) Cohesive harmony and its significance in listener perception of coherence. In Brookshire RC (Ed) Clinical Aphasiology: Conference Proceedings. Minneapolis, MN: BRK Pub.

Armstrong EM (1988) Cohesion Analysis of Aphasic discourse. Unpublished MA(Hons) thesis, Macquarie University, Sydney.

Armstrong EM (1991) The potential of cohesion analysis in the assessment and treatment of aphasic discourse. Clinical Linguistic and Phonetics 5 (1) 39–51.

Armstrong EM (1992) Clause complex relations in aphasic discourse: a longitudinal case study. Journal of Neurolinguistics 7 (4): 261–76.

Armstrong EM (1993) Aphasia rehabilitation: a sociolinguistic perspective. In Holland AL, Forbes MM (Eds), Aphasia Treatment: World Perspectives. San Diego CA: Singular Press.

Bottenberg D, Lemme M, L Hedberg N (1985) Analysis of oral narratives of normal

and aphasic adults. In Brookshire RH (Ed) Clinical Aphasiology Conference
Proceedings. Minneapolis, MN: BRK Pub.

Byng S (1988) Sentence processing deficits: theory and therapy. Cognitive
Neuropsychology 5 629–76.

Coehlo C, Clarkson JV, Elia D (1992) Longitudinal assessment of narrative discourse
in a mildly aphasic adult. Paper presented to the 22nd Annual Clinical
Aphasiology Conference, Durango, CO.

Crystal D, Fletcher P, Garman M (1976) The Grammatical Analysis of Language
Disability: A Procedure for Assessment and Remediation. London: Edward
Arnold.

Davis GA, Wilcox MJ (1985) Adult Aphasia Rehabilitation: Applied Pragmatics. San
Diego, CA: College-Hill Press.

Dressler WU, Pleh C (1988) On text disturbances in aphasia. In Dressler WU, Stark JA
(Eds) Linguistic Analyses of Aphasic Language. New York: Springer-Verlag.

Edwards S, Garman M, Knott R (1993) The grammatical characterization of aphasic
language. Aphasiology 7 (2): 217–20.

Ferguson AJ (1993) Interpersonal aspects of aphasic conversation. Journal of
Neurolinguistics 7 (4): 277–94.

Glosser G, Deser T (1990). Patterns of discourse production among neurological
patients with fluent language disorders. Brain and Language 40 67–88.

Halliday MAK (1985a) An Introduction to Functional Grammar. London: Edward
Arnold.

Halliday MAK (1985b) Spoken and Written Language. Geelong Victoria: Deakin
University Press.

Halliday MAK, Hasan R (1976) Cohesion in English. London: Longmans.

Holland Al (1980) Communication Abilities in Daily Living. Baltimore MD: University
Park Press.

Holland AL (1991) Pragmatic aspects of intervention in aphasia. Journal of
Neurolinguistics 6 (2): 197–211.

Jackendoff R (1987) The status of thematic relations in linguistic theory. Linguistic
Inquiry 18: 369–411.

Kintsch W (1977) On comprehending stories. In Just MA, Carpenter PA (Eds)
Cognitive Processes in Comprehension. New York: Wiley.

Lemme ML, Hedberg NL, Bottenberg DF (1984) Cohesion in narratives of aphasic
adults. In Brookshire RH (Ed.), Clinical aphasiology: Conference proceedings.
Minneapolis, MN: BRK Pub.

Longacre R (1976) An Anatomy of Speech Notions. Lisse: Peter de Ridder Press.

Martin J (1992) English text: System and Structure. Philadelphia PA: John Benjamins
Publishing Company.

Martin JR, Rothery J (1981) Writing project report. Working Papers in Linguistic 2.
Linguistics Dept, Sydney University.

Mattiesson, CMIM (in press). Lexicogrammatical Cartography: English Systems.

Piehler MF, Holland AL (1984). Cohesion in aphasic language. Clinical Aphasiology:
Conference Proceedings. Minneapolis, MN: BRK Pub.

Rumelhardt DE (1985) Notes on a schema for stories. In Bobrow, DG Collins A (Eds)
Representation and Understanding: Studies in Cognitive Science. New York:
Academic Press

Saffran EC, Berndt RS, Schwartz MF (1989) The quantitative analysis of agrammatic
production: procedure and data. Brain and Language 37 440–79.

Shewan CM (1988) The Shewan spontaneous language analysis (SSLA) system for aphasic adults: description, reliability, and validity. Journal of Communication Disorders 21 103–38.

Ulatowska HK, North AJ, Macaluso-Haynes (1981) Production of narrative and procedural discourse in aphasia. Brain and Language 13 345–371.

Ulatowska HK, Weiss-Doyell A, Freedman-Stern R, Macaluso-Haynes S (1983) Production of narrative discourse in aphasia. Brain and Language 19 317–34.

Ulatowska HK, Bond Chapman S (1989) Discourse considerations for aphasia management. Seminars in Speech and Language 10 (4): 298–314.

Ulatowska HK, Allard L, Bond Chapman S (1990) Narrative and procedural discourse in aphasia. In Joanette Y, Brownell HH (Eds) Discourse Ability and Brain Damage: Theoretical and Empirical Perspectives. New York: Springer-Verlag.

Van Dijk TE (1977) Text and Context: Explorations of the Semantics and Pragmatics of Discourse. London: Longmans.

Van Dijk TA, Kintsch W (1978) Macrostructures: An Interdisciplinary study of Global Structures in Discourse Interaction and Cognition. Hillsdale NJ: Erlbaum.

Vermeulen J, Bastiaanse R, van Wageningen B (1989) Spontaneous speech in Aphasia: a correlation study. Brain and Language 36 252–74.

Wagenaar E, Snow C, Prins R (1975) Spontaneous speech of aphasic patients: A psycholinguistic analysis. Brain and Language 2 281–303.

Yorkston K, Beukelman D (1980) An analysis of connected speech samples of aphasic and normal speakers. Journal of Speech and Hearing Disorders 45 27–36.

Chapter 6
An Assessment of PACE Therapy

RALF GLINDEMANN AND LUISE SPRINGER

Introduction

The main goal of any language therapy is to enable the aphasic patient to cope with *everyday communicative interactions*. There is an ongoing debate, however, whether this is best achieved by training specific language abilities and strategies (starting at disturbed single elementary functions) or by communicative stimulation with the complex components of everyday behaviour. Representatives of the different language-oriented approaches have been able to demonstrate transfer of improvement to non-trained problems and to material of similar linguistic structures (e.g. Mayer and Kerschensteiner, Huber, 1978; Basso, Faglioni and Vignolo, 1979; Seron et al., 1979; Wertz et al., 1981; Kearns and Salmon, 1984: Shewan and Kertesz, 1984; Shewan and Bandur 1986; Thompson and Mc Reynolds, 1986; Brindley, et al., 1989; Poeck, Huber and Willmes, 1989; Springer, Willmes and Haag, 1993). The language-oriented procedures concerned with specific aphasic symptoms with the more recent approaches focusing on the hypothesized underlying neurolinguistic mechanisms (Hatfield and Shewell, 1983; Byng and Coltheart, 1986; Lesser, 1987; Howard and Patterson, 1987; Springer et al, 1991a; Springer and Willmes 1993. See Edmundson and McIntosh, Chapter 8, and Edwards, Chapter 7, this volume). Most of the language-oriented techniques focus on linguistic units, structures, regularities or strategies and are based on a (more or less empirically demonstrated) hierarchy of complexity of the linguistic tasks. In all these approaches it is important to select exemplary and symptom/strategy-specific linguistic material and tasks or problems to be practiced. Yet a generalization of improved linguistic performance to everyday communication has hardly ever been demonstrated. In one respect it is methodologically very difficult to investigate the transfer of learning effects in everyday communication. On the other hand, it is often not a requirement of the language-oriented approaches to modify pragmatic abilities.

If the final objective of therapy has to be the improvement of everyday communication, one would object that this goal cannot be attained by controlled linguistic therapy alone. Pragmatic approaches seem to be most applicable to help the patients realize their full residual communicative potential (Wertz, 1984; Aten, 1981; 1986). Even patients with severely impaired linguistic competence often can be surprisingly successful in their communicative competence (Prinz, 1980; Martin, 1981; Holland, 1982; Green, 1984; Feyereisen, et al., 1988; Glosser, Weiner and Kaplan, 1988; Holland, 1991). Therefore, pragmatics oriented aphasia therapists argue that therapy should focus on the use of language in context rather than setting the goal in terms of linguistic units and regularities that have been lost or are inconsistently available (Prutting, 1982; Weniger, Springer and Poeck, 1987). In a pragmatic setting it should be possible to elicit a variety of communicative acts and to develop appropriate verbal and nonverbal strategies to realize these acts. For example, the *Promoting Aphasics' Communicative Effectiveness* (PACE) therapy by Davis and Wilcox (first described 1978) is an approach which tries to stimulate such pragmatic performances.

A main purpose of this chapter is to discuss the advantages and problems of the PACE approach in improving linguistic or communicative abilities. Moreover, we discuss how to modify and combine PACE with symptom specific approaches. We first review the traditional PACE approach and consider it under pragmatic and didactic-therapeutic aspects. Finally, we discuss the general efficacy of the PACE approach and propose necessary conditions for applying it.

Traditional PACE-Therapy

Since the late seventies, the American authors Davis and Wilcox (1980; 1981; 1985; 1986; Wilcox and Davis 1977; 1978) emphasized pragmatic aspects in aphasia therapy. They tried to insert more language functions into their therapy using a context in which language is normally used, such as natural conversation. With this procedure they claim

> for several pragmatic components of communication to occur repeatedly in a standard clinical environment. These components include an expression of a wide range of speech acts, turn-taking between participants, hint-and-guess sequences when communication breakdown occurs, opportunities to make use of variables governing expression and comprehension of given and new information, and opportunities to make use of linguistic, paralinguistic, and extralinguistic contexts (1985: 89).

The procedures in PACE are based on four principles:

1. The clinician and patient participate equally as senders and receivers of messages.

   While the patient and the therapist alternate in the role of initiator or sender of informations and in the role of responder in such interactions, the therapist is no longer the only director or teacher. On the other hand, the patient may become an equal participant in sending and receiving messages. With this principle Davis and Wilcox (1985: 91) try to accomplish three goals: First, to allow the patient to gain experiences with topic or turn initiation as well as topic or turn responding. Second, to enable the therapist to demonstrate the use of different channels and types of communicative behaviour. Third, to ensure that the patient may practice sustaining communicative interaction for more than one turn on the same topic.

2. There is an exchange of new information between the clinician and the patient.

   This technique ensures that the therapist will be unfamiliar, to a certain extent, with the content of the therapeutic discourse. If an utterance includes new information for the clinician, more aspects of natural conversation may occur within the aphasia therapy. As the authors know, it is sometimes difficult to maintain this principle, because therapists normally know their stimulus items very well. Davis and Wilcox (1985: 98) suggest using a larger number of stimuli and changing them frequently to minimize this difficulty.

3. The patient is allowed free choice with respect to selection of communicative channels with which to convey messages.

   This principle deals with the fact that aphasic patients very often are focused on linguistic perfection to an extent which prevents the communicative success of an utterance. Inspired by the observed fact, that 'aphasics probably communicate better than they talk' (Holland, 1977: 173), with this third principle Davis and Wilcox want us to encourage the patients to use all their communicative possibilities, verbal (spoken or written), graphic or gestural. In contrast to this suggestion, in most of the traditional stimulation procedures the communicative channel or mode is limited or asserted by the therapist. In PACE the patient decides (and learns to decide) him or herself, how to be successful in discourse.

4. The feedback from the clinician is based on the client's success in communicating a message and is characteristic of receiver feedback occurring in natural settings.

   This principle stands for the attempts to base the clinicians feedback only on the communicative adequacy and not on linguistic accuracy. In this context Davis and Wilcox (1981: 98) are talking about what they call 'natural feedback'. This means that the therapist may not behave as a teacher who is asking for the right words, although he or she already has comprehended what the patient tries to communicate. Only if the therapist is uncertain as to the patient's message, because a spoken word or a pantomime has been somewhat ambiguous, may he or she ask for clarification, as he or she would do in any everyday conversation. Davis and Wilcox request feedback which is based only on what is actually communicated. If a message is totally confusing, the therapist may ask generally for a new attempt or for more information. If the therapist understands partially, he or she may ask more specifically. And if an utterance is a good approximation, the therapist may ask directly for conformation of the meaning.

To apply these principles Davis and Wilcox suggested a structured core activity on which many variations are possible. In this procedure the clinician and the patient take turns in selecting from a stack of face-down cards with a pictured or written message (objects, actions or stories). The sending participant keeps the selected stimulus card hidden from the view of the partner. After one of the participants has taken one of the cards it is his or her task to transmit the information on this card by following the principle of free choice of communicative modes. With this procedure the principle of communicating new information is implemented in the therapeutic setting.

To ensure that the two participants function equally as senders and receivers of messages, they have to alternate in the different roles item by item. Davis (1986: 251) points out that the clinician does not assume any special role of teacher or director within the parameters of the PACE interaction *per se.*' The clinician never corrects the patients' attempts. His or her only duty is to provide natural feedback to the patient (as described above) and to model the use of channels and strategies in the different roles. Thereby, the therapist tries to influence the patients' behaviour indirectly by modelling. Davis and Wilcox (1981: 180) assert that the described PACE procedure is applicable to all types and degrees of aphasia.

Davis (1980) developed a special rating scale for PACE interactions, which allows the evaluation of the communicative effects of the therapy. Therefore, they take into account the type, as well as the amount, of feedback from the therapist. Although, Davis and Wilcox admit (1985: 112) that the use of this scale is sometimes not without problems, it is a procedure which is easily applied in clinical routine (see Table 6.1).

Table 6.1 Rating Scale for PACE Interaction: Production

5	Message conveyed on first attempt.
4	Message conveyed after general feedback from the clinician.
3	Message conveyed after specific feedback.
2	Message partially conveyed after general and specific feedback.
1	Message not conveyed appropriately despite efforts by the patient and clinician.
0	Client does not attempt to convey the message.

Since PACE therapy was first introduced by Davis and Wilcox, therapy studies have been published which assess the efficacy of the approach. Davis and Wilcox (1985) themselves evaluated the efficacy of the approach in a single case study and a small group investigation with eight aphasic patients in a simple cross-over design (i.e. A vs. BA) where they compared direct stimulation with PACE therapy. The patients' performances were measured before, during, and after the treatment with a role-playing-battery and with the PICA (Porch, 1967) and they found some increase in communicative effectiveness for the PACE approach. A further single case study by Chin Li, et al., (1988), demonstrates the effectiveness of PACE compared to Schuell's traditional stimulation (cf. Schuell, 1974). This patient, who showed naming deficits, was able to use communicative strategies such as verbal circumlocutions combined with gestures. Carlomagno, et al. (1991) investigated the efficacy of PACE including tasks of riddle place, picture description and telling stories. In this group study the eight aphasic patients after PACE therapy used more residual nonverbal strategies to complete or substitute inefficient verbal messages. Pulvermüller and Roth (1991) used different language games in a PACE setting. too. Before and after therapy in a timespan of 3–4 weeks they tested the patients with the Token Test (De Renzi and Vignolo, 1962). Five of the eight investigated aphasic patients showed a significant improvement on a Token Test. However, we wonder whether the Token Test really reflects performance in everyday life. (See Carlomagno (1994) for additional recent review of PACE efficacy.)

Some critical considerations about the traditional PACE should be discussed in terms of linguistic pragmatics and didactic-therapeutical perspectives.

Pragmatic Aspects

Davis and Wilcox (1981: 170 ff.; 1985 1 ff.; 1986; 251 ff.) claim that the therapeutic approach of the PACE method is a *pragmatic* one. In other words, PACE therapy should deal with the *communicative functions of language use within everyday contexts* (Stalnaker, 1970). Davis and Wilcox refer to a theoretical distinction between different contexts (Labov, 1970; Pierce, 1989). The first and second of these contexts refer to all segmental signs (linguistic context) and suprasegmental signs (paralinguistic context) in the same text. Therefore, we may call these two contexts the *co-text* as well. This includes, for instance, all words, sentences, gestures, pantomimes, and prosodic patterns before, during, and after a certain communicative unit. They are related reciprocally with each other in different ways, and they are all influenced by an extralinguistic context, which involves all external and internal components of the *situation* in which a communicative act is realized

(Ervin-Tripp, 1964; Hörmann, 1986). Because all the contextual parameters influence what someone says, how it is said and whether someone is able to understand this utterance in a given situation, we have to take into consideration this important extralinguistic context, as much as possible, in any therapeutic approach that tries to enable a patient to take part in everyday communication.

This holds true especially when we include the fact that we do not only give information while we are communicating. Moreover, we perform *communicative acts*. Therefore, we have to distinguish between the information which is given by a *locutionary act* and the *illocutionary force* of the same communicative act (Austin, 1962; Searle, 1969). Such communicative acts – for example, to reproach someone, to justify, to apologize, to invite someone, or to promise something – are not dependent primarily on communicating new information. All these acts vary within different extralinguistic contexts and are influenced, for instance, by the familiarity with the partner in conversation and the relevance of the interaction; the course-of-interaction-patterns; their hierarchically-structured motives and goals (Argyle and Kendon, 1972), their knowledge about the topics of conversation, about the other participant(s); and about the world, in general.

The PACE setting by Davis and Wilcox which is described above takes little account of all these important parameters of the extralinguistic context. To communicate about a hidden picture card as Davis and Wilcox suggest primarily involves components of the *co-text*. The patient, for instance, has to find or to understand an appropriate verbal or nonverbal sign. If there is more than one sign to process, a syntactic combination between the signs is requested; and if the utterance is a spoken word then an articulation or comprehension of the phonemic structure needs to be provided. If some problems occur that are caused by the patient's aphasic disturbances, hint-and-guess sequences, repairs and revisions need to be used. But the clinical situation itself and the relationship to the therapist are always the same. There is no variation of the social occasion for this interaction; the motivation and the intentions are hardly comparable with those in everyday situations. Beside the given fact that at least one of the participants has problems with aphasic symptoms, there is no need to know something special about the other interlocutor. The patient interacts with the therapist in a very special domain of relevance, because they both only simulate communication under specific conditions. In these terms, from a pragmatic point of view, the PACE setting is highly artificial (Howard and Hatfield, 1987; Perkins and Lesser, 1993).

The missing naturalness becomes more obvious in terms of the economical aspects of the discourse. The therapist, for example, is unnaturally tolerant of the patient who tries to find a lexical unit, a phonemic structure or a syntactic pattern. In the same way, the clinician is concentrating on everything which the patient tries to communicate. In contrast to this, in most everyday situations one must maintain a level of communication that keeps someone's interest in what we say. To understand our criticism it is important to address the following: The patient's improvement in language and communicative skills is dependent upon this therapeutic behaviour, but we do not think that it may be called *natural*. Even role playing sessions, where the participants actually have to imagine more of the extralinguistic parameters, are only a more or less adequate simulation of natural conversations.

If we look at the principle of never correcting a patient, some pragmatically based criticism is appropriate again. We doubt whether this principle is natural, since it is not uncommon that people will mutually correct one another in everyday situations; and this behaviour is not exclusive to a mother-child relationship. This leads to the questions: what does the word *natural* actual mean in social interactions? It has been an important effort of pragmatics research to distinguish between the different specific language uses in the large variety of social situations and the conditions under which conversations and communicative acts take place.

Another criticism is that we can not imagine how a therapist, whose profession it is to deal with language, can be a naturally equal partner with a patient with severe verbal deficits. To alternate in the conveying and receiving role may help to simulate some kind of equal participation, although, in our view the behaviour of the therapist in a PACE setting needs a high standard of therapeutic competence and, thereby, is not natural. In this sense, the PACE setting may be regarded as a special communication game and not as a natural everyday situation. Patient and therapist are equal partners only under the specific conditions of this game. But, in fact, there have to be important differences in communicative competence and the therapeutic requirements.

In fact, if one wants to elicit different speech acts in aphasia therapy it would be appropriate to use the PACE setting and the specific task to communicate within a short conversation about pictured items. But in our experience we have to do with a very limited amount of different types of such acts. We are not sure if these acts are really more diversified than in traditional therapeutic session such as in a situation where patient and clinician try to talk about semantic categories; prepositional references to locative relations; verbal strategies by retelling a story; or saying something about hobbies.

In our view the rating scale for PACE interactions does not sufficiently address the nature of feedback in everyday conversations. If a message is conveyed by the patient after general feedback from the therapist, the performance is to be evaluated by a score of 4 (Davis and Wilcox, 1985: 113). But if the message is conveyed after specific feedback the performance is evaluated by a lower score of 3. On the one hand, this is not sensible because the specific feedback assumes a more precise utterance on the part of the patient beforehand. On the other hand, this use of the rating scale requires the clinician always to give general feedback at first and specific feedback afterwards. In our opinion this illustrates again how *therapeutic* rather than *natural* PACE therapy is.

One of the most obvious results of pragmatic research has been that we urgently have to set aside the conventional perspective which states that verbal interaction is only an event between a speaker and another speaker (Duncan, 1974). In more than two decades of pragmatic research we have come to understand that there is the very important influence of the *listeners' response* in conversation (Stubbs, 1983; Glindemann, 1984; 1987). If aphasia therapy intends to improve communicative effectiveness, we must not only look at the language production or our patients, but it is just as important to have a look at their comprehension and the different types of responses given to indicate comprehension. The rating scale for PACE interactions deals only with scoring the behaviour of the patient in the role of the one who informs us about an item. To evaluate the performance of the patient in the comprehending role, Davis and Wilcox (1985) suggest we count the number of turns prior to message comprehension. This procedure does not take into consideration the different types and the amount of feedback and backchannel behaviours. Therefore, we simply suggest we take the production scale and to substitute the word *conveyed* with the word *understood* (see Table 6.2).

Table 6.2 Rating Scale for PACE Interaction: Comprehension

5	Message understood on first attempt.
4	Message understood after general feedback from the clinician.
3	Message understood after specific feedback.
2	Message partially understood after general and specific feedback.
1	Message not understood appropriately despite efforts by the patient and clinician.
0	Client does not attempt to convey the message.

Didactic-therapeutic Viewpoints

From a therapeutic point of view it is important to identify at which stage of recovery and for what types of disorders PACE therapy is appropriate. The authors of PACE suggest their approach is appropriate for all types of disorders and severities of impairment. Neurophysiologically one assumes that the basic mechanisms of functional recovery in the brain are *restitution*, *substitution*, and *compensation*. These mechanisms are related to different ways with stages of recovery. Consequently, contents and methods of aphasia therapy vary depending on the patient's stage of recovery. In our clinical practice, we distinguish three phases of aphasia therapy: *activation, symptom specific treatment* and *consolidation* (Springer, 1986; Huber, Springer and Willmes, 1993). Restitution of impaired language functions occurs typically during the first months and often leads to nearly complete recovery (Kertesz, 1984; 1993). The overall therapeutic goal during the acute phase is to enhance the evolution of temporarily impaired language functions. In our view facilitation techniques are the best methods for the acute phase (e.g. deblocking, multimodal stimulation, inhibition of automatisms).

When a patient has attained a stable condition systematic approaches are applied. During this stage of linguistic learning, gradual functional reorganization of the impaired language system is assumed to take place (Luria, et al., 1969; Pöppel and von Steinbüchel, 1992). This may be achieved by both substitution and compensation of impaired brain functions. This stage of symptom-specific treatment aims primarily at the relearning of degraded linguistic knowledge and the learning of verbal and nonverbal compensation.

If there is no improvement in language abilities to be achieved, the concern of the last stage is to maintain the relearned language abilities and to support the further social integration of the patient. In this consolidation stage symptom-specific treatment with the individual patient is no longer appropriate. Standard techniques are group therapy (conversation circles, role playing and language games), family counselling, and the integration into a support group.

In the following we discuss PACE as a therapeutic method with reference to these stages of recovery and treatment. In our view the stage of symptom-specific training must be complemented by pragmatic approaches like PACE. Such approaches would activate those communicative abilities still retained by the patients and encourage the transfer of practiced linguistic skills of everyday communication. To prevent misunderstandings PACE should not be the *only* technique in this stage. Instead of concentrating only on compensation, we try to fully utilize resources of language relearning while making use of more specific methods.

In the latter stage of consolidation, language games in a PACE setting may be used in group activities with patients or with relatives. Bongartz, Claussen and Sigle (1990) attempted various tasks in a PACE setting between two interacting groups of three aphasic patients, each with one another. The therapist functioned only as supervisor of the interaction. In four patients the authors found improvement in communicating about a certain position of an object in a picture. One patients' ability to be understood improved. Greitemann and Wolf (1991) used the PACE setting in group therapy, too. They found that even patients with severe aphasia modify their communicative behaviour. The indirect modelling was not successful for most of the patients. The therapists had to focus directly on the adequacy and economy of the compensatory strategies practiced by the patients. Newhoff, Bugbee and Ferreire (1981) investigated interaction patterns of four spouses of male aphasic patients who had taken part in an intensive spouse training programme on the principles of PACE. In the stage of consolidation PACE could support the patients in coping with language deficits that remain after the symptom-specific treatment.

However, PACE therapy does not seem to be the right technique for the early activation phase. It stimulates neither language comprehension nor speech production directly and systematically. Furthermore, it does not yield symptom-specific cues and feedback. In addition PACE does not take into account the accompanying, often very severe, neurophsychological disorders.

In our view the PACE approach is not applicable for all patients or severities of aphasia. PACE therapy is especially contraindicated for patients with severe deficits, semantic and phonemic jargon or recurring utterances; these patients may not benefit from indirect techniques. The same holds true for patients with other neurophsychological disorders which occur in most cases of severe aphasia. For these patients the basic aim of PACE – to stimulate compensatory strategies indirectly – often is not applicable. Nonverbal cognitive disorders, like reduced ability to reorientate and to abstract may prevent a successful modification of the communicative behaviour. The use of gestures and the ability to draw may be limited by ideomotor and construction apraxia. Very often deficits in spoken language production may not be compensated for by the written modality because of various disorders in writing.

In our experience PACE, if it is suitable, has a positive impact on patients' motivation to try out available communicative skills. For example, if patients reject compensatory strategies, PACE is an appropriate method to support communicative gestures (Rao and Koller, 1982). The setting which is more comparable to communication games than to systematic language exercises. Usually these games have a relaxing effect on the patient's behaviour. Nevertheless it is necessary to vary the tasks and materials in order not to be monotonous. The positive effect of motivation holds only as long as the patients' experience a sense of achievement. To summarize this in other words, 'pragmatic therapy does not mean that one should ignore structural aspects' (Penn 1993: 48).

In the following we consider the goals of PACE and the related methodology. Howard and Hatfield (1987: 85) argue that 'some pragmatic therapists confuse questions of the aims of treatment with the means used to achieve those ends.' This is also true for the PACE approach. The basic methodological principles are equally important in communication and in conveying new information with a free choice of communicative channels. At the same time these principles represent the main goals of therapy itself. Because of this identification of aims with methods, stepwise procedures are missing in the conventional PACE approach. A systematic course of therapy including symptom-specific techniques, materials and aids, is rarely provided. The therapeutic proposals are rather general. Even the patient's requirements for verbal accuracy and direct linguistic aids are in contrast to the PACE principles. As Davis and Wilcox (1981: 185) emphasize, to be consistent with the principles of interaction in PACE one should not spend too much time trying to elicit desirable verbalization. In the same way Edelman (1987: 19) points out that 'variables such as word-finding ability and complexity of grammatical structure may not now be appropriate.' PACE does not provide direct methods even in order to develop communicative strategies.

The principle of free choice of communicative strategies and modalities as it is described above will not allow the correction of deficit utterances of a patient. The therapist can only indirectly influence the patient by serving as a communicative model. We had some doubts whether this modelling concept by Davis and Wilcox functions specifically enough to exhaust all possibilities, therefore we investigated the modelling hypothesis (Glindemann, 1991; Glindemann, et al., 1991). The question was whether aphasic patients would follow a therapist's model successfully, would they switch between naming and describing when confronted with line drawing items in a standard PACE setting. The study included 12 chronic stroke patients with varying types and severities of aphasia. Ten patients were able to meet the baseline requirements to name *and* to describe. These 10 patients had to be split into four subgroups. Three patients followed the model given by the therapist completely. In four patients modelling worked only for the naming strategy. After the therapist described the items, the frequencies of describing and naming were at chance level. In one patient we found the opposite pattern favouring the describing strategy. In two patients we found the naming strategy predominated even after descriptions by the therapist. There was no clear correspondence between this grouping of patients and the type of severity of aphasia. A high correction was found between the performances on the naming subtest of the Aaschen Aphasia Test (Huber, Springer and Willmes, 1984) and the modelling of naming (rho 0.83, p < 0.001). But there was a low correlation's for modelling of describing (rho = 0.17, Spearman rank correlations). In conclusion, this study demonstrates that the general linguistic capacity still available in aphasia may be more decisive for the effectiveness of verbal modelling than the indirect intervention by the therapist. Therefore, we suggest the use of explicit instructions and direct feedback to modify communicative effectiveness. In the same way, systematically controlled material has to be used in therapy. The importance of the linguistic structure of certain stimuli and how they may influence the success of communicative attempts in a PACE setting has been emphasized by Glindemann (1990b). Edelmann (1987: 27) also suggests increasing the demands for specificy. This is partially taken into consideration in her own therapy material.

Further Development

We suggest that applying only the PACE approach does not engage the patient enough in relearning language abilities, nor does it go far enough in developing proper compensatory strategies. In the sense of optimizing the communicative capacities that are not, or only mildly, affected in the patient, PACE rather seems to be a purely stimulation approach. Therefore we wondered whether a modified approach, that integrates demands of the symptom-specific and theory-based material and feedback into PACE-therapy, would be more efficacious than the traditional one. In a cross-over design we compared traditional PACE therapy with a modified PACE approach which used training material and feedback in a more structured way (Glindemann and Springer, 1989; Springer, et al., 1991). This modified PACE approach included semantic classification tasks. Instead of only one picture, as in the traditional PACE setting, the patient was confronted with an array of pictures, a subset of which the patient had to sort into semantic classes (such as tools, fruits, vegetable, furniture, and so on). The superordinate category was written on a card. This card, together with the random array of pictures, was given to both the patient and the therapist. The two were separated by a screen (described by Clérebaut, et al., 1984). The screen made sure that subjects were required to convey new information to their partners, which is the essential feature of PACE therapy. Each decision on class membership had to be conveyed to the partner. The therapist gave feedback on the accuracy of classification in addition to the natural feedback of the traditional approach.

Three patients with severe semantic-lexical difficulties were treated over a period of five weeks. These patients showed semantic paraphasias and meaning confusions in word-picture matching, and in the case of one patient, pure word-retrieval disorders and speech apraxia. The efficacy of the two approaches was assessed in five control tests. In order to estimate communicative abilities we used the PACE rating-scale. Language systematic skills were evaluated by means of modified four-point naming scale taken from the Aachen Aphasia Test. The result of the therapy study showed that the modified PACE approach, including semantic classification tasks and deficit specific feedback, was more efficacious in the patients with semantic disorders. Only in the initial treatment period was the traditional PACE approach effective in one patient. It is important to stress that even the communicative skills of the patients with lexical-semantic difficulties improved continuously under the modified approach. The reason for this improvement seems to be rather obvious. Improvement of semantic-lexical abilities leads to better communicative skills. Compensation by nonverbal means may be supportive, but we found no evidence for the view that linguistic-ally-unspecific communicative stimulation leads to substantial improvement of verbal or nonverbal communicative skills in patients with lexical-semantic impairments. No differences were seen between the two approaches in the patient with motor speech planning deficits and word retrieval disorders. As we expected, semantic classification tasks had no significant effect for this patient. Only nonverbal communicative skills improved under both treatment approaches. In contrast, oral naming and verbal communication improved significantly after an additional specific treatment period, in which multimodal stimulation and phonetic techniques were incorporated. This therapy study showed that communicative methods should be complemented with deficit-specific approaches.

Besides this modified PACE approach, in which more language systematic components were incorporated, there are other investigations of PACE emphasizing more pragmatic aspects. In a varied PACE setting the patients had to describe small accidents at Playmobile crossroads which the partner had to reconstruct using an identical set of cars, passers by, and traffic signs behind a paper screen. Glindemann (1990a) demonstrated in three patients (Broca, Wernicke, amnesic aphasia) that problems in turn-taking procedures are secondary caused phenomena. There were no *pragmatic paraphasias* found; rather in terms of the aphasic disturbances the related problems were primarily semantic, syntactic and phonemic. In another study Glindemann (1992) showed that aphasic patients predominantly used conventional strategies of linearization when they have to process macropropositions in a modified PACE setting. The interlocutors first had to identify line drawings of persons from everyday life. In a second step the task of this procedure was to describe where two depicted persons were located in relationship to some objects in a line drawing of a situational frame. The partner again had to reconstruct this representation with the identical material behind a paper screen. Because of aphasic disturbances patients attended more to process-related determinations rather than to content-related aspects of certain persons in the situational frame. In a similar PACE setting where we used two sets of the same picture story, we analysed the relationship between cohesive structures and thematic coherence of utterances (Regenbrecht, Huber and Glindermann, 1992). The degree of severity of the aphasic disturbances in four patients was more decisive for the amount of cohesive ties found than the specific syndromes. In terms of thematic coherence we found no difficulties in selecting the appropriate propositions, but we observed problems in arranging the propositions in the right order of the story. There was no systematic correlation between the errors on coherence and the problems with the cohesive combination or propositions.

Conclusion

PACE can actually be an enrichment for aphasia therapy. PACE is an attractive communicative technique that incorporates some aspects of conversation dyads and pragmatic games. This approach motivates patients to utilize their verbal and nonverbal communicative abilities in order to compensate for aphasic deficits. The indirect and unspecific techniques will hardly utilize all the resources of relearning available. From various pragmatic and methodological points of view the claims of the originators of PACE have to be qualified. PACE is not a technique appropriate for all types and severities of aphasia. It is not suitable in all stages of recovery and the related phases of therapy. Furthermore, it is less pragmatic and natural than the authors emphasize. Nevertheless, we regard the artificiality of the procedures in PACE, and in modified PACE settings, as necessary for therapy to proceed. As we have shown, in order to modify communicative behaviour and language abilities it is partly necessary to isolate certain symptoms and strategies and to apply specific and stepwise procedures. Pragmatic and symptom-specific approaches should be integrated. This means that PACE should not be used in competition with language oriented approaches. Rather, PACE can provide a pragmatic framework in which specific approaches should be integrated or used in addition to PACE.

Acknowledgement

The studies reported were supported in part by a grant from the Deutsche Forschungsgemeinschaft.

References

Argyle M, Kendon A (1992) The experimental analysis of social performances. In Laver J, Hutcheson S (Eds) Communication in Face to Face Interaction Harmondsworth: Pengiun.

Aten JL, Cagliuri MP, Holland AL (1982) The efficacy of functional communication therapy for chronic aphasic patients. Journal of Speech and Hearing Disorders 47: 93–96.

Aten JL (1986) Functional communication treatment. In Chapey, R (Ed) Language Intervention Strategies in Adult Aphasia MD: Williams and Wilkins.

Austin JL (1962) How to Do Things with Words (Oxford Clarendon Press. Oxford).

Basso A, Fagliioni P, Vignolo L (1979) Influence of rehabilitation on language skills in aphasic patients: a controlled study. Archives of Neurology 36: 190–6.

Bongartz R, Claussen JP, Sigle G (1990) Anwendung des PACE-Therapieansatzes bei der Behandlung aphasischer Patienten in einer Gruppentherapie. Sprache-Stimme-Gehör 14: 181–7.

Brindley P, Copeland M, Demain C, Martyn P (1989) A comparison of the speech of ten chronic Broca's aphasics following intensive and non-intensive periods of therapy. Aphasiology 3: 695–707.

Byng S, Coltheart M (1986) Aphasia therapy research: metholodogical requirements and illustrative results. In Hjelmquist E, Nilsson LB (Ed) Communication and handicap. Amersterdam: Elsevier.

Carlomagno S (1994)

Carlomagno S, Losanno N, Emanuelli S, Casadio P (1991) Expressive language recovery or improved communicative skills: effects of PACE therapy on aphasics referential communication and story retelling Aphasiology 5: 419–25.

Chin Li E, Kitselman K, Dusatko D, Spinelli C (1988) The efficacy of PACE in the remediation of naming deficits. Journal of Communication Disorders 21: 491–503.

Clérebaut M, Coyette F, Feyereisen P, Seron X (1984) Une methode de rééduction functionelle des aphasiques: la PACE. Rééduction Orthophonique 22: 329–45.

Davis G A (1980) A critical look at PACE therapy. In Brookshire RH (Ed) Clinical Aphasiology Conference Proceedings Minneapolis, MN: BRK Publishers.

Davis GA (1986) Pragmatics and treatment. In Chapey R (Ed) Language Intervention Strategies in Adult Aphasia. 2nd edn Baltimore MD: Williams and Wilkins.

Davis GA, Wilcox MJ (1981) Incorporating parameter of natural conversation in aphasia treatment. In Chapey R (Ed) Language Intervention Strategies in Adult Aphaia. 1st edn. Baltimore MD: Williams and Wilkins.

Davis GA, Wilcox MJ (1985) Adult Aphasia Rehabilitation: Applied Pragmatics. San Diego CA: College Hill Press

De Renzi E, Vignolo L (1962) The Token Test: a sensitive to detect receptive disturbances in aphasics Brain 65: 665–78.

Duncan SD Jr (1974) On the structure of speaker-auditor-interaction during speaking turns. Language in Society 3: 161–80.

Edelman G (1987) PACE: Promoting Aphasics' Communicative Effectiveness. Bicester, Oxon: Winslow Press.

Ervin-Tripp S (1973) An analysis of the interaction of language, topic, and listener. In Argyle M (Ed) Social Encounters. Readings in Social Interaction. Harmondsworth. Pengiun.

Feyereisen P, Barter D, Goosens M, Ciérebaut (1988) Gestures and speech in referential communication by asphasic subjects: channel use and efficiency. Aphasiology 2: 21–33.

Glindemann R (1984) Wenn 'Sprecher' nicht sprechen und 'Hörer' nicht nur hören. Zur interpretation von Gesprähsshrittrollen. In Cherubim D, Henne H, Rehbock H (Eds) Gespräche zwischen Alltag und Literatur. Beiträge zur germanistischen Gesprächsforschung. Tübingen: Niemeyer.

Glindemann R (1987) Zusammensprechen in Gesprächen. Aspekte einer konsonanztheoretischen Pragmatik. Tübingen: Niemeyer.

Glinemann R (1990a) Welche probleme haben aphasiker beim turn taking. In Mellies R, Ostermann F, Winnecken A (Eds) Beiträge zur interdisziplinären Aphasieforchung. Arbeiten zum Workshop "Klinische Linguistik" Tübingen: Narr.

Glindemann R (1990b) Zum EinfluB des situativen Kontextes und der sprachlichen Struktur von Stimulusmaterial in der kommunikativ-pragmatisch orientierten

Aphasietherapie. Paper presented at the 17th Annual Meeting of the Arbeitsgemeinschaft für Aphasieforschung und-behandlung, Erlangen.

Glindemann R (1991) Modell-lernen in der PACE-therapie. Neurolinguistik 5: 105–15.

Glindemann R (1992) Linearisierungsstrategien auf makropropositionaler Ebene. Befunde von Aphasikern und Sprachgesunden. In Rickheit G, Mellies R, Winnecken A (Eds) Forschung und Intervention bei Sprachstörungen Opladen: Westdeutscher Verlag.

Glindemann R, Springer L (1989) PACE-Therapie und sprachsystematische Übungen – Ein integrativer Vorschlag zur Aphasietherapie. Sprache-Stimme-Gehör 13: 188–92.

Glindemann R Willmes D, Huber W, Springer L, (1991) The efficacy of modelling in PACE-therapy. Aphasiology 5: 425–31.

Glosser G, Weiner M, Kaplan E (1988): Variations in aphasic language behaviours. Journal of Speech and Hearing Disorders 53: 115–25.

Green G (1984) Communication in aphasia therapy; some of the procedures and issues involved. British Journal of Disorders of Communication 19: 35–46.

Habermas J (1981) Theorie des kommunikativen Handelns. Bd. 1: Handlunstrationalität und gesellschaftliche Rationalisierung Frankfurt am Main: Suhrkamp.

Hatfield F M, Shewell C (1983) Some applications of linguistics to aphasia therapy. In Code C, Müller DJ (Eds) Aphasia Therapy London: Edward Arnold.

Holland A (1977) Some practical considerations in aphasia rehabilitation. In Sullivan M, Kommers MS (Eds) Rational for Adult Aphasia Therapy. (Omaha NB: University of Nebraska.)

Holland A (1982) Observing functional communication of aphasic adults. Journal of Speech and Hearing Disorders. 47: 50–6

Holland A (1991) Pragmatic aspects of intervention in aphasia. Journal of Neurolinguistics 6: 197–211.

Hörmann H (1986) Meaning in Context. An Introduction to the Psychology of Language. New York: Plenum Press.

Howard D, Hatfield FM (1987) Aphasia Therapy: Historical and Contemporary Issues Hillsdale: Lawrence Erlbaum Associates.

Howard D, Patterson KD (1987) Methodological issues in neuropsychological therapy. In Seron X, Deloche G (Eds) Cognitive approaches in neuropsychological rehabilitation. London: Lawrence Erlbaum Associates Ltd.

Huber W, Mayer I, Kerschensteiner M (1978) Untersuchungen zur methode und zum verlauf der therapie von phonematischem jargon bei wernicke-aphasie. Folia Phoniatrica 30: 119–35.

Huber W, Poeck K, Willmes K (1984) the Aachen aphasia Test. In Rose FC (Ed) Progress in Aphasiology New York: Raven Press.

Huber W, Springer L, Willmes K (1993) Approaches to aphasia therapy in Aachen. In Holland AL, Forbes MM (Eds) Aphasia Treatment – World Perspectives. San Diego CA: Singular Publishing Groups Inc.

Kearns KP, Salmon SJ (1984) An experimental analysis of auxiliary and copular verb in aphasia. Journal of Speech and Hearing Disorders 49: 152–63.

Kertesz A (1984). Recovery from aphasia. In Rose FC (Ed) Progress in Aphasiology. New York: Raven Press.

Kertesz A (1993) Neurobiological foundations of aphasia rehabilitation. In Paradies M (Ed) Foundations of Aphasia Rehabilitaion. Oxford: Pergamon Press.

Labov W (1970) The Study of Language in its Social Context. Studium Generale 23:

30–87.

Lesser R (1987) Cognitive neuropsychological influences on aphasia therapy. Aphasiology 1: 189–200.

Luria A R, Haydin VL, Tsvetkova LS Vinatskaya EN (1969) Restoration of higher cortical function following local brain damage. In Vinken PJ, Bruyn GW (Eds) Handbook of Clinical Neurology. 3. Amsterdam: North Holland.

Martin AD (1981) Therapy with the jargon aphasic. In Brown JW (Ed) Jargonaphasia. New York: Academic Press.

Newhoff M, Bugbee J, Ferreire A (1981) A change of PACE: spouses as treatment targets. In Brookshire R (Ed) Clinical Aphasiology Conference Proceedings. Minneapolis, MN: BRK Publishers.

Penn C (1993) Aphasia therapy in South Africa: some pragmatic and personal perspectives. In Holland AL, Forbes MM (Eds) Aphasia treatment – World Perspectives. San Diego CA: Singular Publishing Groups.

Perkins L, Lesser R (1993) Pragmatics applied to aphasia rehabilitation. In Paradies M (Ed) Foundations of Aphasia Rehabilitation. Oxford: Pergamon Press.

Pierce R (1989) Linguistic context and aphasia treatment: aphasia and pragmatics. Seminars in Speech and Language. 10 (4): 329–42.

Poeck K, Huber W, Willmes K (1989) Outcome of intensive therapy in aphasia. Journal of Speech and Hearing Disorders. 54: 471–79.

Pöppel E, von Steinbüchel N (1992) Neurophsyological Rehabilitation from a theoretical point of view. In von Steinbüchel N, von Cramon DY, Pöppel E (Eds) Neuropsychological Rehabilitation Berlin, Heidelberg, New York: Springer.

Porch B E (1967) Porch Index of Communicative Ability. Palo Alto CA: Consulting Psychologists Press.

Prinz PM (1980) A note on requesting strategies in adult aphasics. Journal of Communication Disorders. 13: 65–73.

Prutting D A (1982) Pragmatics as social competence. Journal of Speech and Hearing Disorders. 47: 123–34.

Pulvermüller F, Roth VM (1991) Communicative aphasia treatment as a further development of PACE therapy Aphasiology 5: 39–51.

Rao P, Koller J (1982) A total communication approach to aphasia treatment in three chronic aphasic adults. Paper presented at the Seminar – Annual Conference of the International Neurophsychological Society, Pittsburgh, PA.

Regenbrecht F, Huber W Glindemann R (1992) Zum verhältnis von Kohärenz bei aphasie. In Rickheit G, Mellies R, Winnecken A (Eds) Linguistische Aspekte der Sprachtherapie. Forschung und Intervention bei Sprachstörungen Opladen: Westdeutscher Verlag.

Schuell H (1974) The treatment of aphasia. In Sies LF (Ed) Aphasia Theory and Therapy Baltimore MD: University Park Press.

Searle J (1969) Speech Acts: An essay in the Philosophy of Language. London: Cambridge University Press.

Seron X, Deloche G, Bastard V, Chassin G, Hermand N (1979) Word-finding difficulties and learning transfer in aphasic patients. Cortex 15: 149–55.

Shewan CM, Bandur DL (1986) Treatment of Aphasia: a Language-oriented Approach. San Diego CA: College-Hill Press.

Shewan CM, Kertesz A (1984) Effects of speech and language treatment on recovery of aphasia. Brain and Language 23: 272–99.

Springer L (1986) Behandlungsphasen einer syndromspezifischen Aphasietherapie. Sprache-Stimme-Gehör 10: 22–9.

Springer L, Glindemann R, Huber W, Willmes K (1991a) How efficacious is PACE-therapy when 'Language Systematic Training' is incorporated? Aphasiology 5: 391–401.

Springer L, Schlench C, Schlenck K-J (1991b) Reduzierte syntax therapie (REST) als Methode zur therapie von chronischem agrammatismus. Paper presented at the 18th Annual Meeting of the Arbeitgemeinschaft für Aphasieforschung und behandlung, Amsterdam.

Springer L, Willmes K (1993) Efficacy of language systematic learning approaches to treatment. In Paradies M (Ed) Foundations of Aphasia Rehabilitation. Oxford: Pergamon Press.

Springer L, Willmes K, Haag E (1993) Training the use of questions and prepositions in dialogues: a comparison of two different approaches in aphasia therapy. Aphasiology 7: 251–70.

Stalnaker RC (1970) Pragmatics. Synthese, 22 (1/2): 272–89.

Stubbs M (1983) Discourse Analysis. The Soziolinguistic Analysis of Natural Language. (Blackwell, Oxford).

Thompson C, McReynolds L (1986) Interrogative production in agrammatic aphasia: experimental analysis of auditory-visual stimulation and direct-production treatment. Journal of Speech and Hearing Research 29: 193–206.

Weniger D, Springer L, Poeck (1987) The efficacy of deficit-specific therapy materials. Aphasiology 3: 215–23.

Wertz F T (1984) Language Disorders in adults: state of the clinical art. In Holland A (Ed) Language Disorders in Adults. San Diego CA: College Hill.

Wertz RT, Collins MJ, Weiss DG, Kurtze JF, Friden T, Brookshire RH, Pierce J, Holtzapple P, Hubbard DJ, Porch BE, West JA, Davis L, Matovitch V, Morley GK, Ressureccion D (1981) Veterans Administration cooperative study of aphasia: a comparison of individual and group treatment. Journal of Speech and Hearing Research 24: 580–94.

Wilcox MJ, Davis GA (1977) Speech act analysis of aphasic communication in individual and group settings. In Brookshire R. (Ed) Clinical Aphasiology Conference Proceedings. Minneapolis MD: BRK Publishers.

Wilcox MJ, Davis GA (1978) Promoting aphasics' communicative effectiveness. Paper presented to the American Speech-Language-Hearing Association, San Francisco, CA.

Yngve V (1970) On geting a word in edgewise. Papers from the 6th Regional Meeting of the Chicago Linguistic Society. Chicago IL: Chicago Linguistic Society.

Chapter 7
Linguistic Approaches to the Assessment and Treatment of Aphasia

SUSAN EDWARDS

Introduction

If we consider that aphasia is an acquired disorder of language and understand that linguistics is the study of language then it would seem essential that any approach to treat that disorder must be firmly based on and motivated by knowledge which goes beyond the therapist's intuitions as a native speaker. Indeed, in the United Kingdom the study of linguistics is now an essential component of all degree courses leading to a professional qualification in speech and language therapy. The language disorder, aphasia, arises subsequent to brain damage which might also cause disruption or damage to motoric and cognitive functions as well as the language system. It is therefore important for the therapist to be aware of other factors which may influence the linguistic behaviour of an aphasic patient and the type of intervention which is possible. Having assessed the patient, if treatment is considered appropriate, the therapist must select therapeutic strategies suited to each patient. Therapists are dealing with individuals operating within unique social contexts which may be radically different to their previous experiences; we are dealing with individuals who are learning to cope with a variety of deficits and problems. The speech and language therapist, therefore, selects his or her method or methods of intervention from an extensive repertoire, some of which are illustrated in this volume. For some clients the emphasis may rightly be on counselling, for others the appropriate intervention may consist of teaching alternative methods of communication, but for many, intervention will be focused on the linguistic functioning of the aphasic client. For these clients, a systematic analysis of their language is a basic prerequisite for therapy, and the assessment should reveal errors, omissions and mismanagement of the language system as well as highlighting those linguistic functions which remain intact; all of these factors will motivate therapy. The models for linguistic assessment and the relation between linguistic assessment and therapy, (which is far from straightforward – see Edwards and Garman, 1989 for an earlier discussion) will be explored in this chapter.

Crystal (1981) identified two emphases of linguistic concern which he claimed to have considerable clinical importance: the development of 'reliable procedures for the collection, transcription, description and analysis for linguistic data' and theories to account for the data (p.17). In this chapter we will consider both attempts to account for the data, that is providing explanations of aphasic phenomena by way of linguistic theory and the development of procedures to manage data. The main types of data we will consider are those which are obtained in controlled experimental conditions and those comprising spontaneous connected speech. We will consider both in this chapter but focus on the latter. In aphasiology the deployment of linguistic theories of normal language functioning may be used to explain or predict language impairment in aphasic subjects. Aphasic data is taken from a speaker or selected groups, then linguistic explanations are generated for certain features of that data, or theories may be expanded which predict certain phenomena, for example, Kean (1977) offers a phonological account of agrammatism and Grodzinsky (1990) an account based on a linguistic theory known as Government and Binding. Or the approach may come from the other direction, that is taking aphasic data to substantiate or refute theories of language functioning in normal subjects. For example, Linebarger (1989) claims that the patterns of selective preservation and loss observed in aphasics required to parse sentences support her claims for the modularity of the language system.

Although most linguistic interest in aphasia has gone beyond the surface manifestations of language and has been directed towards providing theoretically motivated linguistic explanations for aphasia or has used examples of restricted comprehension or expressive language to test linguistic theories, the area of linguistic research which focuses on data collection of surface forms is of immediate clinical importance. The management of such data is of increasing interest to linguists, highly significant in aphasiology and deserves closer examination. The framework used by Crystal, Fletcher and Garman (1976; 1989) (which is now widely used by British speech and language therapists) was based on a reference grammar (Quirk, et al., 1972) and is concerned with the surface structures used in output. This framework has been found to be especially useful for dealing with naturalistic, informal speech where phrasal structures, as well as clausal structures, frequently occur. Thus, this framework does not assume that the spoken language recorded in the clinic will consist of sentences (as is the case with written language) and therefore seeks an alternative unit for segmentation. This is not to deny, of course, the theoretical importance of the sentence and its constituents but to acknowledge, record and account for the fragments that appear in normal spontaneous connected speech. Careful, detailed analyses of aphasic speech which are based on principled criteria have the potential to reveal aspects of aphasia which are not only theoretically interesting but also clinically important.

We will start by reviewing some theoretical accounts of aphasic symptoms; we will then consider detailed, linguistically motivated protocols for the description of spontaneous aphasic speech and argue for the importance of spontaneous speech data in the clinical assessment procedure. We will evaluate the contribution theoretical explanation and detailed description can make to aphasia therapy and finally, we will present some examples of assessment and therapy from one fluent aphasic speaker.

Theoretical Accounts: Linguistic Theory and Aphasia

Theoretically motivated studies take a different perspective from those studies which aim to build a comprehensive description of surface structures and which we will consider below. Researchers, who approach aphasia from a theoretical rather than a clinical point of view, treat spoken (or written) language as surface manifestation of underlying rule systems; examples of sentence construction or language task performance are given as revelations of the proposed underlying damaged grammars which are deployed in aphasia. Unlike the clinical approach, language functioning is considered more or less as an isolated, although multi-component, system and non-linguistic factors such as physical limitations, emotional effects, the effect of context including the interlocutor or the examiner, are rarely discussed. That is not to say that such research is of no consequence to the clinician but it may be helpful to regard the research findings as details of a portrait seen through a magnifying glass – important details but, as yet, only part of the picture.

The fundamental principle behind any linguistic account of aphasia is that language can be described as a system or series of systems with internal organization consisting of relating units. While the nature of and relationship between these units and how the system may be best accounted for, through a series of rules or a grammar, continues to be a matter of debate, the complexity of this abstract system is now acknowledged to be one of the central interests of the therapist in the quest to make sense of aphasic data. Thus, while over a decade ago, Lesser (1978) noted that a linguistically-orientated student of aphasia would not be content with simplistic descriptions of language functioning such as 'this patient has problems with repetition' (p.23), there can now be few aphasia therapists who have graduated in the last decade who would not share that student's discontent.

Jakobson is generally credited with being the first linguist to attempt to construct a linguistic account of the deficits observed in aphasia (Lesser, 1978). Jakobson's observations (1968) concerned phonological errors, the loss of grammatical forms and the division of aphasia into two distinct types. These types were characterized by syntagmatic or contiguity errors versus paradigmatic or similarity errors. He further proposed that some aspects of aphasia could be accounted for by the Regression Hypothesis, whereby loss of certain features (essentially, phonemic contrasts) mirrors the acquisition of these linguistic contrasts. This notion was largely rejected, at least in extending the contrasts to include syntactic contrasts. For example, Crystal, et al's (1976) approach to therapy with an agrammatic patient was guided by a developmentally-based profile of the patient's expressive speech. The profile used, LARSP, consists of various lexical, phrasal and clausal constructions reflecting aspects of language development. Thus therapy, which follows this profile, is aimed at making progress towards the normal adult targets, following a developmental framework. However, the authors explicitly state that while believing that the developmental framework gives a workable scale of 'grammatical complexity', they are not tied to a developmental hypothesis which includes the notion of regression but are only concerned with successful introduction of graded structures (p.196). However, more recently, Grodzinsky (1990), working within a Chomskian theoretical framework, has suggested that there are at least three possible interpretations of the hypothesis: these concern syndrome differentiation, stage of recovery and degree of severity. While rejecting the first two interpretations, Grodzinsky concludes that the third interpretation, (i.e., that severity of the language impairment in aphasia mimics stages of acquisition), offers a strong empirical hypothesis for evaluationbut that, to date, there is insufficient evidence to accept or reject this hypothesis.

Kean (1977) proposed a linguistic characterization of agrammatism based on generative phonology. Clinical observations record the relative preservation of certain types of words while other words and bound grammatical morphemes tend to be omitted. Rather than offer an explana-tion of the reduction observed in agrammatic speech in terms of the preservation of *open* class words and the omission of *closed* class words, she proposed a phonological explanation. She claimed that omission errors were distributed according to whether an item was a phonological word (and subject to stress and owning certain phonological boundaries) or a *clitic*. In her account, items which are clitics (which include not only bound morphemes but also so-called function words) would be omitted while phonological words would remain. This version was extended and strengthened by the concept of *lexical construal* whereby intact linguistic knowledge interacts with the phonological deficit. Thus, her characterization of agrammatism is considered by some to be at a 'level of representation on the boundary between syntactic and phonological' (Marshall, 1990: xi) and to be theoretical and predictive rather than merely descriptive. The unextended version, while able to predict some features of agrammatism (omission of certain morphemes), did not predict all the features generally considered to be characteristic of agrammatic speakers, such as the omission of certain whole words, paraphasic errors or specific comprehension deficits (Garman, 1982). The extended version still does not account for partial loss of these elements or the diverse patterns of output error found, for example, by Saffran, Berndt and Schwartz, 1989.

Strikingly, none of her examples were taken from real data but constructed to support her theory, an approach still widely favoured in the linguistic literature. Further criticism of Kean's claims are made by Grodzinsky (1990) who characterizes them as, at best, 'non-*ad hoc* partitions of the data' but nevertheless, descriptions, rather than explanations (p.49). He points out that while her claims are supported by the examples she selects, the same claims cannot account for the pattern of agrammatic errors found in languages other than English. In languages which do not employ linear processes (such as the addition of grammatical morphemes signalling plurality, tense, etc.), agrammatics do not omit inflections that would leave non-well formed words: no examples are found in the data. (We have certain analogous cases in English: there is no phonological segment which can be omitted from irregular past forms such as *sang* or irregular plurals such as *women*). The omission patterns in Hebrew aphasic speakers are constrained lexically and, presumably, governed by hierarchical rather than linear processes (p.51). He compares agrammatic errors across languages and particularly compares English, where inflections may be omitted, to Hebrew where comparable omissions do not occur: 'a word must be inflected if it does not have a zero form' (p.58). Grodzinsky further argues that the pattern of omissions (or substitutions) found in agrammatic speech can be explained, and indeed, predicted, by reference to Government and Binding Theory rather than a phonological account which disregards the syntactic context of words. His explanation makes powerful predictions, for example, that prepositions in certain syntactic roles, depending on their syntactic relationship with other elements within the sentence, will be omitted and while others retained. Thus the claim is that the distribution of morphemes (both free and bound) in agrammatic speech has a grammatical rather than a phonological or lexical explanation. We will return to consider what implications this might have for aphasia therapy.

Since Kean's publication, there has been a steady flow of linguistic accounts of aphasia, mainly concentrating on the agrammatic type of output (see, for example, Kean, 1985) offering the therapist a confusing picture and, to date, no clear irrefutable guide to therapy. We can make some sense of the field if we roughly categorize these accounts into those which seek to characterize the underlying system, language competence, and those which characterize how that system is put into effect, the processes. Grodzinsky (1990), viewing the confused accounts of agrammatism, claims that confusion arises because of the different modalities on which writers focus. He divides the various accounts into those which focus on the structural aspects of the language, which may be only descriptive, and those which focus on the processes. His search is for a theoretical account of the underlying language competencies (the systems) and, after reviewing various data, proposes a theoretical explanation for the production and comprehension deficits found in agrammatics which we have briefly considered above.

Linguistic and psycholinguistic influences

Most therapists are more familiar with accounts of the surface forms of aphasia and explanations which are based on the notion of language processing rather than theoretical accounts based on notions of the underlying competence. These models arise from psycholinguistic studies which in turn are rooted in the disciplines of linguistics and psychology (see Lesser and Milroy, 1993). Both of these disciplines are concerned with language: whereas the former is more concerned with description and identification of the system(s), psychology is perhaps more often concerned with the operation of the system(s). However, there is considerable overlap of interest and knowledge with highly relevant research arising from both fields. It is appropriate, therefore, to briefly review the influence of psycholinguistic research, although the topic is dealt with in more detail elsewhere in this volume. (See Edmundson and McIntosh, Chapter 8.)

Processing models offer representation of abstract functions, which may be conceptualized either as sequential activities and offered visually as flow-charts or as units functioning in parallel and represented visually as interconnecting networks. Bates and Wulfeck (1989) provide an example of such an account and like Grodzinsky, they also use cross-linguistic data (including data from English, German, Italian and Serbo-Croatian aphasic speakers) to support their case. Their account differs, however, in that whereas Grodzinsky examines the underlying grammar, they employ a model, of language processing known as the Competition Model based on the sentence processing model developed by Bates and MacWhinney (1982; 1989). Their model has the same properties as other parallel processing models: it depends on parallel activation and conflict resolution. Whereas in the simplified serial models (with which speech and language therapists are now familiar) the processes are conceptualized by a series of stages arranged in linear/vertical fashion (see, for example, Byng, 1988; Byng and Coltheart, 1986); in this model the process is conceptualized as a network of components, likened to logogens. In expressive language, an underlying meaning configuration simultaneously activates all the associated forms as the communication plan takes shape. Decisions are made and the field of possible forms narrowed down until there is one well formed possibility. The competitors within this cohort have various forms and meaning (which includes sensitivity to semantic/syntactic context), ability to inhibit their neighbours and threshold of activation (Bates and MacWhinney, 1982: 355). Information coming into the system may be via form (known as bottom-up processing) or meaning (known as top-down processing); either can activate the logogens. This is, essentially, a lexicalist approach which, extended to aphasia, accounts for the patterns of impaired language in terms of impaired lexical access.

Presumably, the aphasic speaker either lacks the ability to activate the target logogen and thus fails to access the word or, fails to inhibit neighbouring logogens and thus produces an incorrect word. If near neighbours are activated according to form, then a lexical paraphasic error results; neighbours activated by meaning result, presumably, in semantically related lexical paraphasic errors. It is not clear how phonemic paraphasic errors result, although each unit within this system also contains 'context-sensitive' phoneme units which carry inter-morphemic information concerning order of phonemes. Conceivably, these internal units could be mis-activated through abnormal bottom-up processing and produce phonological mis-ordering. Similar intramorphemic context-sensitive units are proposed to explain the resistant positional information retained by aphasics; the knowledge of morpheme ordering and the ability to order constituents within simple phrases and sentences displayed by the subjects studied (Bates and MacWhinney, 1982: 358). If this is considered to be a valuable interpretation of language processing, then there are some immediate implications for therapy. The most obvious would be the need to attach great importance to the patient's lexicon, both in assessment procedures and the therapy programme. Second, these concepts support the practice of testing and subsequently utilizing the relative strengths of phonemic versus semantic cueing in therapy. (See Lesser's chapter (9) on assessing psycholinguistic processes in aphasia.)

Although there are not, as yet, any clear indications as to how these theoretical claims might be applied to clinical procedures, clinical aphasiologists are relatively familiar with the idea of using processing models to test the nature of the breakdown observed. Lesser (1987) advances three different types of psycholinguistic models which might be used in assessment and treatment: a transcoding model of comprehension/production of single written words; a model of the stages of activity involved in naming tasks; and a model of sentence production. The models used are borrowed from psychology, especially from cognitive neuropsychology and a recently published assessment of aphasia (Kaye, Lesser and Coltheart, 1992: see Chapter 9 in this volume), based on experimental data from psycholinguistics, is likely to ensure continued use of this approach for some time. There are also some published accounts of therapy programmes which have been motivated by experimental cognitive neuropsychology. Byng (1988), Byng and Coltheart (1986) and Jones (1986) report on therapy programmes conducted with aphasic patients presenting with impaired language skills. Both studies refer to Garrett's model of sentence production (Garrett, 1982) and base their therapy programmes on the hypothesis that agrammatic patients have an impaired ability to map from the level of semantic to syntactic representation which limits output as well as comprehension of certain syntactic structures.

These reports represent considerable advances in clinical aphasiology in that therapy was theoretically motivated and the writers were able to document some improvement in their patients. Byng also makes a strong case for detailing the programmes used in order to permit replication, and such studies are now appearing (Byng, Nickels and Black, 1991). These innovative approaches have been very influential in the field despite early limitations. For example, in Jones' case, (a report on therapy with a chronic agrammatic patient), only one stage of the processing chain was considered to be important for her subject; it is not clear whether she is proposing an impairment of process, i.e. the mapping from semantic to syntactic representation or an impairment of a certain level of representation, i.e. verb subcategorization, or an impairment of both; the reduced morphology was neither accounted for theoretically nor addressed therapeutically. Byng presents detailed reports on therapy with two aphasic patients which is clearly successful along the chosen parameters. There is some evidence that improvement goes beyond performance on the test, although this is difficult to assess as her criterion for well-formed spoken output is based on the unit of sentence. We should also note that she makes it clear that success of the therapy administered is not dependent on the theoretical interpretations of the disorder.

These comments, however, in no way diminish the importance of studying in detail, certain aspects of an aphasic patient's performance, and publications which give such details add to our clinical knowledge. In clinical practice, however, it is equally important for the therapist to be eclectic when planning intervention; it is unreasonable to expect one theory, one model or one branch of behavioural science to either offer the complete and final explanation or indicate the only course of remediation. For example, Lesser and Milroy (1987; 1993) make a case for combining assessments based on cognitive neurological models with considerations of pragmatics of communication. A comprehensive clinical approach to aphasia must, we would contend, include both some theoretical knowledge of how the language works, how the components of language combine, and a principled methodology for collecting and describing the essential data, i.e. aphasic speech. We will consider some illustrative findings of psycholinguistic research and how these might influence therapy. We will then consider some methods of handling spontaneous speech data and how such assessments might motivate therapy.

Psycholinguistic Investigations and Clinical Observations

It is probably true to say that to date, linguists, like psychologists have directed most attention towards subjects with reduced output, variously described as non-fluent, Broca's aphasics or agrammatics, although some studies do use groups of mixed aphasics. Clearly, subjects with relatively intact comprehension are far better able to participate in psycholinguistic investigations than those aphasics with comprehension deficits. There is considerable evidence that patients with Broca's aphasia, although appearing to understand everyday speech, do have problems comprehending certain utterances where access to meaning can only be achieved by successful syntactic parsing. (See, for example, the discussion in Caplan, 1987.)

Deficits of this kind may only be revealed in psycholinguistic tasks where contextual clues are removed and the subject is required to access the meaning of a series of unrelated, isolated sentences. The experimental material is designed to ensure that the subject is unable to access meaning by employing non-syntactic strategies, for example, by arriving at the meaning of the sentence by applying a word-by-word comprehension strategy in conjunction with world knowledge. Thus, if the object of an experiment is to explore the subject's comprehension of passive structures, then the experimental material will consist of reversible sentences where either of the noun phrases could be interpreted as agent. In these situations, it can be demonstrated that agrammatic patients have difficulty in assigning thematic roles. Similar test protocols have been used to demonstrate that agrammatics have problems with sentences involving co-reference where the listener has to assign reference to pronouns in such sentences as in *John gave him the book* versus *John gave himself the book* (Caplan, 1987; Linebarger, 1989). Such tests uncover specific comprehension deficits in aphasics who had been thought to possess relatively intact comprehension although it should be noted that these deficits are revealed in psycholinguistic tasks rather than in everyday situations.

There have been efforts to explore whether the presence of such sentence processing deficits diminishes an aphasic's ability to comprehend language above the sentential level. Caplan and Evans (1990) investigated the relationship between a sentence parsing deficit and the ability to comprehend discourse. They examined asyntactic listeners' comprehension of a set of narratives controlled for length and information content but contrasting in syntactic complexity. They found that although there was an overall relationship between the level of sentence comprehension of their subjects and the comprehension of discourse, they were unable to demonstrate that their asyntactic comprehenders found the syntactically complex form of narratives more difficult to understand than the syntactically easy forms. Similar findings are common in clinical experience; the patient who has difficulty with selected comprehension tasks may demonstrate an ability to follow discourse and often has relatively intact comprehension within a conversational context.

Linebarger (1989) observes that other apparent anomalies arise when we compare the performance of some aphasic patients on tasks of sentence comprehension with their ability to make grammatical judgements about the same structures. It has been demonstrated that agrammatic patients have difficulty comprehending sentences in which the meaning is dependent upon the syntax, for example, reversible passive sentences, such as, *the woman was kissed by the man* and sentences containing reflexive pronouns such as *the man washed himself* versus *the man washed him*. The same subjects are, however, more able to make accurate grammatical judgements on a number of structures including subject-inversion, empty elements, phrase structure categorization and gapless relative class. Linebarger considers that these findings demonstrate that sentence processing may be computed separately from semantic/pragmatic interpretation and that these two processes be impaired independently. Several explanations are examined, including the loss of or difficulty with accessing closed class words; restrictions of the short term memory; a failure to co-index elements; problems in mapping from the syntactic frame to the semantic interpretation of syntactic roles. If there is a failure to integrate the syntactic and semantic information, it is suggested that it only occurs in agrammatics; Linebarger further notes that an absolute disability cannot be demonstrated.

Linebarger's detailed review of sentence parsing is an excellent illustration of the complexity of investigating comprehension. It is as well to bear in mind that after detailed controlled tests, we still may not know why a subject fails to comprehend. For example, a patient may fail to correctly select reversible passive sentences because he or she is unable to parse, unable to semantically interpret or because of limitations of the short-term memory store. The clinician strives to tease these factors apart in order to target therapy appropriately, but the approach must always be one of testing hypotheses and one that can be adapted in the light of new evidence from the patient. Such investigations are particularly problematic when the patient has fluent rather than non-fluent aphasia. Unlike the extensively studied agrammatic patients some fluent patients present with noticeable comprehension deficits. Linebarger notes that to date there is insufficient evidence to support the notion that these patients have a relatively intact parsing system which parallels their relatively intact syntax in their output, a position well attested in clinical work. We will consider some limited data below which suggest that at least some fluent patients may have similar asyntactic comprehension.

Although clinicians will be expecting to reveal some limitations of comprehension when they test their agrammatic patients, associates of these patients are often quite surprised by such deficits for often, although not always, comprehension seems to be adequate in everyday use. This is because the agrammatic patient is seldom required to decode isolated sentences where the meaning is wholly dependent on parsing ability. He or she is able to infer meaning by using lexical-semantic information and his life experiences. However, although in general terms, comprehension may be adequate, it is also common for the patient to report, and clinicians and family to observe, subtle problems in understanding. These subtle problems may arise from selected loss of understanding of low frequency words or, as above, an inability to parse certain syntactic structures or, presumably the accumulative effect of processing demands of low frequency words and certain syntactic constructions. If we apply the lexical interpretation (as advanced by Bates and Wulfeck, for example) to these findings, we would need to conclude that the aphasic listener is unable to access the contextual information associated with (or contained within) certain conditions. If we exclude lexical deficits and work within a sentence processing model, then we assume that there are limitations, weaknesses or malfunctioning at the level of syntactic frame formulation or maintenance. Part of the clinician's assessment procedure will consist of probes or tests of the available hypotheses.

Having uncovered these problems of comprehension, the clinician needs to judge whether the patient's everyday communicative competence is hindered or whether, by and large, the patient is able to communicate. The clinician's judgement will lead him or her to either further testing and therapy or to select other areas for further testing and remediation. The patient who formerly put a high priority on verbal skills may be highly motivated to improve his or her ability to comprehend language at a complex level. Equally, although the casual observer (which often includes medical professionals), may judge the aphasic's comprehension to be adequate, the partner of the aphasic may report many incidents of daily frustration caused by impaired comprehension. In these cases, the clinician needs to use his or her experience and judgement to decide which components of the disorder are candidates for the intervention programme, to prioritize the components of the programme and devise ways of introducing exercises which maximize each patient's preserved skills and relate to the social context in which the patient now operates. While hypothesis testing is central to the assessment procedure, we also contend that in addition to specific tasks which probe the nature of the aphasic disorder, the assessment must include a detailed description of the patient's spoken language. It is at this point that we advocate a detailed linguistic assessment.

Describing Naturalistic Speech Data

We will consider descriptions and explanations of aphasic data, starting by outlining three types of descriptive studies: descriptive studies of large corpora of aphasic speech which aim to describe all significant aspects of the grammatical system; studies of certain aphasic features (i.e. a subset of the system); cross-linguistic studies which examine the universality of certain features.

An increasing number of linguistic studies have attempted to provide a comprehensive descriptive framework for the characterization of spontaneous, naturalistic aphasic speech. The results of these projects are particularly useful to clinicians, for not only do they extend our knowledge of aphasia and provide frameworks for analysis which can be replicated in clinical work, they also provide potential means of quantifying the effectiveness of therapy. They permit us to describe and quantify the language the aphasic speaker is actually using rather than the aphasic's performance on a number of language tasks. Traditional tests do not provide guidelines which enable the therapist to analyse the naturalistic speech collected in the subtests (for further discussion see Edwards, Garman and Knott, 1993) nor do such test batteries offer criteria which permit consistent quantification or a descriptive framework related to what, in structural linguistics, are generally agreed to be appropriate levels of language description (Hatfield and Shewell, 1983). There are now a number of studies published which provide information about the surface nature of aphasic speech. Some have taken an undifferentiated population (Penn and Behrmann, 1986; Vermeulen, Bastiaanse and Van Wageningen, 1989; Edwards, Garman and Knott 1992) while others, (Saffran, Berndt and Schwartz, 1989; Menn and Obler, 1990) have focused on a particular type of aphasia, agrammatism.

Some of these studies have focused on the development of systematic procedures for the collection and presentation of corpora of spontaneous aphasic speech and offer detailed descriptions of that speech using the profile of the surface level taxonomy developed by Crystal et al., 1976; (for example) Penn and Behrmann, 1986; Edwards, et al., 1992. These studies afford a precision in the characterization of the linguistic symptoms of the population studied (Fletcher 1989) and thus go beyond the traditional clinical descriptions and short illustrations given in standard texts (e.g. Albert, et al., 1981). They present detailed portraits of aphasic speech collected from a number of subjects and thus add to our knowledge of aphasia while challenging some of the traditional notions of classification. In addition, these studies provide protocols for the collection, analysis and quantification of aphasic data which can be used or adapted for clinical means. We will return to discuss the importance of such work.

The second systematic type of linguistic descriptive study comprises studies which examine features of aphasic production, (for example, the reduction of grammatical free and bound morphemes, Goodglass and Menn, 1985), or comprehension, (for example, the ability of subjects to parse passive versus active sentences, Caplan and Hildebrandt, 1988; Linebarger, 1989). Such studies offer the therapist important insights into certain details of production and comprehension in selected groups of subjects and are increasingly seen as providing essential basic knowledge in aphasiology. A third type of study uses cross-linguistic data and may offer a descriptive account of the manifestation of aphasia (or one type of aphasia) in a number of languages (e.g. , Menn and Obler, 1990). These studies may be seen as a bridge between theoretical investigations and the detailed linguistic descriptions of aphasic speech. Therapists working with multilingual clients will immediately see the potential of such cross-linguistic studies as providing a useful reference database. The samples and analyses given by Menn and Obler, for example, provide a good starting point for the therapist's own investigations (and include speakers from 14 different languages), although as we have noted, this study is of agrammatic speakers only. Data from normal controls are also given, so permitting a comparison between features found in aphasic and normal speech. Features detailed in this study are given as proportions as well as raw scores, so it is possible to observe, for example, the difference between the aphasic subject's use of nouns compared with the normal speaker's. For the English subjects, 32 different grammatical categories are tallied and additional information given on major lexical classes and their distribution across the sample taken. Similar details are given for other languages.

However, therapists who are working with a bi- or multilingual population may seek a more formalized approach to assessing the language of their clients. In particular, they may wish to ascertain if and how the client's languages have been differentially impaired. The Bilingual Aphasia Test (Paradis, 1987) is designed to reveal which of the speaker's languages are most accessible post-morbidly and in which language the client should receive therapy (p.19). While containing many familiar tasks which investigate comprehension, repetition, propositionizing, reading and writing, it also seeks to explore separately, phonemic, morphological, syntactic and semantic levels of language functioning. The test is not only available in a number of different languages but aims to take account of specific linguistic characteristics of each language as well as using culturally appropriate material. It therefore provides a valuable clinical tool in our increasingly multilingual societies.

Finally in this section, we should note that as well as providing a useful reference database, cross-linguistic studies may be used to support or refute claims concerning either the fundamental nature of aphasic features and/or language universals (e.g., Bates, Friederici and Wulfeck, 1987; Bates and Wulfeck, 1989; Grodzinsky, 1990). These studies are probably more properly considered as belonging to the theoretical investigation which we considered above.

Descriptive Approaches: Linguistic Assessment of Aphasic Speech

It is axiomatic that a linguistic approach to aphasia therapy starts with a detailed assessment of the language exhibited. This assessment will include a description of the preserved features of language and will not be limited to listing or quantifying errors. Clinically, therapists will wish to assess the production and comprehension of spoken and written language of the majority of the aphasic patients referred. To date, descriptive linguistics has most to offer in the assessment of spoken language, especially spontaneous speech, in contrast to the cognitive neurological approaches which have focused on written language and the production of single words (see Mitchum and Berndt, 1992, for a comparison of the two approaches). The process starts with collecting a sample of spontaneous speech: the therapist is then required to transcribe, segment, code and analyse the sample using a framework for that analysis. The more detailed the framework, the more information gained, although the clinician will need to balance the time taken by the analysis with the information needed for assessment and therapy. Whereas some clinicians may claim that a busy clinic schedule precludes this stage of assessment, there is a strong case to be made that time spent at this stage enables the clinician to target therapy more efficiently. Crystal, et al., (1989) argue that the details provided by their profile are an essential prerequisite for therapy.

> The use of the profile forces the therapist to concentrate on the symptomatology. It is no longer possible using such an approach to restrict oneself to the use of simple labels such as *language delay* or *agrammatism* which we feel to be gross simplifications (p.199).

The current work with agrammatics would certainly lend support to this view.

In addition, descriptive studies based on the sort of detail provided by

Crystal, et al's profiling procedure provide the therapist with a baseline whereby aspects of treatment might be evaluated. Whatever therapeutic approach the clinician selects, these need to measure the patient's progress. Scores on certain tests will provide part of that baseline but the therapist will also want to have some way of assessing whether or not the patient's spontaneous speech has improved. Ideally, the therapist would also be able to indicate the severity of the aphasia in terms of how far the aphasic output deviates from normal speech for, having collected the data and analysed it according to the criteria of the chosen procedure, therapy should be guided by comparing the aphasic performance with that expected from a normal speaker. Unfortunately, although some norms are available for child language, the data on normal adult spontaneous speech are sparse. Additionally, we are aware that context, situation and task influence the type of naturalistic speech data collected for both normal speakers (Garman, 1990) and aphasic speakers (Menn, 1990; Berko Gleason, et al., 1980). Of course, lack of norms do not prevent therapists from identifying lexical, syntactic or semantic errors. All native speakers are able to judge the semantic and syntactic legitimacy of an utterance and linguistic theory depends on this ability.

The traditional test batteries, such as the Boston Aphasia Diagnostic Examination (Goodglass and Kaplan, 1983) or the Western Aphasia Battery (Kertesz, 1982) consist of series of tasks involving the production and comprehension of language. Such tasks typically include the naming of pictured or real objects, repetition and sentence completion. A sample of spontaneous speech is collected via conversation and picture description. Whereas task performance can be scored more or less objectively, the quantification of the speech samples relies on *ad hoc* measures such as *melodic line* and *phrase length*. More seriously, although there is some attempt to measure output in terms of length of utterance, little attention is paid to either describing or quantifying the output in terms of lexical, syntactic or semantic control.

A number of projects have sought to remedy this situation by using or developing a more comprehensive and systematic system of analysis and applying it to relatively large samples of spontaneous speech. Penn and Behrmann (1986) collected samples of unstructured conversational speech from a range of aphasic speakers. Certain syntactic structures were coded following LARSP (Crystal, et al., 1976) and the data analysed using the method of hierarchical cluster analysis. The authors claim that the results, while confirming the traditional dichotomy of fluent versus non-fluent aphasia, demonstrated that subgroups could be identified and that certain features were characteristic of more than one group. The non-fluent group typically displayed a low total number of sentences, a low mean number of sentences per turn and restricted sentence length. Their profiles showed severe restriction of clause, phrase and lexical deployment. In contrast, the fluent group showed greater use of syntactic structures and more sentences per turn. The subgroups were identified by both quantitative measures, for example, number of unanalyzable utterances and qualitative measures of error type. The results demonstrate that syntactic deficits were present in all subtypes and that therefore, it might be more profitable to consider syntactic deficits on a continuum rather than distinctive features of certain aphasia subgroups. When considering these results, we should note that only 36 of the available features logged by LARSP were used in this analysis and it is by no means certain that those features selected captured the extent of the subjects' syntactic abilities. The problem of what should be included in an assessment or profile of an aphasic patient's linguistic abilities is one that concerns the clinician as well as the researcher. One of the objectives of descriptive-type research must be to determine which measures are diagnostic, for various types of aphasic patients (cf. Fletcher 1990 for this type of approach with child language data), and which are predictive. Otherwise, there comes a point where the amount of data is overwhelming and no longer contributes to our knowledge. The pragmatic therapist may decide to collect detailed information on one aspect of the patient's language system such as the lexicon, but such decisions can only be made when the therapist has a fair amount of knowledge about the patient's language system – a tautological situation.

Saffran, et al. (1989) published data collected from agrammatic and normal speakers. Subjects in both groups were invited to retell a well known fairy tale. The speech samples were transcribed, segmented and analysed following specific criteria developed by the authors. The results show a clear difference between the grammatical output of the agrammatic speakers compared with normal controls, but they also indicate that agrammatics display a variety of grammatical deficits. Like Penn and Behrmann, the authors claim that these results are evidence of different subgroups. Unlike Penn and Behrmann who examined a range of aphasic speakers, however, Saffran, et al's subjects were initially selected as agrammatics. However, their subgroups of agrammatics exhibited different patterns of omission and preservation of bound and free morphemes and varying limitations of verb usage, supporting the claims that agrammatism is not one clearly delineated syndrome (Howard, 1985). Details of production revealed by this type of analysis gives the clinician a much clearer picture of his or her patient's linguistic abilities and has obvious implications for therapy.

It is apparent, then, that detailed profiles of an aphasic speaker's output can not only provide valuable clinical material but also increase our knowledge of this disorder. For example, there is mounting evidence, from both psycholinguistic and linguistic research, that syntactic deficits might be characteristic of a range of aphasic speakers and not confined to the agrammatic, non-fluent group: whether the range can best be described in terms of a continuum of severity or whether there are discrete and unrelated deficits, has yet to be established. A project at the University of Reading (co-directed by Michael Garman and the author), is currently investigating spontaneous speech from a mixed group of aphasic speakers (see Edwards, et al., 1991; 1992). The purpose of this project is to extend and refine the descriptive framework LARSP (Crystal, et al., 1989) and apply it to adult normal and aphasic speech; to build up detailed profiles of all the subjects; to obtain details of syntactic and lexical structures used by a range of aphasics and to thus obtain a data reference base on normal and aphasic spontaneous speech. Unlike written language, much of normal adult speech cannot be satisfactorily segmented using the notion of sentence. Furthermore, it is typified by the deployment of a wide range of linking devices which establishes syntactic coherence between units which is one measure of complexity. The focus of the first part of the project, then, has been on the development of explicit, comprehensive and coherent criteria for the transcription, segmentation and analysis of the data and especially the establishment of criteria for identifying units for analysis and the grouping of these units within the discourse. (See Edwards and Garman, 1989; Garman, 1989; Edwards, et al., 1991; 1992 for further details). These criteria must be able to cope with the abnormal output of fluent and non-fluent speech as well as the normal adult speech samples which serve as a basis for comparisons. Until we have satisfactory criteria for this stage of analysis (and our view is that none are currently in existence), we are not able to make meaningful statements about frequency or complexity of utterances or about the management and organization of units within discourse nor are we able to make reliable comparisons between subjects or over time.

Applications and Conclusions

Assessment

We will conclude this chapter by illustrating some of the above points with a brief description of some of the assessment and treatment procedures used with one aphasic patient seen at the Communication Disorders Centre at the University of Reading. (This account of assessment and therapy is illustrative only and therefore certain aspects of the programme have been omitted. Further details to which the linguistic analyses refer will be available in forthcoming publications.) The patient, MG, a 56-year-old man, had suffered a sudden cerebral vascular accident nine months previous to his referral to the Centre. A CT scan located an infarct in the distribution of the left-middle cerebral artery, implicating areas in the cortical and sub-cortical areas, especially left temporal and adjacent posterior parietal lobe. Prior to his stroke, the patient had held a middle management position in a national insurance company; he had a high level of literacy skills and led a full and active social life. Routine standard assessments had persuaded the referring therapist, who continued to be involved with his rehabilitation programme, to describe the language disorder exhibited by this patient as fluent Wernicke's aphasia.

Production

An example of his spontaneous speech, collected soon after his referral to our clinic, is as follows (segmented according to our criteria):

Example

therapist:	do you watch television
MG:	yes
	plenty
	plenty
therapist:	right
	are there any serials
	that you are watching
	at the moment
MG	{F} (not) not very much
	{F} we get {F}
	what does it do
	(I) I
	a (news) news
therapists:	right
MG:	I get in
	I get {F} - the {F}
	come
	set {F}
	{F} I can't do that - - one
	I can do them
	I (can) sentence it
	but it doesn't say them
	anymore
	I can do it
	marvellous
	but I can't say it

Note: *{F} = filled pause; (X) = repeated element; - = brief pause. The segmentation is based on clausal, minor and adverbial constructions. The units are linearized but arranged to convey the grammatical-textual relationship between* *them.*

The assessment of the patient received high priority. The above sample of speech illustrates that the patient had access to a range of word classes and grammatical structures and could make a good attempt at answering the therapist's questions within a conversational context. Incomplete utterances, filled pauses and possible paraphasic errors suggest a lexical retrieval problem. This in turn may be responsible for some of the confusion in his last turn or may portray poor syntactic control. We considered it important to obtain a more detailed description of his output difficulties. This information was obtained by sampling his spontaneous speech as well as collecting data on task performance and by administering certain standardized tests. A spontaneous speech sample was obtained, transcribed, segmented and coded according to our criteria. This enabled us to construct a profile of his lexical, phrasal and clausal usage and provided a baseline whereby we would be able to judge improvement in his natural conversational speech as well as performance on specific tasks. MG's wife was able to obtain some video-recordings of her husband making professional conference presentations prior to his stroke which were used for comparison. Although the majority of the recorded speech was dependent upon his prepared written text, he started the presentation with what seemed to be relatively informal warm-up comments. We need to be cautious when comparing this type of monologic speech and conversational speech, for we are aware of the possibility of contextual/situational influences. However, this text gives us a unique opportunity to make some comparisons between pre- and post-incident speech.

Inspection of the post-incident transcript confirmed the clinical impression we had about speech. Using a modified LARSP framework for analysis and comparing this sample with a pre-incident sample (sample size was controlled following our grammatical criteria), the following features emerged. As an aphasic speaker, he used more incomplete, unintelligible and minor utterances; fewer examples of both noun and verb phrases; fewer bound morphemes signalling person, tense, plurality, possession; a reduced range of phrasal and clausal structures; fewer structures with four or more clausal constituents; less connectivity; a reduced amount of grammatically related structures. The aphasic speech was not noticeably marked by grammatical errors: there were no deviant utterances and one unintelligible (compared with none in the normal data) and five incomplete. However, this analysis revealed that although he did have at his disposal a range of grammatical forms and structures and no obvious omission of grammatical morphemes, as an aphasic speaker, MG was not using the same range of grammatical structures which he had previously deployed.

Investigations of his lexical system were carried out by using a standardized test of naming and by analysing the word-classes used in his spontaneous speech. Testing on the Boston Naming Test (Kaplan, Goodglass and Weintraub, 1983) revealed a severe problem. He initially achieved 13 of the 60 target nouns, achieved a further 14 with phonemic cueing and only three with semantic cueing. He clearly had difficulty with confrontational naming tasks and demonstrated some frank lexical problems within his conversational speech. However, he maintained access to all word-classes. All word-classes were represented in the speech samples although the diversity was reduced: i.e., there were a reduced number of types, especially nouns and verbs. The difference can be illustrated by reduced type/token ratios although, again, we need to be cautious with interpretations of this measure.

Comprehension

A comprehension deficit had been demonstrated by standard assessments but we wished to explore what aspects of comprehension were affected so that we might offer appropriate therapy. We have seen above that there are various components which can be demonstrated within a comprehension loss and that different theoretical explanations might be put forward in explanation (see Pierce, Chapter 10, this volume). The exploration of comprehension abilities therefore covered a number of possibilities and included the following: investigating his ability to use syntax to access meaning; investigating aspects of his semantic system including comprehension of isolated lexemes; noting the effect of short-term memory on comprehension, or at least on comprehension tasks given in clinic; understanding discourse.

His spontaneous speech contained examples of lexical paraphasic errors which were not often self-corrected and so we were uncertain about his comprehension of single words. Given an array of common pictured objects, he had no difficulty in selection, although performance was limited by short-term memory. In the early stages of therapy he had been unable to select more than one object at a time, but this improved, and by the time he was attending our sessions he was able to retain four object names. This was still abnormal and there remained an impression that memory load interfered with comprehension. However, testing on a standardized test of understanding of single words (Brimer, 1982) revealed a poor performance; he achieved a standard score of 84, which puts him in the 18th percentile. His errors included nouns, verbs and adjectives, but as this test is not controlled for word class, these results merely demonstrate that there was marked difficulty in matching single word to meaning and that this difficulty was not reserved for nouns. Further investigations found that he was unable to categorize written or spoken words according to semantic category, neither was he able to relate supra/sub- ordinate terms.

We investigated his ability to use syntactic knowledge in comprehension with a number of tasks. Testing on TROG (Bishop, 1983) revealed that he had problems understanding sentences which had reversible structures (locative terms and passive constructions); embedded sentences and those containing *but not* phrases. Further investigations showed that he had difficulty selecting reversible passive sentences, choosing the reversed role rather than the lexical distracter. He had more difficulty with understanding passive than active sentences and found it more difficult to make grammatical judgements about these sentences even when length of sentence was controlled. These findings would suggest that, like the agrammatic patients reported in the literature, MG showed some difficulty comprehending sentences when meaning was dependant on grammatical structure.

Despite these difficulties, he had retained some ability to make grammatical judgements and was more accurate at saying whether a sentence was grammatically correct than he was judging whether a sentence was semantically acceptable (12/15 compared with 8/15). Performance on repetition tasks also revealed some type of parsing problem although his handling of grammatical information seemed superior relative to his handling of semantic information. It was established that although MG could repeat stage 2 and 3 LARSP structures, he made errors if the sentences contained either syntactic or semantic inappropriacies. When asked to repeat sentences which contained either syntactic or semantic violations, he made more errors repeating sentences with syntactic violations. Although his errors with the syntactically violated sentences tended to be in the direction of correcting the error, an interesting difference emerged. He accurately repeated just under half (6/13) of the sentences which contained semantic errors, but he was able to repeat only (3/13) of the sentences which contained syntactic errors. (We had previously established that he could repeat similar structures when no errors were present). His poor performance on the syntactically contaminated sentences could show that although his ability to parse was impaired, he had retained some ability to recognize ungrammatical structures (and attempted to correct errors) but his recognition of the violation contained within the sentence interfered with his ability to repeat. However, if recognition of an error is reflected in his repetition errors, then his comparatively good performance on repeating sentences containing semantic errors might suggest that he is less aware of the semantic inappropriacy. This suggests that although he was unable to reliably make correct grammatical judgements, he was sensitive to grammatical structures. All these results suggested that despite his fluent output and obvious weak semantic system, there was also some weakness of the grammatical system and that this might be one factor contributing to his comprehension problems.

However, when given the Caplan and Evans comprehension of

discourse tasks (see above), there was no difference in his ability to comprehend the syntactically complex texts compared with the syntactically simple texts (which is in line with the performance of the asyntactic comprehenders in the research report). However, as he only managed to score at chance level on all texts, the only firm conclusion we can draw is that a comprehension deficit is present for discourse as well as for single sentences but that this level of, albeit impaired comprehension, was not adversely affected by increasing the complexity of the syntax. There may be evidence that his restricted memory capacity interfered with his performance on the test of discourse comprehension as his performance varied depending on the type of statement he had to verify. Three types of probes are used in this task. MG produced most errors (13) in response to *event type probes* which are designed to assess the listener's ability to retain the sequential order of the story; he made 10 errors in response to probes designed to assess his ability to make inferences about the story and he made 4 errors judging whether *verbatim probes* were true or false. These differences held irrespective of story type which strongly indicates that the nature of the question had more effect than the type or syntactic complexity of the text.

These investigations confirmed that MG had marked difficulty comprehending language at single word, sentence and discourse level. He could access some meaning using his residual comprehension at each level of processing which enabled him to participate in conversations. He also judged that his performance on the story comprehension test was fair although his demeanour would suggest some intellectual struggle. However, although he claimed to have understood the general theme of each story, when tested on the recall of details, his comprehension was only at chance level.

Earlier in this chapter we considered the hypothesis that certain language deficits in aphasia may arise because of the loss, or reduced, ability to co-index and, indeed, it was found that MG had great difficulty in assigning reference for pronouns. This performance, together with his difficulties with passives, lends support to this hypothesis. His performance was slightly better when given written rather than spoken input, which was in line with the findings of his reduced auditory short-term memory. These investigations using linguistically controlled data and standized tests revealed that there were a number of factors contributing to his poor comprehension. Short-term memory limited his performance on some tasks, he had difficulty interpreting certain grammatical structures, notably passives and pronominals and his semantic system as far as categorization tasks and accessing meaning of some single words were concerned was impaired. At this stage, we can only speculate whether the deficits revealed pointed to a mapping deficit or whether the lexical or grammatical theories proposed to account for agrammatism might be extended to account for MG's deficits. Certain features of grammatical performance, the difficulty with assigning correct meanings to passive structures, pronominals and locatives, reflect reports on agrammatic performance. While we considered our results motivated therapy, they are insufficient at this stage to support any one theoretical position. They do, however, seem to confirm that there were some weaknesses within the management of the grammatical system. This fluent patient certainly exhibited problems with the use of his semantic system and the accessing of lexical items, but the aphasia cannot be accounted for solely at these levels.

Management

MG is representative of a large number of patients seen by aphasia therapists in that he presents with a complex picture of language deficits. He has a keen interest in all stages of assessment and therapy and responds well to explanation and discussion of his language problem. His wife attended every session, contributed to the discussions, made helpful observations and reported that the sessions had increased her insights into the nature of the disorder. Increased knowledge helps redress the balance of power and contributes to the patient's and spouse's self-esteem. Both MG and his wife were soon able to predict which tasks would be difficult and were also able to observe improvement after practising tasks. They also become aware that improvement on a task might not always be maintained once practice ceased. We have demonstrated above that MG had weaknesses at all levels of language production and that there were a number of factors contributing to his damaged comprehension. Therapy tasks were therefore targeted at several areas: here we will briefly outline two of them.

One area of focus was on his semantic system and consisted of two essential parts. First, we drew his attention to the association between high frequency, highly imageable nouns and their possible semantic groupings; second he was encouraged to seek supra-ordinate terms for the groups; third, by linking these two types of tasks, he was encouraged to recall and report on the attributes of the objects. The second type of task involved working with single words and their meanings. This was achieved through seeking synonyms and antonyms and for creating and checking definitions. Baselines were established for all tasks and practice continued until he achieved 80 per cent success. Therapy which concentrated on single words and their meanings was justified by the results of the tests given but also relates to the lexicalist explanation we have considered above. If MG's semantic system could be strengthened, he should theoretically have improved top-down mechanisms available for word access. Retesting on the Boston Naming Test would seem to confirm this. After a ten-week course, he showed a modest improvement on his score (from 13 to 17) but produced more correct responses following semantic cues (9 compared with 3) suggesting that we were establishing stronger semantic associations.

The further area of interest was his syntactic system. We have noted that there was a restricted range of clausal, phrasal and lexical structures in his spontaneous output and some evidence of an impaired parsing facility. We decided that it was inappropriate to focus on his output directly in terms of encouraging specific structures but would concentrate on his reduced parsing ability. Therapy was focused on tasks which required MG to assign syntactic roles to constituent structures within a sentence and to relate syntactic structures and semantic forms. The rationale was that the weakened system(s) would be assisted by making implicit rules which govern word order and convey meaning explicit and available through explanation and practice exercises. He was unable to participate when first exposed to a test of selecting reversible active sentences but with practice achieved an 80 per cent level of performance on related tasks. However, although his clinical performance improved, retesting showed performance to be hovering around the 50 per cent level. Attention has therefore been shifted to other areas of his performance.

These two examples of therapy used with MG are given as examples of applying knowledge gained from the linguistic and psycholinguistic literature to clinical practice and tempering that application in the light of the patient's perceived needs. We have also made a case for sampling the patient's spontaneous speech both to provide a detailed characterization of the surface features used and as a way of charting generalization of task skills to everyday speech. A third sample of speech taken 12 months after MG's referral to the University Clinic gives some substance to an informal judgement of improvement. Examination of data obtained from profiling shows the following features: the proportion of total complete utterances has risen from .70 to .77 (compared with .92 pre-incident); the proportion of noun phrases has increased (but not the verb phrase); the proportion of grammatical-bound morphemes has increased; and there is some increase at stage 4 phrase level. MG still presents with a limited profile of syntactic structures but the trend is towards normality (using his pre-morbid speech sample as control data). His increased use of noun phrases may reflect his modest improvement in naming although the relationship between word access in conversation and word access in naming tasks is not clear. While it remains difficult to relate much to the extensive and at times contradictory findings of theoretical research to clinical practice, therapy continues to benefit by attempting to make these connections. However, applied linguistics is increasingly seen to offer a comprehensive and systematic means of describing and evaluating aphasic speech, and it is probably this area of linguistic research that currently has the most to offer clinical practice. It was once held that linguistics has little to offer treatment in aphasiology (Farmer and O'Connell, 1979). There can be few serious practising clinical aphasiologists who would still agree.

Acknowledgements

I would like to thank the following: my colleagues Paul Fletcher and Michael Garman for their comments on this paper; Raymond Knott for some of the analyses of the MG data; Shelagh Grier for referring MG to my clinic; MG and his wife for their cheerful participation.

References

Albert M, Goodglass H, Helm N, Rubens A, Alexander M (1981) Clinical Aspects of Dysphasia. New York: Springer.

Bates E, Friederici A, Wulfeck B (1987) Grammatical morphology in aphasia: evidence from three languages. Cortex 23; 545–74.

Bates E, MacWhinney B (1982) Functionalist approaches to grammar. In Wanner E, Gleitman L (Eds) Language Acquisition: The State of the Art. Cambridge: Cambridge University Press.

Bates E, MacWhinney B (1989) The Crosslinguistic Study of Sentence Processing. Cambridge: Cambridge University Press.

Bates E, Wulfeck, B (1989) Crossed linguistic studies of aphasia. In Bates E, McWhinney B (Eds) The Crosslinguistic Study of Sentence Processing. Cambridge: Cambridge University Press.

Berko Gleason J, Goodglass H, Obler L, Green E, Hyde M, Weintraub S (1980) Narrative strategies of aphasic and normal speaking subjects. Journal of Speech and Hearing Research. 23: 370–82.

Bishop D (1983) Test for Reception of Grammar. Published privately.

Brimer M (1982) The Listening for Meaning Test. Gloucesteshire: Educational Evaluation Enterprises.

Byng S (1988) Sentence processing deficits. Cognitive Neuropsychology. 5: 629–76.

Byng S, Coltheart M (1986) Aphasia therapy research: methodological requirements and illustrative results. In Hjelmquist E, Nilsson L (Eds) Communication and Handicap. Amsterdam: Elsvier

Byng S, Nickels L, Black M, (1991) Replicating therapy for mapping deficits: remapping the deficit. Paper presented to the conference of the British Aphasiology Society, University of Sheffield.

Caplan D (1987) Neurolinguistics and Linguistic Aphasiology. Cambridge: Cambridge University Press.

Caplan D, Hilderbrandt H (1988) Disorders of Syntactic Comprehension. Cambridge MA: MIT Press.

Caplan D, Evans K (1990) Syntactic structure and discourse comprehension. Brain and Language 39: 206–34.

Crystal D (1981) Clinical Linguistics. London: Edward Arnold.

Crystal D, Fletcher P, Garman M (1976; 1989) The Grammatical Analysis of Language Ability. (1st.; 2nd edn.) London: Edward Arnold.

Edwards S, Garman M (1989) Case study of a fluent aphasic: the relation between linguistic assessment and therapeutic intervention. In Grunwell P, James A (Eds) The Functional Evaluation of Language Disorders. London: Croom Helm.

Edwards S, Garman M, Knott R (1991) Unmasking unmarked sources of evidence: explorations in the grammatical characterization of aphasic speech. Paper presented to the conference of the British Aphasiology Society, University of Sheffield.

Edwards S, Garman M, Knott R (1992) Project report: the linguistic characterization of aphasic speech. Clinical Linguistics. 6: 161–4.

Edwards S, Garman, Knott R (1993) The grammatical characterisation of aphasic language. Aphasiology. 7 217–20.

Farmer A, O'Connell P (1979) Neuropsychological processes in adult aphasia: rationale for treatment. British Journal of Disorder of Communication 14: 39–49.

Fletcher P (1989)Language Pathology. Annual Review of Applied Linguistics 10: 26–36.

Fletcher P (1990) Evidence from syntax for language impairment. In Miller J. (Ed) Research on Child Language Disorders: A Decade of Progress. Boston MA: College Hill.

Garman M (1982) The role of linguistics in speech therapy: assessment and interpretation. In Grunwell P, James A. (Eds) The Functional Evaluation of Language Disorders. London: Croom Helm.

Garman M (1990) Psycholinguistics. Cambridge: Cambridge University Press.

Garrett M (1982) Production of speech: observations from normal and pathological language use. In Ellis A. (Ed) Normality and Pathology in Cognitive Functions. London: Academic Press.

Goodglass H, Kaplan E (1983) Assessment of Aphasia and related Disorders. Philadelphia PA: Lea & Febiger.

Goodglass H, Kaplan E (1983) Boston Diagnostic Aphasia Examination. Philadelphia PA: Lea & Febiger.

Goodglass H, Menn L, (1985) Is agrammatism a unitary phenomenon? In Kean ML (Ed) Agrammatism. New York: Academic Press.

Grodzinsky Y (1990) Theoretical Perspectives on Language Deficits. Cambridge, MA: MIT Press.

Hatfield F, Shewell C (1983) Some applications of linguistics to aphasia therapy. In Code C, Muller D. (Eds) Aphasia therapy. (1st eds) London: Edward Arnold.

Howard D (1985) Agrammatism. In Newman S, Epstein R. (Eds) Current Perspectives in Dysphasia. London: Churchill Livingstone.

Jakobson R (1968) Child Language, Aphasia and Phonological Universals. The Hague: Mouton.

Jones E (1986) Building the foundations for sentence production in a non-fluent aphasic. British Journal of Disorders of Communication. 21: 63–82.

Kaplan E, Goodglass H, Weintraub, S. (1983) The Boston Naming Test. Boston MA: Lea & Febiger.

Kay J, Lesser R, Coltheart M (1992) Psycholinguistic Assessment of Language Processing in Aphasia. London: Erlbaum.

Kean ML (1977) The linguistic interpretation of aphasic syndromes: agrammatism in Broca's aphasia, an example. Cognition 5: 9–46.

Kean ML (1985) Agrammatism. New York: Academic Press.

Kertesz A (1982) Western Aphasia Battery. London: Grune & Stratton.

Lesser R (1978) Linguistic Investigations of Aphasia. London: Edward Arnold.

Lesser R (1987) Cognitive neuropsychological influences on aphasia therapy. Aphasiology 1: 189–200.

Lesser R, Milroy L (1987) Two frontiers in aphasia therapy. Bulletin. London: College of Speech Therapists.

Lesser R, Milroy L (1993) Linguistics and Aphasia. London: Longman.

Linebarger M (1989) Neuropsychology of sentence parsing. In Caramazza A. (Ed) Cognitive Neuropsychology and Neurolinguistics: Advances in Models of Cognitive Function and Impairment. Hillsdale NJ: Erlbaum.

Marshall J (1990) Foreword. In Grodzinsky Y. Theoretical Perspectives on Language Deficits. Cambridge, MA: MIT Press

Menn L (1990) Agrammatism in English. In Menn L, Obler L (Eds) Agrammatic Aphasia: a Cross-linguistic Source Book. Philadelphia PA: Benjamins.

Menn L, Obler L (1990) in Menn L, Obler L (Eds) Agrammatic Aphasia: a Cross-linguistic Source Book. Philadelphia PA: Benjamins.

Mitchum C, Berndt R (1992) Clinical linguistics, cognitive neuropsychology and aphasia therapy. Clinical Linguistics 6: 3–10.

Paradis M (1987) The Assessment of Bilingual Aphasia. Hillsdale NJ: Lawrence Erlbaum.

Penn C, Behrmann M (1986) Towards a classification scheme for aphasic syntax. British Journal of Communication Disorders. 21: 21–38.

Quirk R, Grenbaum S, Leech G, Svartvik J (1972) A Grammar of Contemporary English. London: Longman.

Saffran E, Berndt R, Schwartz M (1989) The quantitative analysis of agrammatic production: procedure and data. Brain and Language. 37: 440–79.

Vermeulen J, Bastiaanse R, Van Wageningen B (1989) Spontaneous speech in aphasia: a correlation study. Brain and language. 36: 252–74.

Part III: Cognitive and Neuropsychological Approaches

This section brings together a collect of chapters which address aspects of treatment from within a broad cognitive framework. The first chapter by **Anne Edmundson** and **Jaqueline McIntosh** provides an introduction to cognitive neuropsychology and how this paradigm has influenced aphasia therapy. They give particular emphasis to the need to work on an individual basis with a view to identifying, in a detective-like fashion, each person's specific impairment. The chapter provides an excellent introduction to this approach which is supported by a careful review of the research literature and by the presentation of a detailed analysis of a case study. The emphasis placed upon single case studies is in line with the emphasis earlier chapters have placed on developing treatment techniques in response to the individual person's needs.

The opening chapter is supported by a brief contribution by **Ruth Lesser**. Ruth describes the psycholinguistically-based approach to assessing individuals with aphasia known as 'psycholinguistic assessments of language processing in aphasia' (PALPA). The theoretical framework for PALPA is derived from cognitive neuropsychology; a clear case is presented for applying psycholinguistic analysis to assessment to support treatment. The PALPA is relatively new and has been identified as an important clinical tool to support the development of treatment derived from cognitive neuropsychological frameworks.

A more traditional approach is presented in the review chapter which follows by **Robert Pierce**. He provides a review of comprehension deficits and critically analyses research exploring a wide range of comprehension deficits, including the treatment of single word comprehension, through the broader approach required to treat narrative comprehension. This chapter shows that the treatment of comprehension is likely to be an important aspect of many therapy programmes.

The two chapters which follow review two related aspects of aphasia therapy from slightly different perspectives. **Evelyne Andreeswky**

135

and **Francoise Cochu** overview therapeutic approaches to reading. The authors indicate that reading remains a highly complex process and that although there are different theoretical approaches to remediating deficiencies, the chapter serves to remind the reader of the importance which must be placed on a functional approach to reading through an emphasis on understanding. This chapter draws upon the pragmatic and communicative perspectives outlined earlier and sets them functionally in the context of cognitive and neuropsychological approaches.

Sergio Carlomagno and **Alessandro Iavarone** discuss different approaches to the treatment of writing deficiencies, while setting therapeutic practice into a cognitive framework which focuses on functional recovery. This chapter describes in helpful detail a number of studies, including the single-case study, which has been given particular emphasis in this text. They show that treatment is often very effective, which highlights the importance for aphasia therapists to offer specific remediation. In reviewing research the authors conclude that many of the successful approaches are strongly cognitively oriented. At the same time it is pointed out that careful consideration should be given to the extent to which individuals with aphasia themselves place importance upon writing over other cognitive and social activities. The requirement to provide writing therapy should be determined by the needs of the individual; this may not always correspond entirely to the range of cognitive deficits which have been identified.

The final chapter in this section is slightly different in that it describes a computer system and presents an evaluation study to assess its value in the treatment of sentence processing impairment. **Alison Crerar** and **Andrew Ellis** point out the longer term contribution microcomputer technology can bring to the treatment of aphasia. Their research is derived from a strong theoretically driven linguistic basis and is an excellent illustration of how modern technology combined with theoretically driven intervention can lead to improvements in those individuals with language processing deficits.

Chapter 8
Cognitive Neuropsychology and Aphasia Therapy: Putting the Theory into Practice

ANNE EDMUNDSON AND JAQUELINE McINTOSH

Over the past few years, some exciting developments have been occurring in aphasia therapy. As a result, the term *cognitive neuropsychology* has become increasingly familiar to aphasia therapists. In this chapter, we will begin with a brief introduction to cognitive neuropsychology, consider how cognitive neuropsychological theory has influenced aphasia therapy, and explore what this approach can offer to the clinical management of people with acquired aphasia.

What is Cognitive Neuropsychology?

As a result of brain damage, many adults suffer from impairments of higher mental functions such as memory, language or perception. The study of such impairments has traditionally been the concern of neuropsychology. Over the years, many neuropsychological syndromes have been described. Each syndrome (for example, Wernicke's aphasia) is defined by a pattern of symptoms (poor auditory comprehension and fluent, paraphasic speech) and is claimed to arise as a result of damage to a particular region of the brain (left temporal lobe). One aim of neuropsychological assessment is to identify the person's symptoms in order to allow a syndrome diagnosis to be made.

While neuropsychology tries to group people together into syndromes, cognitive neuropsychology focuses on the differences between people who present with superficially similar disorders. Cognitive neuropsychologists draw on theories that attempt to explain how the human brain normally performs cognitive functions. Each individual is studied in depth, the aim of assessment being to identify the processing impairments responsible for producing his or her particular pattern of symptoms. A comprehensive introduction to cognitive neuropsychology can be found in Ellis and Young, 1988. For the purposes of this chapter, we shall just briefly outline the main features of this approach.

Cognitive neuropsychology is based upon the general assumption that the mind is a complex processing system. All cognitive functions, such as understanding a spoken word or recognizing a person's face, are claimed to involve a number of different processes each of which is carried out by a specialized processing component or module. A given module receives information from and sends information to other modules in the system, but carries out its own processing independently of the rest of the system. Few claims are made about the locations of the modules within the brain. However, they are assumed to be neurologically distinct, brain damage being able to selectively impair individual modules and/or the connections between them.

By definition, cognitive neuropsychologist study people with damaged processing systems. It is assumed that the information obtained can help to reveal the characteristics of the normally functioning system. The person's performance is understood to reflect a normal system attempting to function without the damaged process(es), and conclusions are drawn about which processes remain intact, which are impaired. The adult brain is assumed to be incapable of developing new processing modules to replace or compensate for those that have been damaged. 'The injured brain may develop new strategies for coping in a particular task or situation, but it must do so using pre-existing structures' (Ellis and Young, 1988: 19).

Although cognitive neuropsychology is still a relatively young academic discipline, a wide variety of neuropsychological impairments have now been studied within this framework. Many of the current theoretical developments in this field are being influenced by advances in technology. Sophisticated brain scanning techniques are allowing further investigation of the relationship between psychological functions and the brain's neurological organization (see for example, Wise, et al., 1991). Advances in artificial intelligence have led to the development of powerful interactive processing theories. These computer models are being lesioned in order to try to simulate the types of impairments observed in people (see Patterson, Seidenberg and McClelland, 1989; Plaut and Shallice, 1993). Perhaps the development that is of most immediate interest to the aphasia therapist is the recognition that cognitive neuropsychology has potential implications for the remediation of acquired cognitive disorders.

Coltheart (1984) suggested that an aim of cognitive neuropsychology should be to develop theoretically motivated remediation programmes for people with neurological impairments. In 1987, Howard and Hatfield described the emergence of this new approach to aphasia therapy in which cognitive neuropsychology provides the framework for the assessment and interpretation of each person's language processing skills and deficits. From this information, a therapy programme is devised, the treatment method being 'founded in a rational analysis of the patient's problem' (Howard and Hatfield, 1987; 105). The approach also places considerable emphasis upon the objective evaluation of the therapy. In the next sections we will consider each of these features in turn. However, it is important to note that, while we have chosen to discuss them separately, the divisions are artificial. Assessment, treatment and evaluation are very intimately interrelated aspects of the therapeutic process.

Cognitive Neuropsychology and Aphasia Therapy

Identifying the Language Processing Impairment

Standardized aphasia batteries such as the Minnesota Test for the Differential Diagnosis of Aphasia (MTDDA) (Schuell 1973) and the Boston Diagnostic Aphasia Examination (BDAE) (Goodglass and Kaplan, 1983) are the tools traditionally used to assess acquired language disorders. These assessments are designed to identify the characteristic symptoms of different aphasic syndromes. In contrast, the aim of cognitive neuropsychologically - based assessment is to explain each person's processing skills and deficits in terms of a model of normal language processing. Figure 8.1 is a diagrammatic representation of one account of single-word processing. It encompasses many aspects of language including understanding spoken and written words, repeating words, reading aloud, speaking, and writing spontaneously and to dictation. Visual recognition of pictures and objects has also been included.[1] The boxes and arrows provide a convenient way of identifying the modules that make up the processing system and describing the relationships between them. Each box in the diagram represents a processing module. The arrows indicate where a particular module receives information from and, having processed it, where it then passes the information to. Such diagrams describe the organization of the processing system but do not indicate how it is suggested to function. The full theory also has to explain what each of the different processing modules does, and which processing modules are normally involved in carrying out a particular language skill (that is, the processing route(s) involved).

Because the characteristics of single-word processing are specified, ways to investigate the functioning of a processing module or a processing route can be devised (see Psycholinguistic Assessments of Language Processing in Aphasia: PALPA (Kay, Lesser and Coltheart, 1992; Lesser, Chapter 9, this volume). Variables such as word-frequency (the frequency of occurrence of words), imageability (the ease with which a word conjures up a mental image of its meaning), and regularity of spelling are suggested to influence processing in specific ways. Clear predictions can therefore be made about the consequences of

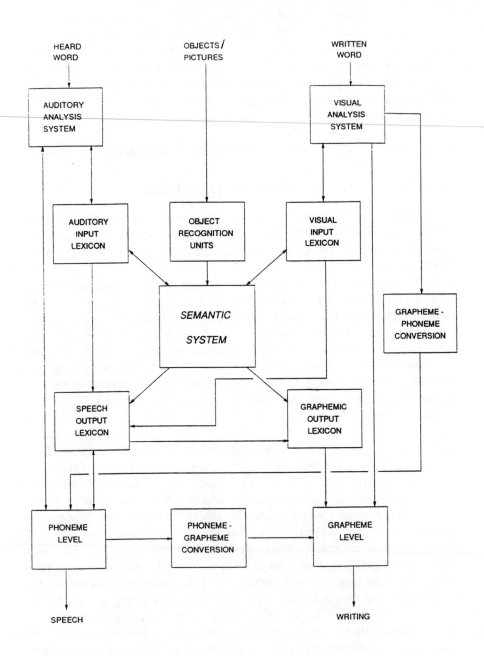

Figure 8.1 Diagram summarizing the processes involved in single word comprehension (spoken and written words), picture comprehension, spoken naming, repetition, reading and writing (based on Ellis and Young, 1988)

damage to different parts of the system. While many cognitive neuropsychological assessment procedures resemble sub-tests in the standardized aphasia batteries, the test materials are carefully controlled to allow the influence of theoretically relevant variables to be investigated.

In contrast to the traditional aphasia batteries which are usually intended to be presented in their entirety, cognitive neuropsychology does not advocate that a particular battery of tests should be presented to all aphasic clients. Because emphasis is placed on the identification of each person's specific processing impairments, cognitive neuropsychological assessment has been likened to detective work.

> From observing how patients interact with their environment and with other people, and by noting the level of language disorder they present with in conversational language, comes the initial hypothesis about the kind of difficulties they have. From the first contact with the patient the therapist needs to bring to that observation clear, logical and rational enquiry in order to observe and follow the clues, like a detective, to determine the source of the deficit (Jones and Byng, 1989; 2).

The language processing theory provides the framework for thinking about language and the ways in which it can be impaired. This framework can guide the therapist to ask clear, logical questions about the language disorder. Rather than trying to describe this process, it is perhaps easier to attempt to illustrate *hypothesis-driven* assessment. In doing so, we shall briefly discuss certain aspects of the model represented in Figure 8.1. Further information about single word processing can be found in Ellis and Young (1988).

From Figure 8.1, it should be apparent that the *semantic system* is central to all aspects of language processing. In very general terms, this is the store of meanings or semantic representations. This particular model assumes that the same stored information is involved in the comprehension of spoken words, written words, objects and pictures, and in the production of spoken and written output.[2] When the functioning of the semantic system is impaired, performance is known to be influenced by variables relating to the meanings of words. For example, confusions may exist between semantically similar words such as DAUGHTER and SON. Differences may also be observed between the processing of high imageability (or concrete) words such as CHURCH, and low imageability (or abstract) words such as RELIGION. The influence of these semantic variables may be apparent both in comprehension and production.

Let us assume that a hypothetical person, Mr X, has been referred with a diagnosis of acquired aphasia. How can a knowledge of normal language processing help the therapist to identify the nature of his language processing impairments? While interacting with Mr X and taking the case history, observation reveals that he can participate in the general conversation and is able to communicate a lot of relevant information. However, when asked specific questions his responses are not always appropriate, suggesting that his auditory comprehension may be impaired. His spoken output is fluent and characterized by frequent paraphasic errors. These are generally real words that are semantically related to the target (for example, referring to his hemiplegic right arm as his 'leg'). He seems to have very little awareness when he has made a semantic error. It also becomes apparent that he is reluctant to try to write with his non-preferred left hand, but he says that his reading is 'not too bad'. An initial investigation reveals that he is able to read out a newspaper headline.

Many questions could arise from these initial observations, including:

1. Why does he make semantic errors in speech?
2. Is his auditory comprehension impaired – if so, what's the problem?
3. Why doesn't he notice when he makes a semantic error?
4. How good is his understanding of written words?

The framework provided by the single-word processing model allows further refinement of the questions. For example, because it is known that semantic errors (Question 1) are likely to arise because of some problem with semantic processing, it could be hypothesized that Mr X's semantic system is impaired. Such an impairment could also have implications for his comprehension (Questions 2, 3 and 4). It would therefore seem logical to question his semantic processing.

Any tasks which are believed to normally involve the semantic system (comprehension of spoken and/or written words and/or pictures; spoken and/or written naming of pictures, etc.) could be used to investigate semantic processing. However, for particularly pertinent information to be obtained, the psycholinguistic variables known to influence semantic processing (semantic similarity; imageability) should be investigated. For example, a word-to-picture matching task should include semantically related distractor pictures. While such a task could be devised specifically for Mr X, a suitable test can be found in the PALPA (Kay, Lesser and Coltheart, 1992; Chapter 9, this volume). This word-to-picture matching task consists of 40 items. For each item the distractor pictures include a close semantic distractor (Target = CARROT; Close semantic = CABBAGE), a distant semantic distractor (LEMON), a distractor that visually resembles the target picture (SAW) and a distractor unrelated to the target (CHISEL). In the spoken word-to-picture version of the test, Mr X correctly identifies the target picture for 30 items and makes ten errors. For seven of these he selects the close or distant semantic distractor, for three the unrelated distractor. When the written word-to-picture version is presented during the following session he makes six errors, all of which involve semantically related distractors.

From this information it would appear that Mr X does not always fully comprehend single words, the pattern of errors suggesting that while he generally knows something about the meaning of the word, he has difficulty distinguishing between semantically similar items. This evidence would lend support to the hypothesis that he has a semantic processing impairment. To investigate this further, other comprehension tasks could be presented. For example, the Synonym Judgement Task (Kay, Lesser and Coltheart, 1992) could be used to ascertain if Mr X's comprehension of words is affected by imageability.

The processing theory also suggests that it may be important to question the precise nature of the semantic processing problem. Brain damage can disrupt the information stored in a processing module (in this case, the semantic representations) or it may impair the procedures by which this information is accessed. Shallice (1987) discusses the characteristics of different semantic processing impairments.[3] One factor to consider is item-consistency. If performance is inconsistent across items (the same word sometimes being understood, sometimes miscomprehended) then this is likely to be evidence for a semantic access deficit: inconsistency suggesting that the relevant semantic information is still available in the semantic system. Consistent performance (the same words always being misunderstood) may be evidence that the stored information is lost or unavailable.

Mr X's performance on the PALPA word-to-picture matching task also raises a further question. Why is his comprehension better when he sees a word written down than when he hears it? Overall, he made slightly more errors in the spoken word-to-picture matching version, some of which were not semantically related to the target. In Figure 8.1, the processing route from *heard word* to the semantic system is distinct from the route for *written word* input. It could be hypothesized that, in addition to the semantic impairment, other aspects of Mr X's auditory comprehension are disrupted. In order to understand a spoken word, you obviously need to be able to hear it, so any peripheral hearing loss needs to be taken into account. The incoming sensory information undergoes *auditory analysis* to identify the phonemes. This information is passed to the *auditory input lexicon*, a store of spoken word forms. Word recognition occurs when the incoming information is matched to the appropriate stored representation in this lexicon, a process which is known to be influenced by word frequency. Access to the semantic representation allows the word to be understood. Specific questions can therefore be asked about Mr X's spoken word comprehension. (For example, can he distinguish phonemes? Can he recognize spoken word forms?) Table 8.1 provides some suggestions about the types of tasks that could be presented in order to try to identify Mr X's auditory processing impairment(s). For more details about such investigations, see Franklin, 1989; Franklin, Turner and Ellis, 1992; and Kay, Lesser and Coltheart, 1992.

It will be remembered that the initial hypothesis was largely driven by the fact that Mr X was observed to produce semantic errors in speech. Assessment of his spoken and/or written output could help to confirm the conclusions drawn so far about his semantic processing, and also investigate any further impairments in output processes. Given his difficulties with writing, it would seem sensible to focus, at least initially, on his spoken output. A suitable assessment would be a spoken *picture naming* task. To successfully name a picture, the processes involved in object recognition (see Figure 8.1) need to be intact. The semantic representation is then accessed, this information being used to access the phonological form stored in the speech *output lexicon*. The appropriate phonemes are activated (*phoneme level*) and, after further processing, the speech sounds are articulated.

Table 8.1 Assessing the processing involved in spoken word comprehension

Stage of processing	Examples of assessments	Variables influencing processing
Auditory Analysis	Minimal Pairs; Same/Different Judgements e.g., /kan kan/ /tan kan/	Number of Distinctive Features different
Auditory Input Lexicon	Lexical Decision e.g., /hand/ /sk3g/ /hind/ /sk3g/	Word-frequency
Semantic System	Word-to-picture matching (semantic distractors) Synonym Judgements	Semantic similarity Imageability

Although Mr X does not appear to have any agnostic (visual object recognition) difficulties, the model would predict that he will have problems with picture naming because of his hypothesised semantic impairment. In order to establish whether any of the other processes involved in spoken word production are impaired, two sources of evidence will be useful: the types of paraphasic errors produced and the effects of cueing. When a picture naming task is presented, Mr X's responses are either the appropriate words, semantically-related words or 'no responses'. This suggests that when he produces a response, he either accesses the correct phonological output representation or that of a semantically-related word. This would be consistent with the hypothesized semantic impairment, insufficient or incorrect semantic information being sent to the speech output lexicon. As we noted earlier, when Mr X makes a semantic error he usually thinks that he has produced the correct word. One explanation for this lack of self-monitoring could be the fact that Mr X's comprehension of semantically similar words is poor.

When Mr X failed to name the picture, he was given a phonemic cue (the first phoneme of the target word). This occasionally helped him to produce the word. It would appear that when inadequate semantic information is sent to the speech output lexicon, the phonemic cue sometimes provides sufficient additional information to allow the appropriate phonological output form to be accessed (see Howard and Orchard-Lisle (1984) for discussion of the effects of phonemic cueing).

All of the evidence obtained so far suggests that, with the exception of semantic processing, the processes involved in spoken word production are functioning adequately. To confirm this hypothesis, converging evidence could be sought from tasks such as reading or repetition which also require a spoken response. The model in Figure 8.1 suggests three different processing routes can be used for reading aloud (see Barry (1989) for details). After the letters have been identified by the visual analysis system, the *sub-lexical* reading route relies on a sounding-out strategy (grapheme-phoneme conversion) to build up a plausible pronunciation for the letter string. This route allows novel letter strings (unfamiliar words, or non-words such as SHIG) to be read aloud. Regularly spelt words (like CAT) will also be pronounced correctly, but irregular words will produce errors (for example, YACHT being read as /jatʃt/). Assessment of Mr X's reading aloud demonstrates that he is quite good at reading non-words, indicating that his sub-lexical reading route is functional. However, because he is able to read both regular and irregular words accurately he is obviously not relying on this reading route when reading words.

In order to read irregular words aloud, the letter string has to be recognized by the visual input lexicon, and the pronunciation of the word 'looked up' in the speech output lexicon. This can occur either via the semantic system (the *semantic* reading route) or directly (the direct *lexical* route). As both spoken picture naming and the semantic reading route rely on semantic information accessing the phonological output form, if Mr X is using the semantic reading route, he should also make semantic errors in reading. This is not the case. His word reading is accurate and much better than his picture naming, indicating that he must be using the direct lexical route to successfully access the stored phonological representations. This evidence would support the hypothesis that there are no additional processing impairments disrupting his spoken output.

From this hypothetical example it should be apparent that the theoretical framework is being used to guide both the assessment and the interpretation of the findings. Many aspects of Mr X's language processing were suggested to be functioning adequately, but the same approach is equally applicable to aphasic people with diverse processing impairments. By thinking logically about what the language processing problems might be, the therapist can ask specific questions about what the person is able to do and what they have difficulty with. From thinking about the processing that would be required to carry out a particular task (naming pictures, reading non-words, etc.) suitable assessments can be selected or devised to investigate the aspect of processing that is being questioned. As one processing module may be involved in a number of different tasks, converging evidence about its functioning can be obtained by investigating performance on a number of different tasks.

Successful performance indicates that the processing necessary for the task is functioning adequately. The interpretation of the findings becomes more complicated when errors are produced or the person is unable to attempt the task; the therapist then has to work out why the difficulties arise. Any language assessment will also involve cognitive processes such as memory and attention which are not as yet incorporated into cognitive neuropsychological theories of language processing. For example, in order to perform Same/Different minimal pair judgements (see Table 8.1), in addition to discriminating between the different phonemes, the two forms have to be retained in short-term memory and then compared. Poor performance on this task would therefore not necessarily indicate a problem with auditory analysis *per se*. Language processing models therefore have their limitations. While they are useful guides, to interpret the assessment findings the therapist is also required to think logically about aspects of processing outside the bounds of the theory.

A further limitation of cognitive neuropsychological models is that they are underspecified. First, the functions of the processing modules are not fully understood (for example: How is the semantic system organized? How is this information accessed?) Second, the models fail to reflect the complex interrelationships that must surely exist between the different aspects of processing (a limitation addressed by the highly interactive connectionist computer models of processing). Some attempt to represent this is seen in the two-way arrows between certain processing modules (see Figure 8.1). For example, the arrow between the auditory input lexicon and the semantic system indicates that in addition to receiving information from the auditory input lexicon, the semantic system can send information to the auditory input lexicon and so influence the functioning of this module.

So far, all of our discussion has focused on single-word processing models. Psycholinguistic models of sentence processing have been shown to provide useful frameworks for the investigation of aphasic language impairments (for example, see Schwartz (1987) for details of a model of sentence production). For the processing of larger units of language (text, discourse, etc.), the cognitive neuropsychological literature currently has little to offer. However, Byng, Kay, Edmundson and Scott (1990) suggest that the principles of the approach can also be applied when investigating aspects of language processing above the single word. By thinking logically about any task, it can be broken down into a sequence of stages (processes), each of which can then be investigated.

As our discussion has been restricted to language processing, it is perhaps worth mentioning at this point that the relationship between language processing abilities and communicative effectiveness is not well understood. For example, one aphasic person with severely impaired language processing abilities may have very limited communication while another may be an effective communicator. When using the results of cognitive neuropsychologically based assessments to help to specify treatment aims, the therapist must therefore consider both the hypotheses about the language processing skills and impairments and the person's communication abilities (See Chapter 4 and 5 this volume). We will return to this issue again later in the chapter.

Treating the Language Processing Impairment

In the previous section, we suggested that cognitive neuropsychology provides a logical framework to guide the investigation of acquired language disorders. How can the information obtained aid the therapist to develop effective language remediation programmes?

The cognitive neuropsychological approach assumes that language remediation will be most effective when it is directed at a specific language processing problem. When adopting this approach, it can be tempting to keep on assessing the language abilities in more and more detail. How much assessment is it necessary to carry out before decisions can be made about therapy? Howard and Hatfield (1987) suggest that the hypothesis about the language processing impairment(s) need only be sufficiently detailed to motivate therapy. Once therapy is initiated, the treatment effectively becomes the assessment tool. The person's response to the therapy programme can confirm the hypothesis about the impairment or indicate that this needs to be revised. As we noted earlier, it is therefore somewhat misleading to discuss assessment and treatment as distinct aspects of the therapeutic process.

How can information about the language impairment be used to motivate therapy? The relationships between language impairments and successful remediation procedures are still only understood at a very simplistic level. Hypotheses about the integrity of a person's language processing system do not, in themselves, identify the focus for therapy (if only they did!). Nor do they specify how the treatment should be carried out (Howard and Hatfield, 1987; Caramazza and Hillis, 1993). What they can do, however, is provide information which helps the therapist to make these decisions. A programme of therapy aiming to target a specific aspect of the aphasic person's language processing abilities can then be developed.

It is currently assumed that information about the intact and impaired language processing skills will indicate which therapy approach is likely to be most appropriate. The treatment approaches that have been evaluated in single-case therapy studies fall into three categories: *Facilitation, Reorganization* and *Relearning* (Howard and Hatfield, 1987). Facilitation is defined as a treatment procedure that aims to enable or improve access to intact information when the locus of the processing deficit lies in an access procedure. Reorganization involves processing being re-routed through intact components to bypass the processing deficit. The new processing route is different from the one that would normally be used, but the end result is the same. Relearning incorporates either the learning of lost items or information, or re-establishing lost rules or procedures. It is perhaps worth pointing out that, while aphasiologists have been using all of these different therapy approaches for many years, the terminology is still not used consistently in the literature. This can be the source of some confusion (See also Carlomagno, and Iavarone, Chapter 12, who discuss reorganization and reestablishment in the treatment of writing.)

Each of these three approaches will be illustrated with examples drawn from single-case therapy studies. In each case, the treatment procedure was shown to be an effective way to remediate the hypothesized language processing impairment. Issues relating to the evaluation of the therapy will be discussed in the next section.

Facilitation

Scott (1987) reports a therapy study carried out with a dysphasic man called AB. From the assessment results, Scott hypothesized that AB's ability to access stored semantic representations was impaired. AB was poor at comprehending both spoken and written words. In word-to-picture matching tasks he often selected semantically related distractors (such as choosing a picture of a FORK for the target word SPOON). When the assessments were repeated, his performance was found to be inconsistent. AB responded correctly to items that he had previously made errors to, and vice-versa. AB's performance suggests that he was able to access general semantic information (such as the semantic category). Access to the item-specific information necessary to distinguish between semantically related items was less reliable. This pattern would be predicted by Warrington's theory (1975), which states that general semantic information is accessed before specific information.

Scott devised a programme of therapy which aimed to facilitate AB's ability to access the stored word meanings. AB attended three therapy sessions a week for a period of three months. The therapy tasks were all standardly used comprehension tasks involving pictures and/or spoken words (such as picture categorization, word categorization, word-to-picture matching). However, in order to try to enable AB to access very precise knowledge about words and pictures, the tasks were carefully graded. Initially, each task simply required AB to access general semantic knowledge (for example, classifying a set of words into Animals and Non-animals). Scott monitored AB's progress and modified the tasks as necessary to allow him to produce a successful response. As the therapy progressed, the tasks required access to increasingly specific semantic information about the words and pictures (for example, classifying animals in terms of their main habitat: Land, Sea or Air).

When AB was reassessed the therapy was shown to have produced a number of effects. As well as improving AB's comprehension of pictures and spoken words, significant changes were also found in his ability to comprehend written words. This modality had not been treated in the therapy. Although the therapy had focused on AB's comprehension of words and pictures, his ability to produce spoken output (picture naming) had also significantly improved.

An example of a different facilitation technique is to be found in a series of single-case studies reported by Marshall, et al., 1990. To illustrate the treatment procedure, we shall just discuss one man, RS. Like all of the subjects in the study, RS was poor at naming pictures. In order to try to identify the deficit underlying this problem, his ability to comprehend single words was investigated. Assessment revealed that he had no difficulty understanding the meanings of pictures and high imageability words, indicating that the semantic processing of high imageability items was relatively intact. Phonemic cues were found to assist his picture naming, suggesting that his difficulty was in using the intact semantic information to access the speech output lexicon.

Converging evidence to support this hypothesis was obtained from reading aloud. RS was very good at reading single words aloud. The fact that he could read irregular words accurately suggests that RS was looking up the pronunciation of the word in the speech output lexicon, rather than trying to sound it out sublexically. When reading aloud, he was able to access the speech output lexicon directly from the visual input lexicon (the *direct lexical* reading route). The phonological output representations therefore appeared to be intact, RS having difficulty accessing this information from the semantic system.

The therapy aimed to reinforce the links between the semantic representations and the phonological output representations, and so hopefully improve access to the speech output lexicon from semantics. A task was devised in which RS was presented with one picture and five written words. One of the words was the name of the picture, the others were all semantically related to the picture. RS had to read all of the words aloud (activating their phonological output representations) and then select the correct name for the picture (accessing the semantic representations of the picture and the words). After six hours of treatment over a period of two weeks, RS's ability to name the treated pictures was found to have significantly improved.

Reorganization

Bruce and Howard (1987) also describe a treatment procedure that aimed to overcome problems with spoken word-finding. As the five subjects in this study were all aided by phonemic cues, it could be hypothesized that they all had difficulties with accessing the phonological output representations of words. Rather than trying to directly facilitate access, Bruce and Howard attempted to reorganize the language processing and so bypass the deficit.

The treatment procedure was based on phonemic cueing. Phonemic cues produce an immediate effect, often helping the person to find the spoken word on that particular occasion. Unfortunately, no long-term benefits of phonemic cues are evident (Patterson, Purell and Morton, 1983). However, if someone is able to generate his or her own phonemic cues, a self-cueing strategy can help them to spontaneously access the phonological form. This would logically seem to require a number of processing skills. In addition to being aided by phonemic cues, the person needs to be able to access information about the first letter of the word he or she is unsuccessfully trying to say. The person also requires knowledge about grapheme–phoneme conversion to enable him or her to convert the letter into a phoneme, and so produce the equivalent of a phonemic cue.

For this study (1987), Bruce and Howard identified aphasic people who were often able to indicate the first letter of the spoken word that they were trying to find, but were unable to then sound it out. The study investigated their ability to learn to use a computer aid to carry out the grapheme–phoneme conversion stage, and so cue themselves. Each subject received five treatment sessions in which he or she was trained to select the first letter of the target word on the computer keyboard, listen to the computer-generated phonemic cue, and then attempt to produce the spoken word. All learned to use the computer aid. The results showed that four subjects were significantly better at naming pictures when they were using the computer aid than when they were just given extra time to try to find the word spontaneously. One subject showed a dramatic improvement in spoken word-finding during the course of the treatment. Post-treatment, he was able to successfully self-cue himself on many of the items by saying the initial phoneme of the target word aloud without using the aid.

Relearning

De Partz (1986) discusses a treatment procedure carried out with SP, a dysphasic native French speaker who was very poor at reading. When reading aloud he made semantic errors and was unable to use the sub-lexical sounding out strategy to build up pronunciations of words. De Partz hypothesized that SP's reading errors were arising because he was relying on the semantic reading route (deep dyslexic reading). In order to improve his reading skills, she developed a therapy programme that aimed to re-establish SP's sub-lexical reading route.

De Partz observed that when SP saw a written letter he often said aloud a word that began with that letter. He was therefore taught to associate a written letter with a relay word that he could say aloud. For example, SP selected the French word *allo* for the letter A. Having established a relay word for each letter of the alphabet, SP was taught to lengthen the first phoneme of the word as he said it, and segment off this sound. SP worked through a series of stages in which he learnt to produce just the appropriate phoneme for each letter, and eventually to blend phonemes together and so read aloud letter strings.

After nine months of intensive therapy, re-assessment showed that SP was significantly better at reading. The few reading errors he produced were nearly all regularizations (for example, the French word CESSE read as /kɛs/ instead of /sɛs/), confirming that he was using grapheme–phoneme conversion when reading. Such errors were successfully remediated in a subsequent therapy programme in which he was specifically retaught rules about French orthography (for example, how the pronunciation of a consonant changes when it occurs in the context of different vowels).

From this example of relearning it can be seen that the different therapy approaches are not mutually exclusive. To enable SP to relearn and re-establish the lost information about grapheme–phoneme correspondences, a reorganizational strategy was used. In order to pronounce single letters, SP was taught to use his knowledge about whole word pronunciations. Only later in the therapy was he directly retaught some of the more complex conversion rules that he had lost.

Evaluating the Effects of the Treatment

It should be apparent from the examples discussed above that cognitive neuropsychology has not revolutionized the treatment methods used to remediate aphasic language. Such treatment techniques have been used for many years and, from clinical experience, aphasia therapists know that they can be very successful. However, for theoretical and practical reasons, we are faced with the challenge of objectively demonstrating the effectiveness of aphasia therapy.

The evaluation of therapy is a central feature of the cognitive neuropsychological approach (Howard and Hatfield, 1987). As we have described, assessment leads to the development of hypotheses about the individual's specific language processing impairment(s). This, in turn, allows the aims of the therapy and the treatment techniques to be clearly specified. If appropriate measures of performance have been obtained pre-therapy, re-assessment post-therapy can determine the effectiveness of the treatment procedure. In addition to describing the therapy effects, a theoretical account of how these changes in language processing were achieved can be attempted.

While changes in language processing may result from a specific treatment programme, they can also occur for a variety of other reasons. They may, for example, arise as a result of spontaneous recovery of function, or from general aspects of the therapeutic process such as the supportive relationship that has developed between the aphasic person and the therapist. To evaluate the effects of a treatment programme, studies must therefore be designed to control for such factors. Some of the features of single-case therapy studies will be briefly outlined. For further discussion of these issues, see Coltheart (1983); Howard and Hatfield, (1987); and Willmes, Chapter 15, this volume.

The language processing skills of acquired aphasics are known to show spontaneous improvements, particularly in the first few months following the CVA. Considerable spontaneous recovery may occur but the length of time that it continues and the factors that influence it are still not fully understood (Basso, 1992). To control for spontaneous recovery, subjects selected to participate in single-case therapy studies are generally at least six months post-CVA. In addition, pre-therapy baselines (repeated assessment on the same measure across a period of time) can be taken. The treatment phase of a study often takes place over a number of months, but for practical reasons, the pre-therapy baselines may be obtained across a relatively short period of time. In such cases, the pre-therapy baselines would indicate whether or not the person's level of performance fluctuated significantly across sessions (important information in itself) but would not adequately control for the effects of spontaneous recovery. Further evidence allowing spontaneous recovery to be conclusively ruled out could be obtained by examining the nature of the changes observed post-therapy.

Cognitive neuropsychology allows clear predictions to be made about the therapy effects. From consideration of the hypothesized processing impairment(s) and skills and the therapy aims, it is possible to identify tasks on which performance should improve as a result of the therapy, and those on which changes should not occur (unrelated control measures). Where the changes are found to be confined to predicted improvements this would seem to be clear evidence favouring the hypothesis that the change was attributable to the therapy programme. Spontaneous recovery and/or improvements occurring as a result of the general therapeutic process would be difficult to reconcile with such results. An example might be useful to illustrate this point. As we discussed in the previous section, Scott (1987) devised a therapy programme focusing on the comprehension of spoken words and pictures, with the aim of improving AB's ability to access semantic information. It was therefore predicted that the therapy should improve AB's performance on assessments such as spoken word-to-picture matching. Because the semantic system is so central to language processing, it is quite difficult to think of tasks which would not be predicted to change as a result of improvement in semantic processing. As unrelated control measures, Scott selected automatic speech tasks (for example, reciting the alphabet) and a variety of other measures including written *lexical decision* (a task used to assess written word-recognition). Post-therapy, AB's performance had improved on spoken word-to-picture matching but not on the unrelated control measures, hence it was concluded that the changes had arisen as a result of the remediation.

An important factor to consider when evaluating the effectiveness of therapy is whether or not the effects generalize. Generalization can occur in a number of ways. If a particular set of items has been treated during the therapy, the observed improvements may be restricted to just the treated items (item-specific effects) or may generalize to untreated items. Scott (1987), for example, divided the words/pictures in the baseline assessments into two sets: one set was used in the different therapy tasks (the treated items), the other was not exposed during the therapy (untreated items). Depending on the specific aims of therapy, it may be possible to predict that the treatment effects could also generalize to other language skills. Scott aimed to improve semantic processing. While her treatment procedure involved only comprehension (input) tasks, as the semantic system is also involved in producing spoken output, the therapy might logically be predicted to generalize to tasks such as spoken picture naming. Pre-therapy baselines were therefore obtained both on comprehension tasks and on a picture naming task. Post-therapy, AB's ability to name pictures of treated items had significantly improved, indicating that the therapy effects had generalized from input tasks involving semantics to an output task. There was also some evidence of generalization to naming *untreated* items. Although he was still poor at producing the correct name for untreated items, the pattern of errors changed. Pre-therapy, he generally produced either an unrecognizable response or no response. Post-therapy, many of the naming responses were semantically related words.

From this brief discussion it should be apparent that in order to objectively evaluate therapy, appropriate measures of performance need to have been obtained pre-therapy. Unfortunately, it is generally too late to decide to try to evaluate the therapy once it has been carried out. By thinking logically about the hypothesized language problem, the aim of the therapy and the treatment procedure, questions can be asked of the therapy. For example, Will auditory comprehension improve? Will the effects be restricted just to the treated items? Will working on comprehension generalize to spoken output/naming? Only by thinking through the evaluation in advance is it possible to ensure that the necessary information will have been obtained about the person's pre-therapy language abilities.

When this approach is compared to the type of study that has traditionally been used to investigate the effectiveness of aphasia therapy, cognitive neuropsychologically based single-case studies can be seen to have a number of advantages. In the group efficacy studies, the subjects within the group have generally had diverse language impairments and very little information is provided about the therapy they received. To identify changes in language skills, very general measures such as standardized aphasia batteries have commonly been used. It is perhaps not surprising that these studies have produced equivocal results (Howard, 1986).

A limitation of single-case therapy studies is that their findings only indicate that the treatment procedure was effective for one individual. For this research to have relevance to theoretical advances in aphasia therapy and to clinical practice it has to be assumed that a treatment procedure will produce similar effects when carried out with other aphasics. It is therefore essential to replicate the therapy with other people with similar language processing impairments and so establish that the findings do indeed generalize (Coltheart, 1983). Replication helps to identify which processing skills have to be intact for the procedure to be effective, and clarifies which language processing impairments can be effectively remediated by the treatment procedure. As this approach is still in its infancy, it is only very recently that replications of single-case therapy studies have begun to be reported in the literature (see, for example, Le Dorze, Jacob and Coderre, 1991; Nickels, Byng and Black, 1991; Nickels, 1992).

Many of the other problems faced by single-case study research are common to all attempts to evaluate the effectiveness of aphasia therapy. For example, a statistically significant improvement on a particular assessment is generally taken as evidence that the treatment programme has been effective. When designing any therapy study it is therefore essential to ensure that the baseline measures contain sufficient items to allow changes to be statistically identified (see Willmes, Chapter 15). However, statistically significant improvements in performance are not necessarily clinically significant improvements. The fact that someone can name 75 per cent of pictures post-therapy compared to 25 per cent pre-therapy does not indicate that the treatment has significantly influenced his or her ability to communicate verbally. This issue is intimately related to the need to ensure that treatment effects generalize from the clinic to the real world (see Worrell, Chapter 4). In order to demonstrate that the therapy has resulted in functionally significant changes, methods attempting to measure such changes need to be developed. One such method may be Rating Scales, designed to evaluate whether or not the treatment has produced observable changes in communication (Peach, 1992; Audit: a manual for Speech and Language Therapists, 1993). As yet, few aphasia therapy studies (either single-case or group) have attempted to build such evaluation into their experimental designs.

We have described the features of the cognitive neuropsychological approach to aphasia therapy, emphasizing the interaction between assessment and treatment of the language impairment and the evaluation of the effectiveness of the therapy. The examples discussed were drawn from the many single-case therapy studies that have now been published. Such studies have provided objective evidence that a variety of acquired language impairments can be successfully remediated. These include disorders of semantic processing (Scott, 1987; Behrmann and Lieberthal, 1989); reading (De Partz, 1986; Byng and Coltheart, 1986; Scott and Byng, 1989); writing (Hatfield, 1983; Behrmann, 1987; De Partz, Seron and Van der Linden, 1992); and sentence processing (Byng and Coltheart, 1986; Jones, 1986; Byng 1988). For the remainder of the chapter we shall focus on further clinical implications of these research findings.

Cognitive Neuropsychology: Clinical Application

In many disciplines, theoretical research can appear to be rather remote from its real-life practical applications. The distinction between *research* and *practice* is not so apparent for clinically based research. Many of the studies we have referred to were carried out by aphasia therapists working within standard clinical settings. However, unlike many aphasic people, the subjects of the single-case studies are often quite a long time post-onset, highly motivated, physically well and not significantly handicapped by other neuropsychological impairments. The studies could therefore appear to suggest that cognitive neuropsychology is only applicable to certain very specific forms of clinical practice. In addition, because the studies aim to demonstrate the efficacy of language remediation the reports emphasize the subject's language disorder, particularly those aspects directly related to the remediation being discussed. This may give the erroneous impression that decisions about cognitive neuropsychologically-based remediation are driven purely by the hypothesized language processing impairments rather than by consideration of both the aphasic person's language and communication abilities. As often only one short period of treatment is reported it can also be difficult to see how this fits into the overall management programme.

While many of the aphasics in a clinical case load would not make ideal research subjects, that does not mean that cognitive neuropsychological principles will not be relevant to their rehabilitation. In Britain, the College of Speech and Language Therapists' quality assurance document (Communicating Quality, 1991) specifies that the therapist should aim to provide his or her aphasic clients with a service that meets their linguistic, psychological and interpersonal needs. The general aim of rehabilitation should be to enable the aphasic person to regain, as far as possible, 'communicative independence and self determination, and achieve a fulfilling life-style' (p. 146). Management should include the provision of advice and support for both the client and his or her carers. The therapist should be aware of the person's global needs (such as financial hardship, physical problems, etc.), liaising with and referring on to other professionals as appropriate. A variety of different therapy approaches should be offered including, where appropriate, direct language remediation aiming to reduce the language impairments. It is to this aspect of rehabilitation that cognitive neuropsychology can make a major contribution.

Aphasia is a diverse and complex disorder with implications that extend far beyond language processing. As the therapeutic relationship develops, the therapist's knowledge about the aphasia and the person with aphasia will increase. Many other factors will also change over time. Recovery of language skills will occur spontaneously, as a result of remediation, or a combination of the two. The aphasic person's insight into his or her language and communication problems may change, strategies may be developed to overcome specific difficulties in daily life, changes will occur in the aphasic person's or the family's adjustment to the effects of the stroke, and additional factors may be introduced (the partner, for example, suddenly being made redundant). Rehabilitation must be a dynamic process, the therapist and the aphasic person constantly reviewing and revising the short and long-term aims in the light of the changing situation. The way in which the aims are translated into a practical programme of rehabilitation will be influenced by variables such as the clinical setting and the therapist's own skills and experience.

Although many factors will influence the clinical decisions, it is assumed that it is of paramount importance that the therapist has an understanding of the aphasic person's language processing skills and impairments. A language processing framework can be used to interpret information about every aphasic individual's language, the ther-apist maintaining a balance between the need to specify precisely the person's language processing abilities and the need to provide appropriate and effective overall management. As we attempted to demonstrate earlier, the therapist's observations can guide the initial investigations. Interpretation of the findings allow preliminary hypotheses to be developed about the integrity of the language processing system. Many factors will determine the extensiveness of further investigations and hence the amount of detail in which the hypotheses can be specified. These will include the reason for the referral, the person's physical health/cognitive status, etc., and the findings obtained from the initial assessment. If, however, the decision is taken to directly remediate a particular language difficulty, the therapist must ensure that the pre-therapy assessment provides adequate information to allow the therapy to be objectively evaluated.

When all relevant factors have been considered, it will be concluded for many (but by no means all) aphasic people that direct language remediation should be an aim at that particular stage in their rehabilitation. The therapist then has to think logically about the hypothesized processing impairments and the therapy aims and use his or her own ingenuity to devise and evaluate a treatment programme aiming to reinstate impaired language skills using facilitation, reorganization or relearning techniques. The longitudinal case study of PC (Jones 1989) clearly demonstrates how cognitive neuropsychologically-based assessment and treatment can be successfully integrated into the total management of an aphasic individual.

At the time of his stroke, PC was 51 years old and employed as a machine operator. He lived with his wife and two grown-up children. His family were already adjusting to a major change in family roles because his wife, who had previously devoted her time to running the family home, had recently set up a thriving business. For many reasons, the family situation was not easy after PC's stroke. He resented having to remain at home while the rest of the family went out to work each day, his feeling of isolation being exacerbated by his wife's business success. All of the family, but in particular his daughter, found it difficult to come to terms with PC's stroke.

The study describes Jones' involvement with PC and his family throughout the first year post-onset. During this time PC attended individual therapy sessions as an outpatient. Their first contact was two weeks after his stroke. He presented with fluent, empty speech interspersed with jargon (strings of real words and neologisms). Initial observations and informal assessments revealed that his comprehension of written language was superior to his auditory comprehension. However, while he sometimes required repetitions, his auditory comprehension generally appeared adequate in a conversational setting. He had no spontaneous written output. Cognitive neuropsychologically-based investigations of PC's auditory comprehension revealed some difficulty with phoneme recognition (Auditory Analysis System). His semantic processing was found to be adequate for the comprehension of single words and pictures, but he had difficulties using this information to access the phonological output forms of words. In naming tasks, all responses were neologisms.

As PC's auditory comprehension was functionally adequate, this was not felt to be a priority for direct remediation. His family were advised to use simple written language to supplement their spoken language when they wished to convey specific information (a communication strategy which became superfluous as his comprehension improved). The expressive language difficulties were PC's major concern and a source of severe frustration. For example, PC felt that the family in general avoided communicating with him. He said that his wife generally finished his sentences for him, often not as he had intended. In contrast to his considerable verbal output difficulties, PC demonstrated a sophisticated level of gesture.

We have selected PC's expressive language problems to illustrate how, in reality, language processing deficits, functional communication skills, and the psychosocial situation are all highly inter-related and can not be considered in isolation. Jones adopted a three-pronged attack to these problems. First PC was encouraged to capitalize on his gestural abilities and make use of gesture to communicate with family and friends. Second, to address the many psychosocial issues that were becoming apparent, Jones established and maintained contact with PC's family via the telephone and home visits. Much of the therapy session time was spent counselling PC, and a number of home visits were carried out to enable the whole family to discuss the situation. Third, a remediation programme aiming to facilitate PC's ability to use semantic information to access the phonological word forms was developed. After ten weeks of therapy, reassessment showed that his performance on a picture naming task had improved. Although only half of the words had been specifically treated, he no longer produced any neologisms. All of his responses were either correct or phonologically related to the target. The fact that no improvements were found to have occurred on other language tasks, such as repetition and non-word reading, demonstrated that the changes could not simply be attributed to spontaneous recovery. PC's wife also noted improvements in his spontaneous output, reporting that his conversation was much less empty of content.

The case study also demonstrates how the therapy aims changed over time. As PC was now producing considerably more output, much of which bore a phonological resemblance to the target, it was decided to specifically target his auditory comprehension problems. Jones hypothesized that improved phoneme identification would enhance both his auditory comprehension and repetition abilities, and possibly ultimately allow him to monitor and self-correct his phonological speech errors. Reassessment after six weeks of therapy again demonstrated specific therapy effects. PC was by then six months post stroke and his spontaneous speech showed continued improvements. Over the next four months, therapy targeted both spoken and written output. The final therapy phase described in the study concentrated on encouraging PC to use appropriate strategies when faced with word-finding problems in spontaneous speech. Although we have specifically described how the focus of the language remediation changed over time, all aspects of the situation and the remediation were constantly reviewed and revised.

To summarize the situation one year post-stroke, considerable improvements had occurred in PC's expressive language. He still had some spoken word-finding difficulties but was described as being able to communicate 'very well indeed'. He was able to play an active part in his wife's business and gave a speech at his daughter's wedding. Strategies had been developed to enable PC to deal with day-to-day problems such as coping with money when he went shopping, and many of the psychosocial problems were resolving. For example, although Jones felt she should have handled better the daughter's grief at the 'loss' of her father, the father–daughter relationship greatly improved as PC became better able to communicate. PC and his wife also found considerable support from a social group which arranged monthly activities (theatre trips, etc.) for a group of aphasic people and their families.

While therapy will often aim to directly remediate language processing impairments, the use of a cognitive neuropsychological framework to guide and interpret assessment does not preclude the therapist from employing pragmatically based treatment approaches such as compensatory strategies and non-verbal communication systems. This is demonstrated clearly in Jones' study. PC was encouraged to use gestures, and later, a variety of communication strategies to help him to overcome his word-finding difficulties. A further example illustrating how the cognitive neuropsychological and pragmatic approaches can be combined in clinical practice can be found in our single case study detailing TW's therapy (Edmundson and McIntosh, 1991).

TW had a stroke when she was 70 years old. She was a very sociable woman with supportive family and friends. Six months post-onset, TW had good comprehension of spoken language. Spoken output was fluent, but she frequently faced word-finding problems. She occasionally produced phonemic errors but usually was simply unable to attempt to say the word. Reading and writing were also impaired. TW had considerable insight into her aphasia and was very frustrated by her difficulties. At her request, the reading and writing problems were investigated. A cognitive neuropsychological framework was used to guide the assessment, and treatment programmes were developed to directly target aspects of her reading, and later her writing, difficulties. Evaluation indicated that the treatments had reinstated her ability to read and to spell treated words. Functional improvements also occurred.

In addition to the individual therapy, TW was attending weekly group therapy sessions. Careful observation of TW's word finding difficulties during these sessions led to the hypothesis that, like PC, TW had adequate semantic knowledge about words (she could both understand and give semantic information about a word that she was unable to produce) but had difficulty accessing the speech output lexicon (phonemic cues aided her spoken word production). In structured group tasks she was able to use a number of compensatory strategies to convey information (gesturing, pointing, providing a description or an alternative word) but rarely used such strategies spontaneously. It was also noted that while others perceived her to be a good communicator, TW was very critical about her expressive language abilities and dismissed any response other than the intended target word. The word-finding problems were often intrusive, and TW abandoned the topic of conversation to describe and discuss her anomia.

From the preliminary hypotheses about TW's word-finding difficulties, it was apparent that language remediation should focus on access to the phonological output representations. However, when the other factors were also considered, it was felt that such therapy would have further reinforced her need to always find the correct word. As a number of compensatory strategies were potentially available to her, it was decided that, at that particular time, it would be more appropriate to aim to enhance her ability to successfully communicate information. Pre-therapy assessment (Synonym Judgement Task (from Kay, Lesser and Coltheart, 1992) and baselines on the Boston Naming Test (Kaplan, Goodglass and Weintraub, 1983) confirmed the initial hypotheses about TW's processing impairments. Given the therapy aim, pre and post-therapy measures would ideally have captured TW's ability to spontaneously use strategies in natural communicating situations. In reality, a somewhat simplistic attempt was made to try to monitor her communicative effectiveness. In addition to scoring the Boston Naming Test in the standard way, TW's response to each item was transcribed in full, allowing us to investigate her attempts to communicate information agout pictures that she was unable to name. It was hypothesized that while the therapy would not increase the number of pictures named on the Boston Naming Test, the quality of her responses might change. In addition to the picture naming test, a spoken language sample (retelling the Cinderella story) was also obtained.

The therapy was carried out in the group setting, the aim being to teach and encourage TW to use compensatory strategies in word-finding situations. Whenever a group activity involved spoken word-finding, suggestions were made to TW about the strategies she could use if she found she was unable to retrieve the target word. Emphasis was placed on successful communication of the message, the group setting providing opportunities for feedback and self-monitoring. After ten weekly therapy sessions, reassessment on the Boston Naming Test revealed that there was a significant increase in the number of items she attempted to communicate information about when she was unable to name them. There was also a significant improvement in the communicative effectiveness of her responses (as rated by a group of speech and language therapists). TW's use of compensatory communication strategies was further consolidated during the next ten weeks of group therapy. At the end of this period her ability to retell the Cinderella story was reassessed. Her performance had improved on a number of parameters including content, inclusion of detail, and completion of ideas. These subjective judgements were felt to lend support to the fact that TW was learning to use compensatory strategies to circumvent her word finding difficulties.

Conclusions

The aim of this chapter was to describe the cognitive neuropsychological approach to aphasia therapy and illustrate its clinical application. While cognitive neuropsychology does not provide all the answers, we would argue that the framework it offers for the investigation and remediation of acquired language disorders is applicable to all people with aphasia. In the clinical setting, language remediation is rarely (if ever) divorced from management of the person's communication needs and psychosocial adjustment. Case studies demonstrate the flexibility of this logical, hypothesis-driven approach. The therapist's challenge is to tailor the assessment, treatment and evaluation to the individual, integrating the investigation and remediation of the language disorder into the total management of the person with aphasia.

Notes

1. It should be noted that this model is not the definitive account of single-word processing; other models make slightly different claims about the organization and functioning of the language processing system. However, while the specific details of the models may vary, they all share the same basic characteristics.
2. Others suggest that there are multiple semantic systems. For example, Warrington (1975) states that word meanings are stored in a verbal semantic system, with information about objects and pictures being stored in a visual semantic system.
3. It should be noted that access and storage deficits are the subject of considerable theoretical debate. See, for example, Rapp and Caramazza (1993) for further discussion of this issue.

References

Audit: a Manual for Speech and Language Therapists. (1993) London: College of Speech and Language Therapists.

Barry C (1989) Acquired disorders of reading and spelling: a cognitive neuropsychological perspective. In Code C (Ed) The Characteristics of Aphasia. London: Taylor and Francis.

Basso A (1992) Prognostic factors in aphasia. Aphasiology 6: 337–48.

Behrmann M (1987) The rites of righting writing: homophone remediation in acquired dysgraphia. Cognitive Neuropsychology, 4, 365–84.

Behrmann M, Lieberthal T (1989) Category-specific treatment of a lexical-semantic deficit: a single case study of global aphasia. British Journal of Disorders of Communication 24: 281–99.

Bruce C, Howard D (1987) Computer-generated phonemic cues: an effective aid for naming in aphasia. British Journal of Disorders of Communication 22: 191–201.

Byng S (1988) Sentence processing deficits: theory and therapy. Cognitive Neuropsychology 5: 629–76.

Byng S, Coltheart M (1986) Aphasia therapy research: methodological requirements and illustrative results. In Hjelmquist E, Nilsson LB (Eds) Communication and Handicap. Amsterdam: North-Holland, Elsevier

Byng S, Kay J, Edmundson A, Scott C (1990) Aphasia tests reconsidered. Aphasiology 4: 67–91.

Caramazza A, Hillis A (1993) For a theory of remediation of cognitive deficits. Neuropsychological Rehabilitation 3: 217–34.

Coltheart M (1983) Aphasia therapy research: a single-case study approach. In Code C Muller DJ (Eds) Aphasia Therapy. London: Edward Arnold

Coltheart M (1984) Editorial. Cognitive Neuropsychology 1, 1–8.

Communicating Quality: Professional standards for Speech and Language Therapists. (1991) London: College of Speech and Language Therapists.

De Partz MP (1986) Re-education of a deep dyslexic patient: rationale of the method and results. Cognitive Neuropsychology 3: 149–77.

De Partz MP, Seron X, Van der Linden M (1992) Re-education of a surface dysgraphic with a visual imagery strategy. Cognitive Neuropsychology 9: 369–401.

Edmundson A, McIntosh J (1991) Emerging intervention: a longitudinal case study of a dysphasic client. In: Proceedings of the British Aphasiology Society Symposium 'Therapeutic Approaches in Aphasia'. Newcastle-upon-Tyne.

Ellis AW, Young AW (1988) Human Cognitive Neuropsychology. London: Lawrence Erlbaum.

Franklin S (1989) Dissociations in auditory word comprehension: evidence from nine fluent aphasic patients. Aphasiology 3: 189–207.

Franklin S, Turner JE, Ellis AW (1992) ADA Comprehension Battery. London: Action for Dysphasic Adults.

Goodglass H, Kaplan E (1983) Assessment of Aphasia and Related Disorders. 2nd edn. Philadelphia PA: Lea and Febiger.

Hatfield FM (1983) Aspects of acquired dysgraphia and implications for re-education. In Code C, Muller DJ (Eds) Aphasia Therapy. London: Edward Arnold.

Howard D (1986) Beyond randomised controlled trials: the case for effective case studies of the effects of treatment in aphasia. British Journal of Disorders of Communication 21: 89–102.

Howard D, Hatfield FM (1987) Aphasia Therapy: Historical and Contemporary Issues. London: Lawrence Erlbaum.

Howard D, Orchard-Lisle V (1984) On the origin of semantic errors in naming: evidence from the case of a global aphasic. Cognitive Neuropsychology 1: 163–90.

Jones EV (1986) Building the foundations for sentence production in a non-fluent aphasic. British Journal of Disorders of Communication 21: 63–82.

Jones EV (1989) A year in the life of PC and EVJ In: Proceedings of the British Aphasiology Society Conference 'Advances in Aphasia Therapy in the Clinical Setting'. Cambridge.

Jones EV, Byng S (11989) The practice of aphasia therapy: an opinion. College of Speech Therapists Bulletin 449: 2–4.

Kaplan E, Goodglass H, Weintraub S (1983) Boston Naming Test. Philadelphia PA: Lea and Febiger.

Kay J, Lesser R, Coltheart M (1992) Psycholinguistic Assessments of Language Processing in Aphasia (PALPA). Hove: Lawrence Erlbaum.

Le Dorze G, Jacob A, Coderre L (1991) Aphasia rehabilitation with a case of agrammatism: a partial replication. Aphasiology, 5, 63–85.

Marshall J, Pound C, White-Thomson M, Pring T (1990) The use of picture/word matching tasks to assist word retrieval in aphasic patients. Aphasiology 4: 167–184.

Nickels L (1992) The auto-cue? Self-generated phonemic cues in the treatment of a disorder of reading and naming. Cognitive Neuropsychology 9: 155–82.

Nickels L, Byng S, Black M (1991) Sentence processing deficits: a replication of therapy. British Journal of Disorders of Communication 26: 175–99.

Patterson KE, Purell C, Morton J (1983) Facilitation of word retrieval in aphasia. In Code C, Muller DJ (Eds) Aphasia Therapy. London: Edward Arnold.

Patterson KE, Seidenberg MS, McClelland JL (1989) Connections and disconnections: acquired dyslexia in a computational model of reading processes. In Morris RGM (Ed) Parallel distributed processing: implications for psychology and neurobiology. Oxford: Clarendon Press.

Peach RK (1992) Efficacy of aphasia treatment: what are the real issues? Clinics in Communication Disorders 2: 7–10.

Plaut DC, Shallice T (1993) Deep dyslexia: a case study of connectionist neuropsychology. Cognitive Neuropsychology 10: 377–500.

Rapp BA, Caramazza A (1993) On the distinction between deficits of access and deficits of storage: a question of theory. Cognitive Neuropsychology 10: 113–41.

Schuell HE (1973) Differential Diagnosis of Aphasia with the Minnesota Test. 2nd edn. Minneapolis MN: University of Minnesota.

Schwartz MF (1987) Patterns of speech production deficit within and across aphasia syndromes: application of a psycholinguistic model. In Coltheart M, Sartori G, Job R (eds) The Cognitive Neuropsychology of Language. London: Lawrence Erlbaum.

Scott C (1987) Cognitive Neuropsychological Remediation of Acquired Language Disorders. MPhil Thesis, London: City University, (unpublished).

Scott C, Byng S (1989) Computer assisted remediation of a homophone comprehension disorder in surface dyslexia. Aphasiology 3: 301–20.

Shallice T (1987) Impairments of semantic processing: multiple dissociations. In Coltheart M, Sartori G, Job R (Eds) The Cognitive Neuropsychology of Language. London: Lawrence Erlbaum.

Warrington EK (1975) The selective impairment of semantic memory. Quarterly Journal of Experimental Psychology 27: 635–57.

Wise R, Chollet F, Hadar U, Friston K, Hoffner E, Frackowiak R (1991) Distribution of cortical neural networks involved in word comprehension and word retrieval. Brain 114: 1803–17.

Chapter 9
Making Psycholinguistic Assessments Accessible

RUTH LESSER

This chapter reviews the development of a resource for undertaking the psycholinguistically based assessment of aphasic patients, known as Psycholinguistic Assessments of Language Processing in Aphasia (PALPA) (Kay, Lesser and Coltheart, 1992). This is a relatively new approach to examining such patients, in that it comprises 60 sets of materials from which therapists can select in order to test hypotheses that they have formed from earlier observations of the patient. It is, therefore, very different from a standard battery which is to be used in its entirety. It also capitalizes on a new way of understanding patterns of behaviour through interpreting them as the symptoms of functioning and malfunctioning modules and linking processes. (The reader may find it helpful to read Edmundson and McIntosh, Chapter 8, in conjunction with this chapter.)

The approach used in PALPA is based on an assumption made in cognitive neuropsychology that the mind's language system is organized in modules which serve different functions, and that brain damage can impair these modules to some extent selectively. The exact specification of these modules and their operation and interactions are far from clear at the present stage of development of the theory, and PALPA is conservative in the framework which it has taken as a model. It distinguishes modality distinct inputs and outputs, and phonological, lexical, morphological and semantic domains. Its emphasis is on single-word processing, and, although one section is concerned with sentence comprehension, it does not extend to the domain of discourse. It therefore has obvious limitations of scope. It is neutral as to whether processing occurs in sequenced stages, in cascade form or interactively, but draws essentially on the relatively simple model of the functional architecture of language processing first illustrated by Patterson and Shewell (1987). A variant of this model is illustrated and discussed in Figure 8.1, Chapter 8.

Such models were first developed in respect to reading, particularly reading aloud, i.e. the mental processes involved in going from print to pronunciation. Following this, this type of processing analysis was extended to other language behaviours, such as repeating and understanding words, naming and writing to dictation. From their pedigree of experimental studies in cognitive psychology with normal subjects, the processing models and a prima-facie plausibility as a basis for analysing the patterns of retained and impaired abilities in aphasic patients, on the assumption that such patients had normal processing abilities with which brain damage had selectively interfered. Evidence from brain-damaged patients has now been incorporated into the model, changing its orientation from psycholinguistic to *cognitive neuropsychological*. With this development the potential relevance of this type of analysis to clinicians working with aphasic patients has become increasingly attractive.

For clinicians, however, there is a practical problem in drawing on such theories. The literature in which psycholinguistic studies appear is, in general, not accessible to aphasia therapists, who work under a pressure which generally does not allow them to browse through the psychology and linguistics sections of libraries.

Until recently, therefore, the principal analysis of aphasia available to clinicians has been the neuroanatomically based model which underlies the classification of the aphasias by the Boston Diagnostic Aphasia Examination (BDAE) (Goodglass and Kaplan, 1983). The practical relevance of neuroanatomical models of aphasia for aphasia therapists is at present unclear; only a limited proportion of patients can be unambiguously classified according to BDAE criteria, and the extent to which this can be reliably related to the neuroanatomy of an individual person is uncertain. Moreover neuroanatomical information may not be available to aphasia therapists, whose main sources of medical referrals of patients in General Hospitals are physicians and general practitioners rather than neurologists. When brain scans are available for an individual patient they are usually CT or MRI scans, which have inherent limitations in identifying the extent of the *functional* lesion in the brain. The implications for therapy from a neuroanatomically-based model such as that underlying the BDAE are, therefore, restricted; they depend on observations of language behaviour rather than neuroanatomical data. Consequently, a neurologically-based model of aphasia is somewhat limited in its appeal as an interpretive tool to the majority of aphasia therapists.

There seemed to be scope for applying the newly-developing psycholinguistic analyses to patients in aphasia clinics. The problem was essentially the relative inaccessibility to practising clinicians of, first, a comprehensible theoretical model and, second, materials through which to apply it. The first has been partly remedied by the publication of graphically specific lexical processing models by Patterson and Shewell (1987) and Ellis and Young (1988). The second has been the justification for the development of PALPA. The purpose of this chapter is to briefly summarize PALPA and to illustrate some of its clinical applications.

It must first be emphasized that PALPA is not intended to be an exhaustive set of materials, just as it is not one which it would be appropriate to use in its entirety with a single patient. It is a resource to which the assessor will wish to add further materials for pursuing hypotheses about the nature of an individual's disorder, or into which he or she will wish to dip selectively to test a hypothesis formed about the nature of the patient's assets and restrictions. Furthermore, as we have already acknowledged, it is inherently limited in that it considers only one aspect of the complex business of assessing aphasic disorders as a preliminary to making decisions about therapy and management. It deals only with language as a mental process, and not with language as a social construct or medium of communication. For these, different kinds of investigations are required, for example, measures of functional communication or conversational analysis

Content of PALPA

PALPA assessments fall into four groups, three of which are concerned with lexical processing (auditory, semantic, orthographic) and one with sentence comprehension. The materials are controlled for as many relevant variables as possible – frequency of words in the language, number of phonological distinctive features, imageability, regularity of spelling, length, reversibility. Where possible the same materials are used in several tasks to facilitate cross-modality comparisons. Each group of measures is illustrated in turn below.

Auditory Lexical Processing

One of the problems in examining aphasia is that no single task can be assumed to be testing only one process. Every task taps a chain of events; tasks aimed at examining input necessarily incorporate outputted responses, and vice versa. In examining auditory lexical processing, therefore, PALPA not only varies the type of input according to whether it involves the lexicon or not (the latter as in nonwords), or can be performed without semantics or not, but it also uses different types of responses as alternatives. Examples of these are choosing pictures, selecting written words or spoken repetition. The interpretation of the test results therefore generally depends on extracting the commonalities from a number of measures rather than from the scoring of a single test. The provision of alternative responses, however, also means that a task can be selected whose required responses are within virtually every patient's capabilities, for example, patients who cannot repeat spoken words may be able to take picture-choice tests.

Auditory processing is examined in part through tasks which require the patient to decide whether pairs of nonwords (or words), distinguished by minimal distinctive features, are the same or different. The nonword task is aimed at testing the intactness of the patient's auditory phonological analysis; people who fare badly on this task, and whose pure-tone hearing is adequate, may have *word-sound deafness* (Franklin, 1989). The influence of lexical information on this test can be assessed by a comparable task using real words. An alternative version of this word minimal pair task is provided, to check on the robustness of the results by comparing different types of responses. This version uses a reading choice response, and may be a preferable test for patients with poor auditory working memory but relatively good reading. Two other tasks may throw some light on the patient's auditory phonological processing, provided that he or she can recognize single letters. These two tasks use a mixture of words and nonwords so that lexical and nonlexical processing can be compared. They are aimed at testing the ability to segment the heard stream of sounds into phonemes and match them with a letter representing the first or last sound. All items are controlled for length, syllabic nature and (where they are real words) part of speech used for phonological discrimination i.e. all are CVC nouns.

A test of auditory lexical decision (deciding whether spoken items are real words or not) is aimed at providing some information as to the patient's phonological input lexicon, in association with the word minimal pair discrimination test. This may help in detecting whether the patient is *word-form deaf* (has a reduced ability to recognize spoken words as familiar). The lexical decision tasks used in PALPA allow for various influences to be detected (imageability, frequency and morphology). The auditory lexical decision tasks have a parallel for use in reading, in order to test whether the difficulty is restricted to one modality or is central, in which case some more general impairment of lexical-semantics may be suspected. The influence of type of response can be examined further by also giving the same word and nonword items for repetition.

Lexical decision can be undertaken, in theory, without processing meaning. A task which contrasts with this, necessarily involving the patient in processing meaning, is a picture-word matching task in which the words are phonologically minimally distinctive (e.g *fan* and *van*, with a more distinctive word *man* as a second distractor). Patients who perform worse on this task than on the non-picture tasks may have *word-meaning deafness* (if the difficulty is restricted to auditory input) – difficulty in accessing meaning from the spoken medium. Alternatively, a central lexical-semantic disorder could produce a similar result, although processing semantics through reading will also be affected in this case (see below).

Picture and Word Semantics

PALPA includes a number of measures of central lexical-semantic abilities, using various modalities to test for the centrality of the disorder, including oral and written naming and reading. There are spoken and written versions of tasks asking the patient to decide whether pairs of words mean the same (synonym judgement); this material is controlled for imageability, since some patients succeed better with high imageability words than low, and this is useful information to apply in designing therapy approaches. The effect of imageability can also be tested through a list of words to be read aloud and repeated with or without a brief interval of delay. Close and distant semantic distractors are used in spoken and written versions of a word-picture matching task and spoken-to-written word matching task. The picture tasks also use visual distractors; these may detect the difficulties of patients who have visual as well as semantic problems.

Word Reading

Like auditory input, reading is also tested through a number of tasks, some requiring reading aloud, some silent. Information on the early modules in reading is sought from examining the detection of mirror-reversed letters, upper and lower case letter matching, and the ability to associate letters with their spoken names. The written lexical decision task has four versions: the easy version includes illegal letter strings; another is controlled for imageability and word frequency; in another the nonwords are real words with inappropriate suffixes (e.g. *facey*), whilst a fourth verson uses words controlled for regularity of pronunciation and includes pseudohomophones like *jale*. These latter may be accepted as real words by some patients with the symptom complex of *surface dyslexia* if they draw on their phonological lexicons because of deficient orthographic lexical processing. A task of defining written homophones tests whether or not patients can access meaning directly via the orthographic input lexicon; errors here also suggest that the patient is accessing meaning only through pronunciation. Other tasks also examine this kind of *inner speech*, through asking the patient to find rhyming words (written or for picture names) and to judge whether pairs of words or nonwords sound the same.

In order to test for one feature of *deep dyslexia*, patients are asked to read aloud a list of nonwords; another feature is examined through varying grammatical class. The effect of length on reading aloud is examined in respect both of number of letters (an orthographic factor) and number of syllables (a phonological factor). Regularity of spelling is, of course, an important factor in the detection of the reading difficulties which are included in the symptom complex of surface dyslexia, and PALPA includes tests which compare the number of errors made in reading words which follow regular grapheme-to-phoneme correspondences and those which do not.

Spelling

PALPA includes eight tests of written spelling to dictation, which allow for comparison with the reading tasks and with tasks of similar auditory input but which have spoken responses. One test examines the effect of word length, another of regularity of sound-spelling correspondence (as a means of detecting *surface dysgraphia*); another is controlled for imageability and frequency, to detect for central and lexical influences on the production of letter strings. A test is also provided of the ability to write nonwords to dictation. A test of spelling regular and exception homophones (like bare/bear) after definition examines whether the patient can use the contextual information provided by the definition; if the patient does not, then exceptionally spelled homophones may be spelled as if they are regular, thus giving a spelling inappropriate for the definition. The remaining three spelling tasks look at the effect of grammatical class and appropriateness of morphological suffixes.

Sentence Processing

There is to date no popular model of sentence comprehension such as that which underlies the psycholinguistic cross-modality model of lexical processing (see Figure 8.1). The tests in this section of PALPA have therefore been based on an eclectic survey of theories of the disorders which underlie semantic-grammatical problems in aphasia. These include difficulty in mapping between syntactic and semantic operations such that thematic roles cannot be extracted, a dependency on canonical word order for comprehension, a specific difficulty in the grammatical use of function words and inflections, and problems in handling 'gapped' sentences where underlying subject–object relations are not made overt in surface structure.

Some of the lexical tests described in the previous sections are relevant to the patient's knowledge of grammar and morphology, in that they examine the influence of part of speech on repetition, reading aloud and spelling, and of sensitivity to appropriateness of grammatical suffixes. PALPA also attempts to throw some light on the patients' grammatical and semantic abilities at the level of sentence contexts. It does this only for comprehension, and this examination needs to be complemented by an analysis of the production of sentences (see, for example, Byng and Black, 1989; Saffran, Berndt and Schwartz, 1989).

Sentence comprehension is examined by means of picture-choice (see Black, Nickels and Byng, 1991, for a review of the stages involved in such a task). The sentences predominantly use a set of six animate referents, in order to reduce lexical complexity, and the patient is first tested for recognition of these six referents. The variables controlled for in the sentences include pragmatic reversibility, active/passive mood, verb/adjective predication, length and presence of notional gaps in sentences (which according to some linguistic theories indicate the presence of proforma at D-structure level or traces at S-structure level). Examples of such gapped sentences are, 'The girl's asking what to eat' and 'The girl's suggesting what to eat'. In the first sentence the gapped subject of 'to eat' is the same as the subject of the sentence, whereas in the second it is not. Gapped sentences may present difficulties for some patients, which may be explicable in terms of empty NPs as in Binding Theory (see Caplan and Hildebrandt, 1988, for a description of this theory in the context of aphasia), though the authors of PALPA do not necessarily subscribe to the psychological validity of this linguistic theory.

By comparing comprehension of reversible and nonreversible sentences in active and passive versions, some light may be thrown on how much the patient's extraction of thematic roles is dependent on pragmatics and canonical word order. The use of nonreversible sentences with converse relations like *buy/sell* and *give/receive* is aimed at being able to compare the extraction of thematic roles where the roles are more diverse (donor, recipient, etc) and are not cued by word order. A semantic measure is also included in the test of sentence comprehension, i.e. directionality of motion in some of the verbs used (as in *lead* and *follow*); this is included to see the extent to which increasing semantic difficulty affects sentence comprehension.

The sentence comprehension test has both auditory and written versions for cross-modality comparisons. The same sentences are also used for reading aloud and for repetition, the latter as one means of assessing auditory working verbal memory. The use of a subset of grammatical words (locative prepositions) in context is examined in another picture-choice test, again with auditory and written versions. This test is also aimed at testing whether reversibility of word order affects comprehension. It also incorporates the dimension of living-thing/abstractness; the referents it uses are living things (*chicken on egg*), inanimate objects (*box under bucket*) and abstract shapes (*square in circle*). Some patients may find the last kind of phrases hardest.

Applications for Therapy

The aim of PALPA is to help the therapist to form a reasonably comprehensive picture of an individual patient's assets and difficulties in terms of processing models as they are at present developed. It is from such an overall picture, together with the many other aspects of the patient's needs culled from case history taking and analysis of the patient's communicative needs and abilities, that the therapist will decide whether or not direct intervention is appropriate, and if so, what form a programme will take. There is no one-to-one indication for therapy from the results of a single PALPA test, nor even from a compilation of them supporting the hypothesis of the nature of the patient's processing disorders. For example, even if the pattern of PALPA results suggests that a patient might have a word-sound deafness, it does not follow that a therapy programme should be designed at remedying this directly. It might be more appropriate in the individual circumstances to advise a caring relative on strategies to improve the patient's contextual comprehension, including facilitating lip-reading. It is also part of the therapist's skill to decide (if direct intervention is indeed indicated) whether the aim will be to restore the damaged function by using tactics aimed at stimulation, reorganization or the substitution by prosthetic strategies to achieve a similar functional result.

There is, however, an increasing number of studies which show how the application of psycholinguistic modelling has assisted therapists in designing effective programmes, whether it be to improve naming, reading, spelling or sentence production (see Lesser and Milroy, 1993, for a review). One considerable advantage of mapping a patient's abilities onto a psycholinguistic model is that not only can it suggest ways of supplementing a damaged component by drawing on intact (or more intact) abilities, but it can also indicate what functions would *not* be predicted to improve from therapy targeted elsewhere. Such functions can then be used as controls to test whether any improvement occurring after a period of therapy is general or is specific to the targeted ability.

Conclusion

PALPA must be seen to be relatively modest in its aims. It does not claim to assess in any way the social and interactive aspects of communication, for which other techniques must be used (see Worrall, Chapter 4). Even within the psycholinguistic realm of language processing, it does not claim to be a complete resource; therapists will feel the need to add their own supplementary measures to explore individual patients' abilities, and to use PALPA materials in a flexible way, for example, for oral spelling as an alternative to written spelling, in order to test the hypotheses they have established. The authors have acknowladged, in a forum in the journal *Aphasiology* (in press), several ways in which PALPA needs to evolve.

PALPA is meant, however, to be a practical clinical resource in making more widely available to therapists a means of forming a theoretically consistent picture of their patients' abilities, from which they can then take the next step of deciding on *whether* or *what* therapy. Response to such therapy may itself result in further hypotheses which other tasks in the PALPA resource may help to examine.

Acknowledgements

This research was funded by MRC Project Grant number G8401834N to Ruth Lesser, Max Coltheart and Janice Kay (1984–9). Full-time researchers on the project were Janice Kay assisted by Karen Barr.

References

Black M, Nickels L, Byng S (1991) Patterns of sentence processing deficit; processing simple sentences can be a complex matter. Journal of Neurolinguistics 6:79–101.

Byng S, Black M (1989) Some aspects of sentence production in aphasia. Aphasiology 3:241–63.

Caplan D, Hildebrandt N (1988) Disorders of Syntactic Comprehension. Cambridge MA: MIT Press.

Ellis AW, Young AW (1988) Human Cognitive Neuropsychology. Hove: Lawrence Erlbaum Associates.

Franklin S, (1989) Dissociations in auditory word comprehension: evidence from nine fluent aphasic patients. Aphasiology 3:189–207.

Goodglass H, Kaplan E (1983) The Assessment of Aphasia and Related Disorders. Philadelphia PA: Lee and Febiger.

Kay J, Lesser R, Coltheart M (1992) Psycholinguistic Assessments of Language Processing in Aphasia. Hove: Lawrence Erlbaum Associates.

Lesser R, Milroy L (1993) Linguistics and Aphasia: Psycholinguistic and Pragmatic Aspects of Intervention. London: Longman.

Patterson K, Shewell C (1987) Speak and spell: dissociations and word-class effects. In Coltheart M, Sartori G, Job R (Eds.) The Cognitive Neuropsychology of Language. Hove: Lawrence Erlbaum Associates.

Saffran E, Berndt RS, Schwartz MF (1989) The quantitative analysis of agrammatic production: procedure and data. Brain and Language 37:440–79.

Chapter 10
Comprehension

ROBERT S. PIERCE

Auditory comprehension deficits in aphasic patients are common. They range from severe deficits, including difficulty in the understanding of common single words, to mild deficits, reflecting only the impaired processing of more extensive discourse. At the more severe levels, there are two reasons for treating auditory comprehension deficits.

First, a patient with some comprehension of spoken language is better off than one who has little or no language comprehension. Imagine moving to Germany for the rest of your life. Would you prefer to understand some German or no German? The globally impaired aphasic patient who develops some comprehension skills typically has a better awareness of what is going on around him. Accordingly, it becomes easier for those in his or her environment to provide care. Even if a successful expressive system does not develop, this reason alone provides sufficient impetus for treatment. Second, improved comprehension skills serve as a prerequisite for improved expression. It is virtually impossible to develop a successful augmentative communication system with a globally aphasic patient who has no usable comprehension skills. Improving comprehension in a Wernicke's aphasic patient with florid neologistic jargon can lead to a reduction in jargon, even when no direct therapeutic attention has been devoted to expression.

Treatment of auditory comprehension can also be relevant at the other end of the continuum. One of the professors at Kent State University, who had had a stroke, is trying to return to the classroom. He can prepare and present well organized lectures. However, difficulties remain in his ability to understand questions asked by students. Given the importance of comprehension disorders in the course of recovery from aphasia, this chapter reviews much of what is known about this impairment.

Single Word Comprehension

For patients with severe deficits, it is typical to begin treatment by emphasizing comprehension of single words. Probably the best guideline for selecting which words to treat is frequency of occurrence (Shewan and Bandur, 1986). Frequently occurring words are usually comprehended more successfully than are less common words. While frequency of occurrence correlates significantly with the semantic domains of familiarity and meaningfulness (Toglia and Batting, 1978), it is important to remain sensitive to individual variations. Words that are highly familiar and meaningful to one person may be less familiar to another. Obviously, established norms for frequency of occurrence (e.g., Francis and Kucera, 1982) cannot account for these variations. However, they remain a useful general guideline for word selection.

The semantic domains of concreteness and imagery impact on normal individuals' notion of word meanings somewhat independently from frequency of occurrence (Togia and Battig, 1978) and may similarly affect aphasic patients (Goldstein, 1948). Words that rank high on these domains may make better choices for early intervention than words ranking lower on these domains. An unresolved issue is how far treatment should go along these continua. While it is common to work on frequently occurring words, it is probably less common to directly treat the comprehension of less frequently occurring words. Treatment focus usually progresses to the level of sentences and commands with less emphasis placed on the meaning of individual words. Given the importance of word meanings to the comprehension of sentences and narratives (an issue to be explored later), a continued emphasis on single word comprehension may reap benefits.

Apart from the general influences of frequency of occurrence and concreteness, some patients show differential comprehension abilities for specific word categories. While verbs are frequently more difficult to comprehend than nouns, different levels of impairment may be evident for categories such as foods, living things, and man-made objects (McCarthy and Warrington, 1990). Globally impaired patients may retain the ability to recognize famous and familiar people and landmarks (Van Lancker and Klein, 1990). The clinician should be alert to these patterns.

Semantic Knowledge

Single word comprehension is often treated by asking a patient to point to a picture from an array of choices based on the spoken word. If the patient selects the correct picture, we feel that the word has been comprehended. However, we do not necessarily know what that comprehension consists of; that is, what the patient knows about the word. Some years ago, Goodglass and Baker (1976) indicated that some aphasic patients have holes in their semantic knowledge. That is, they know some aspects of a word's meaning but not others. Representative of this research is a study by Butterworth, Howard and

McLoughlin (1984). They found that aphasic patients were able to select the correct picture from an array of five as well as did normal individuals when the pictures were semantically unrelated. However, the aphasic patients' performance became significantly impaired when asked to select from an array of five semantically related pictures. In other words, they could 'comprehend' the word *saw* when presented with the pictures *apple, shoe, car, horse,* and *saw,* but not when presented with *hammer, drill, screwdriver, axe* and *saw.* These authors felt this differential performance reflected superficial semantic processing. Aphasic patients appreciate sufficient semantic information about a word to allow them to select from unrelated choices but not more detailed semantic information which is needed to choose among related items. More recently, Germani and Pierce (1995) demonstrated that aphasic patients identified more important semantic features of words with greater accuracy than they identified less important features. Furthermore, their comprehension accuracy of the less important features correlated significantly with their general comprehension and naming skill levels.

One way to conceptualize the issue of semantic knowledge is the notion of context-independent and context-dependent attributes (Greenspan, 1986). Context-independent attributes are always activated regardless of the context, and comprise the core meaning of a word. Context-dependent attributes are activated only when emphasized by the context, and comprise the sense of a word (Anderson, 1990). For example, the semantic representation activated for the isolated word *piano* is relatively consistent with the sentence, 'He played a beautiful sonata on the piano', but may not contain some of the attributes highlighted by the sentence, 'I sprained my back moving the piano.' While there is some evidence that context-independent attributes lose their independence (and thus must be activated by the context) in patients with dementia of the Alzheimer's type (Pierce and Townsend, 1990), it is not known whether this occurs in patients with aphasia. If it does, then treatment directed towards the contextually-facilitated activation of these attributes may lead to the re-establishment of their independent activation and subsequently to more full, detailed semantic representations. Germani (1994) provided some evidence that a word's lower important features are activated more successfully in aphasic patients if the word occurs in a sentence that emphasizes those features than if it occurs in a neutral sentence.

Contextual Influences

We often assume that presenting words in isolation constitutes the easiest level of a comprehension task. However, aphasic patients' performance can be enhanced by adding contextual information to the stimulus presentation. Clark and Flowers (1987) found that items such as, 'Which one is the book that you read?' were responded to more accurately than either 'Which one is the book?' or 'Which is the one you read?'. Sentences like 'The girl was peeling an onion (banana). What was she peeling?' were responded to more accurately when the contextually predictive sentence 'The girl was crying' either preceded (Pierce and Beekman, 1985) or followed (Pierce, 1988) the target sentence. The predictive nature of the contextual information contributes to enhanced performance in a manner not accomplished by simply repeating the target sentence (Pierce, 1988). It is conceivable that context improves performance because it activates some semantic attributes that are not realized normally, leading to a fuller semantic representation (Schwanenflugal, 1991).

Treating Single Word Comprehension

Improving aphasic patients' comprehension of individual word meanings is an important treatment goal. Word selection can be based on frequency of occurrence in conjunction with personal interests and familiarity. Depth of word knowledge should be emphasized and contexts can be used to highlight specific semantic features.

Sentence Comprehension

When aphasic patients are presented with sentences to comprehend, many issues other than the meaning of individual words become important. Syntax, sentence length, speaking rate, quantity of information, and memory can all influence performance.

Syntax

Regardless of their overall level of functional comprehension skills, most aphasic patients have difficulty deriving meaning from a sentence's syntax (Peach, Canter and Gallaher, 1988). However, not all syntactic constructions are of equal difficulty. A general hierarchy of syntactic difficulty (from easiest to hardest) is negation, gender, reflexives, prepositions, tense, word order, and relative clauses (Butler-Hinz, Waters and Caplan, 1990; Lesser, 1974; Naeser, et al., 1987; Parisi and Pizzamiglio, 1970; Pierce, 1979; Sherman and Schweickert, 1989).

Some patients are clearly debilitated by their impaired comprehension of syntax. For example, our professor, mentioned earlier, has considerable difficulty understanding prepositions, tense, word order, and wh-questions. This limits his ability to quickly and fully understand what is said to him. Accordingly, treatment has emphasized this particular skill.

However, many aphasic patients are not particularly affected by their syntactic comprehension problems. Despite limited processing of syntax, these patients perform well on auditory comprehension tests (such as the complex materials subtest of the Boston Diagnostic Aphasia Examination, Goodglass and Kaplan, 1983) and function adequately in daily communicative interactions, such as conversations. The reasons for this discrepancy may relate to two very important differences in processing demands generated by natural communication environments versus traditional assessment/treatment environments.

First, treatment environments often present a considerable amount of new information at one time. For example, when presented with the item 'Mary gave the book to John. Who has the book?', the patient must process each of the main lexical items (Mary, give, book, John) as well as the word order relationship (Mary was the agent and John the recipient). This can overload the patient's processing capacity and syntactic comprehension usually suffers (Peach, Canter and Gallaher, 1988). In contrast, in more natural environments, much of the information in this utterance would be *given* information. That is, the patient would already know some of it, such as who Mary and John were and that something happened to a book. This would be the case if the item was in response to the inquiry of 'What happened to the book I had left on the table?' when John and Mary were the residents of the house. Since much of the target utterance would be given information, the patient could devote more processing resources (attention) to the new information, allowing for more successful processing of that information. It has been demonstrated that aphasic patients are able to comprehend reversible active and passive sentences more accurately when this type of prior knowledge is provided in the form of preceding narratives (Cannito, Jarecki and Pierce, 1986; Hough, Pierce and Cannito, 1989; Germani and Pierce, 1992).

However, similar beneficial effects are not evident when only a single prior sentence context is provided, presumably because it does not provide sufficient exposure to the key lexical items to alleviate forthcoming processing demands (Pierce and Wagner, 1985). Note that this type of context does not predict what the word order interpretation in the target sentence should be but only serves to free up processing resources to facilitate the making of that determination.

The second difference between natural and treatment environments is that natural contexts are often predictive. That is, the information that is known actually predicts the meaning reflected by the syntax. For example, the patient may be wondering what Mary did with the book when he heard,'Mary gave the book to John.' In this case, the context predicts that Mary is the agent and that someone else (John) is the recipient. It is well documented that aphasic patients benefit from this type of predictive context; whether the prediction is based on world knowledge (Caramazza and Zurif, 1976; Deloche and Seron, 1981) or information in the surrounding linguistic/extralinguistic environment (Caplan and Evans, 1990; Germani and Pierce, 1992; Hough, Pierce and Cannito, 1989; Pierce, 1988; Pierce and Beekman, 1985; Pierce and Wagner, 1985). Because syntactic comprehension deficits do not always markedly impair a patient's functional comprehension skills, they can often be assigned a low priority in treatment.

Length and Amount of Information

Kearns and Hubbard (1977) provided a hierarchy of difficulty for commands based on such factors as length, amount of information, the fact that verbs are often more difficult than nouns, and grammatical complexity (see Table 10.1). The impact of increasing length on comprehension depends on what is contributing to the length. Sentences that are made longer in order to reduce the syntactic complexity are usually easier to understand than their shorter, more grammatically complex counterparts (Goodglass, *et al.,* 1979). However, if length is increased by adding nonredundant information, such as with Token Test type commands, then performance deteriorates for some, but certainly not all, patients (Curtiss, *et al.,* 1986).

Table 10.1 A hierarchy of auditory comprehension tasks from easiest to more difficult, based on Kearns and Hubbard (1977). Those items with the asterisk represent four levels of significantly different performance accuracy.

Point to one common object by name.

*Point to one common object by function.

Point in sequence to two common objects by function.

*Point in sequence to two common objects by name.

Point to one object spelled by examiner.

Point to one object described by the examiner with three descriptors. (Which one is white, plastic, and has bristles?).

Follow one verb instruction (Pick up the pen.).

Point in sequence to three common objects by name.

Point in sequence to three common objects by function.

Carry out two-object location instructions (Put the pen in front of the knife.).

*Carry out, in sequence, two verb instructions (Point to the knife. Turn over the fork.).

Carry out, in sequence, two verb instructions, with time constraint (Before you pick up the knife, hand me the fork.).

*Carry out three verb instructions (Point to the knife. Turn over the fork. Touch the pencil.).

Memory

Intuitively it seems that memory must play a role in language comprehension. However, determining what that role is and how to assess/treat it remains elusive. Aphasic patients frequently have reduced memory spans for series of digits or words (Tandridag, Kirshner and Casey, 1987). Martin and Feher (1990) demonstrated in aphasic patients that sequential memory span relates to the ability to comprehend commands of increasing length based on nonredundant information (similar to Token Test type commands) but not to the comprehension of sentences containing more complex syntax. Furthermore, performance on the Token Test does not particularly relate to the comprehension of more natural stimuli such as narratives (Brookshire and Nicholas, 1984; Wegner, Brookshire and Nicholas, 1984). The conceptualization of memory as a retention span for nonredundant items is severely limited in its ability to account for more natural language comprehension.

Recognizing that comprehension entails both retention of information and the continued processing of new information, Daneman and Green (1986) developed a working memory test that taps both of these elements. However, aphasic patients' performance on a reading version of this type of memory test did not relate to their comprehension of newspaper articles (Grogan and Pierce, 1991). One reason for this result may be that, although the working memory test taps both retention and processing, the sentences used in the test were thematically unrelated to each other. In contrast, typical narratives have a thematic coherence that contributes to their ability to be understood. (These issues are discussed in the next section of this paper.)

It has been argued recently that the primary role of memory in language comprehension occurs if the listener must backtrack over a spoken message in order to process it after the fact (McCarthy and Warrington, 1990; Waters, Caplan and Hildebrandt, 1991). Certainly, because of their comprehension impairment, aphasic patients may not be able to keep up with the demands of on-line processing and would need to retain information for retrospective processing. This may be similar to what a normal individual goes through when learning a second language. In the early stages, it is extremely difficult to retain information that one could not process in order to 'get back to it'. However, as language skills improve, more of the information is understood. Accordingly, improving language skills may make more sense than trying to improve memory processes *per se*. Until such time as memory is better conceptualized and its relationship to language processing clarified, the role of direct memory training in aphasia treatment should be limited.

Speaking Rate and Pauses

Aphasic patients benefit from a reduced speaking rate and the place-
ment of pauses at syntactically logical locations in a sentence (Lasky,
Weidner and Johnson, 1976; Weidner and Lasky, 1976), although these
effects may be inconsistent (Nicholas and Brookshire, 1986). The
reasons for this benefit may relate to the previously mentioned analogy
of learning a second language. It is a common perception of the
second language learner that native speakers of the second language
talk too fast. Perhaps more to the point, the learner listens too slowly.
Limited proficiency makes it difficult to process as quickly as the
language is produced and to identify where one word and/or processing unit (e.g, clause) ends and the next begins. A reduced rate and
appropriately placed pauses makes it easier to identify the boundaries
of processing units and to process that information on-line, without
having to retain it for retrospective processing.

Treating Sentence Level Comprehension

When treating sentence comprehension, clinicians should continue to
consider frequency of occurrence/familiarity of the vocabulary and
contextual support of particular target words in the sentences.
Sentences that emphasize the inter-relationships among word meanings (e.g., sentence completion items with multiple choice response
sets) may make more appropriate stimuli than those highlighting
syntactic relationships. Syntactic structures that have a high semantic
component, such as negation, locative prepositions and pronouns may
deserve more emphasis than word-order relationships. The difficulty of
these latter constructions is often offset by naturally occurring contextual influences and may contribute little to functional comprehension
performance.

Narrative Comprehension

Many of the factors that have already been discussed continue to influence comprehension at the narrative level. However, there are other
aspects of processing that impact on the comprehension of narratives
which have little influence at the single word and sentence levels.
These processes are reviewed in this section. A more detailed analysis
of narrative comprehension in aphasic patients is contained in Pierce
and Grogan (1992).

Developing the Text Base

The process of narrative comprehension involves several steps (van Dijk
and Kintsch, 1983). The first is the development of a text base; that is,

conversion of the information contained in the sentences within the narrative to a set of propositions (a meaning element containing one predicate and one or more arguments). These propositions are typically arranged in a hierarchical arrangement such that the more central or important information occurs towards the top of the hierarchy and the less important information is placed towards the bottom. Patterson and Pierce (1991) demonstrated that higher level aphasic patients retain a sensitivity to this hierarchy and recall propositions from the third level of a hierarchy less accurately than from the first and second levels. This result may help explain an interesting finding by Wegner, Brookshire and Nicholas (1984). They found that aphasic patients comprehended details more accurately from noncoherent narratives than from coherent narratives. The noncoherent narratives contained several different topics, each of which would have had a limited amount of information and thus a hierarchical structure with mostly higher level propositions. In contrast, coherent narratives have one topic containing a greater amount of information and, therefore, a hierarchy with more propositions contained at lower levels. These lower level propositions (details) would be more vulnerable to reductions in retention and/or recall.

Narratives are typically expected to be coherent. Coherence is based on the perception of relationships among the proportions in the text base. These relationships are based on such features as causality and shared goals, plans, and actions (see Graesser and Bower, 1990). While many relationships are evident, others require the listener to make inferences. Accordingly, comprehension accuracy is influenced by the number and complexity of the inferences required to associate propositions (see Graesser and Bower, 1990). I am not aware of any information on aphasic patients' abilities to make different types of inferences (e.g., causal versus shared goals). However, there is evidence that aphasic patients are affected by the degree of inference required. Brookshire and Nicholas (1984) found that detail statements in narratives that required a minimum of inferencing were not any more difficult for aphasic patients to comprehend than were directly stated details that required no inferencing. In contrast, detail statements that required greater inferencing were significantly more difficult to comprehend than directly stated details (Nicholas and Brookshire, 1986).

The narrative comprehension process is greatly influenced by the listener's knowledge base. Several terms are used to refer to this knowledge base, such as domain knowledge, mental model, and situation model. In general, this notion refers to what the listener knows about the narrative's topic. In addition, listeners have mental schemata (or scripts) and superstructures about the usual nature of specific events, such as ordering in a restaurant or reading newspaper articles versus scientific studies. The application of this knowledge impacts on narrative comprehension in several ways. The listener's knowledge provides a structure that facilitates the formation of a text base. Knowledge also increases coherence because it makes inferencing easier; that is, the ability to see relationships among propositions is enhanced (see Graesser and Bower, 1990). In addition, a strong knowledge base may alleviate potential problems with the text for aphasic patients such as violations in cohesion (Huber, 1990) and violations in the sequential ordering of given/new information (Cannito, Jarecki, and Pierce, 1986). The beneficial influence of contextual knowledge on aphasic patients' processing of specific semantic and syntactic information was reviewed in the previous sections of this paper.

Several studies have demonstrated that knowledge in the form of schemata and superstructures are relatively intact in higher level aphasic patients (Armus, Brookshire and Nicholas, 1989; Ulatowska, *et al,*, 1983). Concerning domain knowledge, Krackenfels and Pierce (1995) has provided some initial data showing that aphasic patients comprehend narratives on topics that they know something about more accurately than those on which they know little.

The information obtained from the text base is combined with the listener's current knowledge to expand his or her knowledge base. Accordingly, responses to questions about a narrative will reflect what the patient learned from the narrative in addition to what they already know. This can make it difficult at times to be certain what source of information a patient is using to respond to questions. Typically, in both treatment and assessment, our interest is in how well a patient can derive information from the narrative. However, this ability remains unknown if the patient can respond to questions based solely on prior knowledge (Nicholas, MacLennan and Brookshire, 1986).

Developing the Gist

After forming the text base, the second step in narrative comprehension is developing the gist or main idea/theme of the narrative. This ability appears to be relatively intact in higher level aphasic patients both for narratives (Brookshire and Nicholas, 1984; Nicholas and Brookshire, 1986) and for monologues and conversational dialogues (Katsuki-Nakamura, Brookshire and Nicholas, 1988). This capacity can be capitalized on in that providing thematic cues often enhances recall of detail information (Patterson and Pierce, 1991).

Treating Narrative Comprehension

Important variables to consider when treating aphasic patients' comprehension of narratives include domain knowledge, saliency, inferencing demands, length and familiarity. Start with narrative topics with which the patient is most familiar and progress to those with which he or she is less familiar. Start with questions about main ideas of the narrative and progress to questions about details (progressing from more to less central or important details). Start with directly stated information and progress to information that requires inferencing by the listener (progressing from minimal to more complex inferences). Vary narrative length and familiarity of the vocabulary.

Conclusion

Almost all aphasic patients can benefit from treatment of comprehension deficits. While treatment usually proceeds from targeting single words to sentences and then to narratives, it is important to recognize that this hierarchy is not a pure one. Words are often better understood in certain sentences than in isolation and sentences are often better understood as part of a narrative than on their own. Our profession's knowledge of the factors that influence comprehension at different levels is expanding and this should enhance our treatment efforts.

References

Anderson RC (1990) Inferences about word meanings. In Graesser AC, Bower GH (Ed) Inferences and Text Comprehension. New York: Academic Press.

Armus S, Brookshire R, Nicholas L (1989) Aphasic and non-brain-damaged adults' knowledge of scripts for common situations. Brain and Language 36:518–28.

Brookshire R, Nicholas L (1984) Comprehension of directly and indirectly stated main ideas and details in discourse by brain-damaged and non-brain-damaged listeners. Brain and Language 21:21–36.

Butler-Hinz S, Waters G, Caplan D (1990) Characteristics of syntactic comprehension deficits following closed head injury versus left cerebrovascular accident. Journal of Speech and Hearing Research 33:269–80.

Butterworth B, Howard D, McLoughlin P (1984) The semantic deficit in aphasia: the relationship between semantic errors in auditory comprehension and picture naming. Neuropsychologia 22:409–26.

Cannito M, Jarecki J, Pierce R (1986) Effects of thematic structure on syntactic processing in aphasia. Brain and Language 27:38–49.

Caplan D, Evans K (1990) The effects of syntactic structure on discourse comprehension in patients with parsing impairments. Brain and Language 39:206–34.

Caramazza A, Zurif EB (1976) Dissociation of algorithmic and heuristic processes in language comprehension: evidence from aphasia. Brain and Language 3:572–82.

Clark AE, Flowers CR, (1987) The effect of semantic redundancy on auditory comprehension in aphasia. In Brookshire RK (Ed) Clinical Aphasiology. Minneapolis MN: BRK Publishers.

Curtis S, Jackson C, Kempler D, Hanson W, Metter E (1986) Length vs. structural complexity in sentence comprehension in aphasia. In Brookshire RK (Ed) Clinical Aphasiology. Minneapolis MN: BRK Publishers.

Daneman M and Green I (1986) Individual differences in comprehending and producing words in context. Journal of Memory and Language 25:1–18.

Deloche G, Seron X (1981) Sentence understanding and knowledge of the world: evidence from a sentence-picture matching task performed by aphasic patients. Brain and Language 14:57–69.

Francis WN, Kucera H (1982) Frequency Analysis of English Usage: Lexicon and Grammar. Boston MA: Houghton Mifflin Co.

Germani M (1994) Semantic attribute knowledge in aphasia: the effects of context. Paper presented at the annual convention of the American Speech–Language–Hearing Association, New Orleans, LA, November.

Germani M, Pierce R (1992) Contextual influences in reading comprehension in aphasia. Brain and Language 42:308–19.

Germani M, Pierce R (1995) Semantic attribute knowledge in adults with right and left hemisphere damage. Aphasiology 9: 1–21.

Goodglass H, Baker E (1976) Semantic field, naming, and auditory comprehension in aphasia. The Assessment of Aphasia and Related Disorders. Philadelphia PA: Lea & Febriger.

Goodglass H, Blumstein S, Gleason J, Hyde M, Green E, Statlender S (1979) The effect of syntactic encoding on sentence comprehension in aphasia. Brain and Language 7:201–9.

Graesser A, Bower G (Eds) (1990) Inferences and Text Comprehension. New York: Academic Press.

Greenspan S (1986) Semantic flexibility and referential specificity of concrete nouns. Journal of Memory and Language 25:539–57.

Grogan S, Pierce R (1991) Influence of working memory on newspaper text comprehension in aphasia. Paper presented at the annual convention of the American Speech-Language-Hearing Association, Atlanta, GA, November.

Hough M, Pierce R, Cannito M (1989) Contextual influences in aphasia: effects of predictive versus nonpredictive narratives. Brain and Language 36:325–34.

Huber W (1990) Text comprehension and production in aphasia: analysis in terms of micro- and macrostructure. In Joanette Y, Brownell H (Eds), Discourse Ability and Brain Damage: Theoretical and Empirical Perspectives. New York: Springer-Verlag.

Katsuki-Nakamura J, Brookshire R, Nicholas L (1988) Comprehension of monologues and dialogues by aphasic listeners. Journal of Speech and Hearing Disorders 53:408–15.

Kearns KP, Hubbard D (1977) A comparison of auditory comprehension tasks in aphasia. In Brookshire R H (Ed), Clinical Aphasiology. Minneapolis MN: BRK Publishers.

Krackenfels D, Pierce R (1995) The effect of familiarity on narrative comprehension in aphasia. Paper presented to the Clinical Aphasiology Conference, Sun River, OR, June.

Lasky E, Weidner W, Johnson J (1976) Influence of linguistic complexity, rate of presentation, and interphrase pause time on auditory-verbal comprehension of adult aphasic patients. Brain and Language 3:386–95.

Lesser R (1974) Verbal comprehension in aphasia: an English version of three Italian tests. Cortex 10:247–63.

Martin R, Feher E (1990) The consequences of reduced memory span for the comprehension of semantic versus syntactic information. Brain and Language 38:1–20.

McCarthy RA, Warrington EK (1990) Cognitive Neuropsychology: A Clinical Introduction. New York: Academic Press.

Naeser M, Mazurski P, Goodglass H, Peraino M, Laughlin S, Leaper W (1987) Auditory syntactic comprehension in nine aphasia groups (with CT scans) and children: differences in degree but not order of difficulty observed. Cortex 23:359–80.

Nicholas L, Brookshire R (1986) Consistency of the effects of rate of speech on brain-damaged adults' comprehension of narrative discourse. Journal of Speech and Hearing 29:462–70.

Nicholas L, MacLennan D, Brookshire R (1986) Validity of multiple-sentence reading comprehension tests for aphasic adults. Journal of Speech and Hearing Disorders 51:82–7.

Parisi D, Pizzamiglio L (1970) Syntactic comprehension in aphasia. Cortex 6:204–15.

Patterson J, Pierce R (1991) Memory for narrative discourse in adults with mild language impairment following left or right cerebrovascular accident. Paper presented at the annual convention of the America Speech-Language-Hearing Association, Alanta, GA, November.

Peach RK, Canter GJ, Gallaher AJ (1988) Comprehension of sentence structure in anomic and conduction aphasia. Brain and Language 35:119–37.

Pierce R (1979) A study of sentence comprehension of aphasic subjects. In Brookshire RH (Ed) Clinical Aphasiology. Minneapolis MN: BRK Publishers.

Pierce R (1988) Influence of prior and subsequent context on comprehension in aphasia. Aphasiology 2:577–82.

Pierce R, Beekman L (1985) Effects of linguistic and extralinguistic context on semantic and syntactic processing in aphasia. Journal of Speech and Hearing Research 28:250–54.

Pierce R, Grogan S (1992) Improving listening comprehension of narratives. In Peach R (Ed) Clinics in Communication Disorders: Aphasia. Reading: Andover Medical Publishing.

Pierce R, Townsend M (1990) Context independent and dependent semantic representations in dementia. Paper presented to the American Speech-Language-Hearing Association, Seattle WA, November.

Pierce R, Wagner C (1985) The role of context in facilitating syntactic decoding in aphasia. Journal of Communication Disorders 18:203–14.

Schwanenflugel P (1991) Contextual constraint and lexical processing. In Simpson G (Ed) Understanding Word and Sentence. New York: North-Holland.

Sherman J, Schweickert J (1989) Syntactic and semantic contributions to sentence comprehension in agrammatism. Brain and Language 37:419–39.

Shewan C, Bandur D (1986) Treatment of Aphasia: A Language-oriented Approach. Austin TX: Pro-Ed.

Tandridag O, Kirshner HS, and Casey PF (1987) Memory functions in aphasic and non-aphasic stroke patients. Aphasiology 1: 201–14.

Toglia MP, Battig WF (1978) Handbook of Semantic Word Norms. New York: John Wiley & Sons.

Ulatowska H, Freedman-Stern R, Doyel A, Macaluso-Haynes S, North A (1983) Production of narrative discourse in aphasia. Brain and Language 19:317–34.

van Dijk T, Kintsch W (1983) Strategies of discourse comprehension. New York: Academic Press.

Van Lanker D, Klein K (1990) Preserved recognition of familiar personal names in global aphasia. Brain and Language 39:511–29.

Waters G, Caplan D, Hildebrandt N (1991) On the structure of verbal short-term memory and its functional role in sentence comprehension: Evidence from neuropsychology. Cognitive Neuropsychology 8:81–126.

Wegner M, Brookshire R, Nicholas L (1884) Comprehension of main ideas and details in coherent and noncoherent discourse by aphasic and nonaphasic listeners. Brain and Language 21:37-51.

Weidner W, Lasky E (1976) The interaction of rate and complexity of stimulus on the performance of adult aphasic subjects. Brain and Language 3:34-40.

Chapter 11
Reading Theories and Their Implications for Rehabilitation

EVELYNE ANDREEWSKY AND FRANCOISE COCHU

Introduction

Learning and rehabilitation strategies for the acquisition of a given skill are often based on theories of the skill itself rather than on theories relevant to its acquisition (or reacquisition). This is notably the case in reading, and the way one teaches reading merely reflects on which view of reading one adopts. Nevertheless, therapists should be aware of both the theoretical foundations of reading and of its acquisition or reacquisition. Nowadays, reading mechanisms are mainly conceptualized as reading processes, within the information-processing framework of *cognitive* approaches to mind and behaviour (See related chapters in this volume by Edmundson and McIntosh, Chapter 8; Lesser, Chapter 9 and Carlomagno and Iavarone, Chapter 12). – Certain approaches deal also with the acquisition of such processes. But we are far from understanding our cognitive mechanisms (in spite of a great number of interesting investigations into these mechanisms) – and even further from understanding their acquisition. Therefore we should keep in mind that our reading therapy practices are theoretically supported mainly by assumptions.

Therapeutic practices depend on postulated differences (here again assumptions) between reading acquisition and reacquisition. Reacquisition is taken either as an equivalent to learning to read, or as involving the development of new strategies to achieve the same result. Whichever the case, reacquisition is by no means uniquely dependent on its theoretical support, since even a therapy based on a wrong theoretical approach may allow some recovery. As we all know, most school children learn how to read no matter which way they are taught. This emphasizes the importance of psychological factors in reading acquisition such as the desire to behave as other children do, confidence in teachers, and so on. Similar factors intervene in adult rehabilitation – confidence in the therapist doubtlessly being one of the most effective. This leads us back, by a totally different route, to the importance of a sound theoretical grounding for the therapist, who in turn earns the trust and motivation of his or her patients.

This chapter deals with the relationship between reading theories and rehabilitation strategies, highlighting the fact that the emergence (or re-emergence) of a sophisticated skill such as reading is a very complex phenomenon, and should be understood as such. Specific therapeutic examples illustrate these relationships. The chapter is divided into two sections: traditional reading and rehabilitation approaches, and cognitive approaches.

From Reading Theories to Rehabilitation Practices – Traditional Approaches

Therapeutic strategies have always been based on conceptual approaches to the skill which is to be recovered. From the Middle Ages to the eighteenth century, language being at that time mainly conceptualized in terms of tongue motion, aphasia therapy aimed at stimulating the tongue (Howard and Hatfield, 1987). Obviously, such strategies seem ridiculous nowadays and have done so for a long time, if literature such as that of France's Molière (1666), Act II, Scene 5) '...so this is why your daughter is dumb' is anything to go on. But such therapies were coherent with contemporary theoretical approaches to the ability in question. The same applies today, as will be illustrated in this section which is devoted to traditional approaches to reading and rehabilitation.

In order to signpost for the reader the universe in which theoretical reading approaches can be assessed, we shall try to introduce these approaches and the theories (which can be psychological, neurological, linguistic or others) from which they are derived, through organizational poles.

Viewpoints on reading and language range between *analytical* poles, which privilege an understanding of reading in terms of *elements* and *synthetic* poles, focusing on global functional aspects of this skill. We shall consider only approaches which have directly induced methods and strategies of reacquisition. It must be understood that all conceptualization of reading cannot be directly linked to a therapeutic approach. This is, for example, the case of the localizationist theories of the last century such as that of Gall's phrenology.[1] If one conceptualizes the intellectual activities as deriving from cerebral centres, there is indeed nothing much to be done after the destruction of a given centre, if it is, for instance, devoted to reading; in such a framework, reading therapy (at least in absence of assumptions upon cerebral reorganization) should be granted as useless. In other words, one cannot altogether claim that a given function is linked to a definite and specific localization and admit the possibility of recovering such a function if its neural substrata is definitively impaired.

Several organizational poles highlight both the traditional conceptualizations of reading and the reading acquisition and reacquisition methods linked to these conceptualizations, the main poles being the Gestalt theory vs. molecular psychology; behaviourism and reflexology; neurolinguistics vs. pragmatics.

Gestalt-theory vs. Molecular Psychology

The localizationistic *static* approaches (which do not favour language therapy) were ousted at the end of the past century by Freud (1953/1891), Jackson (1878), and more recently by Goldstein (1948), Luria (1966), and others, to be replaced by less strongly mechanistic theories, integrating in the neurophysiological domain more recent contributions from psychology or linguistics.

Goldstein, as Jackson before him (cf. Ombrédane, 1951), had conceptualized – on a *dynamic* mode – the components of language mechanisms (as well as those of the other higher cortical functions) as being constantly reorganized. For him – adapting the Gestalt approaches to perception - these reorganizations provide support for the sequence of our different activities, in as much as they facilitate at each moment the main mechanism (the figure) of the ongoing activity in regard to others (the background). This conceptual frame leads to a functional interpretation of aphasia and alexia; these pathologies reflect problems created by the underlying lesion, which endanger both the temporal adjustment of the language mechanism reorganization and the precision of interrelations between figure and background mechanisms. This Gestalt-like approach leads to the insight that a given level of language is quite different from a simple combination of its lower level elements. We do not speak by combining sounds into words. Therefore, Goldstein rejected those re-education procedures for reading aloud, which consisted of improving the uttering of isolated phonemes, the reading aloud of single letters or nonsense syllables; that is to say exercises concerning single elements. Appropriate exercises were, for him, those which favour the perception of interrelations, and notably in written material, the perception of patterns; that is to say of *gestalts*. This is, for instance, the case in exercises such as retrieving out of a text, as quickly as possible, given items, information or structures.

The other pole, the analytical approach to reading, relying primarily on grapheme–to–phoneme conversion (b, a → /ba/), is well known in quite a number of elementary schools as the main teaching approach. In this framework, the mastery of written material is attained first by the mastery of elements, that is letters (graphemes), then by the combination of these elements into syllables and their conversion into phonemes.

These steps, and the underlying analytical reading model, are often incorporated in traditional rehabilitation strategies, with adaptation of exercises to specific problems of patients. The therapy implicitly assumes that the task is to relearn missing information that might enable patients to progress from simple to complex levels. The rehabilitation stresses the need for complete mastery of isolated written segments at a given level, before moving on the upper levels. This is the case, for example, with the Ducarne (1986) range of progressive exercises, each one being adapted to a specific reading problem. This progressive process takes into account the hierarchy of written levels (letters, syllables, words, sentences) and that of internal progression – from the most simple to the most elaborate – of the items belonging to a given level. For example, vowels being considered easier to utter than consonants, they are the ones that initialized the exercises of reading letters aloud. The same kind of hierarchical view works in Luria's (1970) specific exercises aiming at recovering the ability to identify alphabetical characters: patients are required to analyze the *internal structure* of these characters (such as, for the character H, two vertical segments, and one horizontal in between).

The (more or less implicit) theoretical framework underlying these therapies is derived from strongly analytical approaches, in both experimental psychology and neuropsychology. Indeed, first it is in keeping with the traditional psychological hierarchical view of reading and language, and second, with neuropsychological specific approaches to language mechanisms, taken from the *dissociations-fractionations* that one may rely upon to interpret pathological behaviours. Observing selective reading disorders (cf. Shallice, 1988), has led some researchers to infer a set of single components of an underlying modular reading system. For instance, on the one hand, there are patients (surface dyslexics) who read aloud relying only on *spelling–to–sound* regularity (and therefore are neither able to correctly utter irregular words, nor to understand them). On the other hand, other types of patients (i.e. deep dyslexics) rely mainly on *semantic* means, since they are unable to read either letters or non-words, and they often produce semantic errors, that is, uttering semantically related words instead of the lexical items to be read – such as *church* instead of *cathedral* – when reading aloud (such errors are obviously rooted in semantic processes). Therefore the assumption of the existence of two routes, *spelling–to–sound* (or phonological) vs. semantic (or lexical), in the normal reading system. (See also Carlomagno and Lavarone on the application of this processing model to writing.)

Such a dissociation framework is likely to provide a large set of single modular components to characterize reading and language. This is congruent with the main stream of psychological approaches to language and behaviour, which recognizes no other methods for analyzing a complex unity than that of reducing it to its simple elements. The results of this attitude conform more than ever today to what was for Vygotsky (1986) the psychology of the 30s, 'a grandiose atomistic panorama of the disarticulate human mind', justifying therefore our label: *Molecular Psychology,* for these approaches which mimic hard science – namely Molecular Biology – reductionism.

Behaviourism and Reflexology

American behaviourism and Russian reflexology, although developed long before the information processing framework, may be linked to some of the approaches belonging to this framework. Behaviourism derives from the efforts of psychology to establish itself as an objective science, analyzing observable facts (in contrast to introspection). Whatever is studied experimentally is perfectly outlined, controlled, measurable and quantifiable; it concerns stimuli, responses and their relations (in terms of, for example, the number of trials needed to obtain a given response). This theory, claiming the importance of breaking a task down into its simplest elements, has given rise to many step-by-step methods to relearn language in general, and specifically reading. Since such methods are easily programmable, some attempts to use microcomputer-based therapy programs have been proposed, e.g. Katz and Nagy, 1983; (see Katz, Chapter 14, this volume).

The underlying S–R (stimulus–response) theories are mainly physiological: behaviours are somehow the products of a chain of reactions, or reflexes, in terms of neural stimulation, of reinforcement or inhibition of cortical or subcortical connections, leading directly or not – there may be hidden intermediate responses (called *mediational*) – to observable responses. All forms of aphasia therapy being attempts at behaviour modification, Skinner's theory (1938) of *operant conditioning,* which stresses the importance of reinforcement in producing language behaviour, is useful for rehabilitation (cf. Code and Müller, 1989). As Seron (1979: 103–23) points out, 'it also has the potential advantage that by precise specification of the aims and methods of therapy and the aphasic's reaction to it, we can learn more on how to do therapy.'

Reflexology, and Pavlov's approach to the cortex as a 'mosaic of functions ... integrated within a complex dynamic system made up of elements in interaction', foreshadows the latest developments of *connectionism* (e.g. Rumelhart, McClelland and the PDP Research Group, 1986; Sharkey, 1993). Reflexology has been of major theoretical importance in supporting neuro-physiological justifications of language therapy;

elements in interaction are indeed likely to be reorganized in some different form (in the framework of the above mosaic metaphor) if one of them has been impaired. A. R. Luria's (1966) dialectic attempts to understand the higher cortical functions by designing therapies of these functions, and *vice versa*, have resulted in both new interpretations of reading mechanisms and new reading re-education methods.

The postulated possibility of a reorganization of the functional system of reading notably induced Luria to try the reconstitution of the reading ability of patients unable to recognize words, out of unusual ways of proceeding to read. Such a way is to follow, with the finger, the form of the written items to read.[2]

Another example of therapeutic practice similar to this exercise and again rooted in unusual ways of reading, aims to provide a new route for grapheme–to–phoneme links. Through training, a motor stimulus (i.e., a gesture) is associated to a perceptual stimulus (i.e., a grapheme). Such an association created between these stimuli facilities the reorganization of grapheme–to–phoneme correspondences – and therefore improves the patient's lexical responses.

Neurolinguistics vs. Pragmatics

The Chomskian linguistic revolution (Chomsky, 1957) awakened growing interest in formal aspects of language and notably in syntax. Its linguistic approaches led to the formalization of the description of language, just as hard science formalizes the description of its object. These upheavals metamorphosed psycholinguistics and its conceptualization of language mechanisms. Formalization has notably favoured the analytical modular and hierarchical approaches (cf. Fodor, 1983) of the language system, its phonological, syntactic, or semantic modules – and, accordingly, of its pathologies.

Many aphasiologists (such as Goodglass and Gardner in the USA, Hécaen in France, de Bleser in Germany, etc.), interpreting the aphasic's problems in terms of psycholinguistically supported components of language, have developed a *neurolinguistic* approach to aphasia. In the UK, Marshall and Newcombe (1966), observe that semantic features (the postulated elements of the meaning of words) underlie paraphasics errors, since patients often produce paraphasias differing only on a single semantic feature from the target word; the same line of reasoning has been also presented for errors involving phonological features.

The support of linguistics has become inescapable in therapy, offering aid in the design of therapeutic strategies. Specific neurolinguistic approaches to reading therapy (i.e., de Bleser and Weisman, 1981) deal with a range of linguistic problems. For instance, transformational grammar has been used to define a scale of difficulty for sentence reading, enabling appropriate therapeutic exercises to be built, beginning with sentences representing the simplest grammatical construction. On a more general account, therapeutic exercises should be elaborated to meet each specific linguistic problem – the aim of these exercises being to enable patients to deal with such problems. For instance, the handling and overuse of a given standard syntactical structure is considered as allowing both the memorization and the recognition of such a structure.

Pragmatics is devoted to the study of interactions between language and context. It has been developed to try to explain the properties of communication with which linguistic approaches cannot deal. (See Armstrong, Chapter 5, this volume.) Pragmatic therapies aim at enabling patients to make optimal use of all available resources in communication (cf. Albyn Davis, 1989; Carlomagno, 1994). As regards reading, pragmatic therapeutic strategies try to direct attention to extra-linguistic contexts (which may constitute a *prestimulation*, such as a related picture presented before a paragraph to be read. Such a pres-timulation interacts with the reading mechanisms. This was shown to facilitate understanding for severely impaired alexic patients (cf. Pierce and Beckman, 1977). Exercises such as global analysis of a text before trying to read it, enable the patient to grasp its general structure, its main keywords. These exercises may appear as rather similar to pre-stimulations, in that they express a way to contextualize reading out of the text itself.

Pragmatic therapeutic strategies, more generally, aim at developing an active attitude in the patient toward recovering reading abilities. The awareness of the aims of each reading exercise increases the patient's motivation to reach specific goals, such as detecting a given item or retrieving given information in a text. Such goals, which do not require word-by-word reading, could indeed be both directly useful in dealing with texts and (as any kind of prestimulation) indirectly powerful in recovery.

From Cognitive Reading Theories to Rehabilitation Practice

Information Processing vs. Emergence of Meaning

In the era of information processing, the computer metaphor for the mind is prevalent, and a given behaviour (such as reading) is taken to be the output of cognitive processes. *Cognitive science*, a federation of linguistic, cognitive psychology, artificial intelligence, etc., is a *joint venture* to explore the complexity of our cognitive information processing system, and of its range of behaviours.

Cognitive neuropsychology is specifically involved in this joint venture. It assumes that patients operate with a normal cognitive system in which one or more of the components are no longer available (See Edmundson and McIntosh, Chapter 8, this volume). This implies a modular cognitive system made up of a set of rather independent and autonomous components – the kind of errors that patients make being interpreted as reflecting which processes remain available for them or not. The study of aphasia and alexia, and the designing of rehabilitation, has triggered interactions between cognitive science and neuropsychology. Processing models of normal reading could indeed provide an understanding of alexic behaviours in terms of the output of some subset of processes. One of the earliest information processing reading models, the *logogen* (Morton, 1969), built to theoretically support normal subject's psycholinguistic data (resulting namly from lexical decision tasks) is an example of active interactions between normal and pathological reading approaches. Designed to explain normal reading phenomena, it has been very useful in the investigation of alexic phenomena – these investigations resulting in turn in greater sophistication in the model (such as Fig 11.1 (b) vs. Fig 11.1 (a).

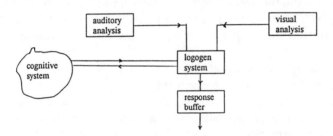

(a)   *Logogen* model (first approach)

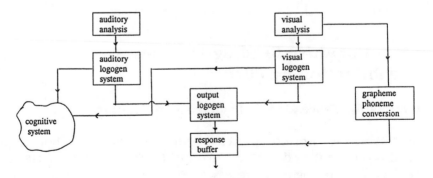

(b)   *Logogen* model (coping with pathological data)

Figure 11.1

In these figures, reading processes appear as external to cognition. The cognitive system in the framework of logogen-like boxes (modules) and arrows is separate and represented as a fuzzy-box. Reading processes are taken to be devoted to perceptual low-level processing, such as letter identification, spelling, etc., that is, all the routines which, by enabling word-recognition, link the perceptual to the cognitive domain through access to word meaning. A concept, the mental lexicon (a kind of store-house for these meanings) has been developed to specify the interface between the two domains (Henderson, 1987). Retrieving the meaning of a given written word from the mental lexicon, first requires a morphological recognition of this word, conditioning access to the representation of its meaning in the lexicon. This representation is then available to feed the cognitive system – as an input to linguistic processes – hence providing the raw material required to build the meaning of sentences and texts (the bricks of linguistic constructions being word meanings) in this information processing framework. The main duty of reading processes is therefore to provide these bricks to the cognitive mechanisms. This explains why both reading models and therapies primarily focus on single word processing (Seron and Deloche, 1889). (See Chapter 12 for applications of such models to writing rehabilitation.)

Such assumptions take for granted the modularity of reading processes, and may appear as more appropriate to support linguistic theories than to support reading behavioural data. Indeed, some of this data is not in keeping with these assumptions; first, a number of usual examples seem to rely on interactions between written word perception, and cognitive-linguistic levels of processing, preventing us from separating the perceptual domain from the other ones. Second, a number of pathological reading data are not compatible with the postulated interface between the linguistic domain and the perceptual one, i.e. the mental lexicon. Rather, this data favours an interactive conception of written language understanding and calls on an emergent view of reading comprehension. We will review some of these arguments and discuss their relevance in rehabilitation.

Emergence of Meaning

Recognition of a given written word out of purely morphological processing, such as letter perception, is assumed to be a prerequisite for retrieving its meaning in the lexicon. Such recognition is therefore taken as perceptual low-level processing, that is a perceptual module on the one-way road to higher cognitive levels.

The example in Figure 11.2 is neither in favour of such a view, nor of an encapsulate perceptual processing approach, since to perceive either *went* vs. *event* or *clear* vs. *dear* (in other words, to perceive different words in front of *identical* handwritten drawings), obviously implies many cognitivo-linguistic high-levels of processing, even at this seemingly earliest stage of letter perception.

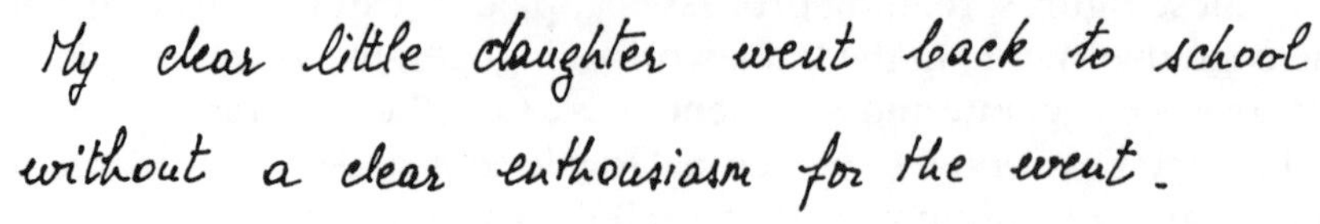

My dear little daughter went back to school without a clear enthousiasm for the event.

Figure 11.2 Examples of hadwritten ambiguities.

This example raises a difficult problem. It clearly demonstrates that handwritten perception and the cognitivo-linguistic domain are inter-dependent (therefore, the identification of a given handwritten word is not merely a pattern recognition problem, i.e., Parisse, Rosenthal and Audrewsky, 1987). This interdependence is not restricted to the case of handwriting, as we may infer from deep-dyslexic patients' identical behaviour when confronted with handwritten or printed material. Indeed, deep dyslexic behaviour[3] provides a range of data which seems to specifically reflect the interdependence of perceptual and cognitive processing, since patients cannot rely upon morphological processing such as grapheme–to–phoneme conversion, which shadows this inter-dependence in normal reading.

Let us recall that deep dyslexic behaviour (cf. Coltheart, Patterson and Marshall, 1980) is evidently not clear cut. It usually involves all of the following range of data: inability to read aloud and/or recognize alphabetic characters, non-words or function-words. Patients read aloud and understand content-words, while often making semantic errors (utterance of some item more or less synonymous to the given written one). Such behaviour highlights (in a rather straightforward way) interesting reading mechanism properties, which together with examples such as the above handwritten one, call on conceptualization of reading in terms of interdependent processing. A functional frame-work for such processing could be a gradual emergence of meaning – a framework which has already been widely developed (cf. for instance, Winograd and Flores, 1986; Andreewsky, 1991). Within this framework, deep-dyslexic's behaviour appears to specifically reflect some starting reading processes.

It is the case of the so-called semantic errors which suit the logic of a gradual emergence of meaning, since these errors may be accounted for as reflecting a stage of fuzzy–meaning – that is a first stage in the emergence of word meaning.

It is also the case for the deep-dyslexic's syntactic impairments. Analogies can be drawn between the starting processes logically required to trigger the emergence of the meaning of sentences, and those which are reflected in the pathological data (Andreewsky, 1986). Patients have a rather good understanding of usual sentences, insofar as meaning could be inferred from the set of the content-words of these sentences; however, deep dyslexics have severe impairments with sentences whose meaning strongly depends upon their syntactical structure and their *function words* (for instance sentences such as: 'the square is *upon* the circle', 'the square is *under* the circle' cannot be matched with the appropriate picture; *passive forms* are understood as if they were active ones, etc). Such impairment may be considered as a failure of the syntactic component of language as a whole. Nevertheless, when reading a sentence, patients utter a given written word only if it occurs as a content-word in this sentence; for instance, a grammatical ambiguity – such as, in French: *sous (penny vs. below)*, or *car (bus vs. because)* – is uttered or not, depending on its grammatical label in the sentence to be read (cf. Andreewsky and Seron, 1975). Such a specific grammatical disambiguation is necessary to discriminate, for instance, nouns from auxiliaries, as in 'John *can* leave a *will*' vs. 'John *will* leave a *can*.' It is a step which could hardly be isolated in the framework of the traditional syntactic component of language. This step only triggers a first idea of these words; their full understanding, to consider the handwritten example in Figure 11.2, should indeed be interactively linked to the understanding of the whole sentence. Nevertheless, the patient's reading behaviour implies both the presence of such discriminations, and the absence of other syntactical cues; these discriminations, given their logical requirement to properly trigger content-words, should constitute a very first step for sentence understanding, in which a preliminary draft of the sentence meaning is defined out of the set of the sentence's content-words. Such a theoretical interpretation of deep dyslexia leads us to search for (and to find) an analog of deep dyslexia for speech dictation or repetition, which we label *Deep Dysphasia* (Michel and Andreewsky, 1983).

Deep-dyslexic behaviour reflects an understanding restricted to this first draft; this is coherent to a gradual emergence of meaning framework, since such a draft may be accounted for as indicative of a stage fuzzy meaning – that is a first step in the emergence.

In terms of such a framework, reading therapies must take into account the ongoing steps of the emergence of the meaning of sentences and texts, in order to improve and refine the understanding of deep-dyslexic patients (and similar patients). Some of the appropriate tasks are semantic association, short-text reporting and the whole set of exercises available for speed-reading training. As in deep-dyslexia, speed-reading should be interpreted as reading restricted to the first steps of understanding (Andreewsky, et al., 1980). Speed reading exercises (some of them being available on microcomputers) have indeed been shown as helpful for deep-dyslexic patients[4]. However, they do not help in the patient's problems with function words, which often remain difficult to resolve.

A number of patients (such as surface dyslexics) demonstrate no evidence of any written understanding; it is often necessary to start the rehabilitation using a spelling mechanism which has been spared to trigger the very first steps of reading. But patients relying mainly on an impaired and slow phonological strategy are severely disturbed, since such a strategy prevents understanding. These patients could be encouraged through speed reading exercises to develop new reading strategies, starting with some emergence of meaning. Such exercises help them to restore the initialization of the emergence processes. Following this, patients could fall back on phonological strategies which can now be used to discover cues for refining understanding. In fact, most alexic patients, who are often also aphasic, present a complex pattern of deep and surface dyslexic behaviors. Such patients show evidence of some limited understanding (when, for instance, they are producing semantic errors) as well as some preserved ability to identify letters and to use phonological strategies – the latter being potentially useful to interact with and to improve the former.

Our examples clearly imply that reading mechanism components, be they perceptual or cognitive, are strongly interacting and therefore interdependent. In spite of attempts to reduce these mechanisms to independent modules (or components), reading remains a highly complex phenomenon. Reading therapy should be coherent with the framework of this complex functional system, keeping in mind that therapy is not devoted to restoring any isolated processing module, but rather to dealing with the main function of the whole reading system – that is understanding.

Notes
1. Gall's theory was far from being orthodox. Gall was even excommunicated by Rome, and his books forbidden. He aimed to forge an alternative theory to metaphysics or vitalism, which were the only possible explanations accepted at that time for intellectual abilities.
2. Such a theoretical approach to word recognition has not only helped alexics, but has also been successful in the very different domain of automatic handwritten recognition (computers being to date almost alexics as regards handwritten texts!). The powerful computer system conceived by the Russian mathematician S. Guberman: Newton (Apple Corp.), is able to deal with handwritten input data and has been designed in the theoretical light of this Luria's re–education exercise (Guberman, 1991; Guberman and Andreewsky, in preparation).
3. We may recall (cf. supra) that deep dyslexic behaviour is taken to derive from processes restricted to one (main) normal reading route. But the deep dyslexic pattern of data is nevertheless difficult to account for in terms of such a one way route to the mental lexicon. An *interdependent processing* framework is a more relevant approach to the logical coherence of this pattern; therefore the theoretical relevance of this framework.
4. Dr M. Desi, Head of the Neurological and Neuropsychological Rehabilitation Center, Centre Hospitalo-Universitaire, 94275 Le Kremlin-Bicêtre, France, personal Communication.

References

Albyn Davis G, (1989) Pragmatics and cognition in treatment of language disorders, in Seron X, Deloche G (Eds) Cognitive Approaches in Neuropsychological Rehabilitation. 317–53.

Andreewsky E, (1986) Quelques questions inhérentes à la compréhension du langage, in Le Moigne JL (Ed) Intelligence des mécanisles, mécanismes de l'intelligence. Paris: Fayard. 213–28.

Andreewsky E, (Ed)(1991) Systémique et Cognition. Paris: Dunod.

Andreewsky E, Deloche G, Kossanyi P, (1980) Analogies between speed reading and deep dyslexia, in Coltheart M, Patterson K, Marshall J (Eds) Deep Dyslexia. London: Routledge and Kegan, 307–25.

Andreewsky E, Seron X (1975) Implicit processing of grammatical rules in a classical case of agrammatism. Cortex: 379–90.

de Bleser R, Weismann H (1981) Uebergang von Struktürübungen zum spontänen Dialog in der Therapie von Aphasikern. Sprache–Stimme Gehör 5:74–9.

Carlomagno S (1994) Pragmatic Approaches to Aphasia Therapy. London: Whurr.

Chomsky N (1957) Syntactic Structures. The Hague: Mouton.

Code C, Muller DJ, (1989) Perspectives in aphasia therapy: an overview. In Code C, Muller DJ (Eds) Aphasia Therapy (2nd edition). London: Cole and Whurr.

Coltheart M, Patterson K, Marshall J (Eds) (1980) Deep Dyslexia. Routledge and Kegan.

Deloche G, Andreewsky E, Desi M (1981) Lexical meaning: a case report, some striking phenomenon, theoretical implications. Cortex, 17:147–52.

Ducarne de Ribaucourt B (1986) Rééducation sémiologique de l'aphasie. Paris: Masson.

Fodor JA (1983) The Modularity of Mind. Cambridge, MA: MIT Press.

Freud S (1953/1891) On Aphasia. London: Imago Publishing Co. Ltd.

Goldstein K (1948) Language and Language Disturbances. New York: Grune & Stratton.

Guberman GA (1991) Vision par ordinateur et Gestalt–théorie, Revue Internationale de Systémique, 5 (2):157–70.

Henderson L (1987) Word recognition: a tutorial review. In Coltheart M (Ed) Attention and Performance XII: The Psychology of Reading. 171–200.

Howard D, Hatfied FM (1987) Aphasia Therapy, Historical and Contemporary Issues. London: Lawrence Erlbaum Associates.

Jackson JH (1978) On affections of speech from disease of the brain, in Brain 1:304–30.

Katz RC, Nagy VT (1983) A computerised approach for improving word recognition in chronic aphasic patients, in Brookshire R H (Ed), Clinical Aphasiology Conference Proceedings, Minneapolis MN: BRK.

Luria AR (1970) Traumatic Aphasia. Mouton: La Haye.

Marshal JC, Newcombe F (1966) Syntactic and Semantic Errors in Paralexia, Neuropsychologia, 169–76.

Michel F, Andreewsky E (1983) An analog to deep dyslexia in auditive modality. Brain and Language 18 (2):212–23.

Molière (1666/1934) Le Médecin malgré lui, Paris: Garnier.

Morton J (1969), Interaction of information in word recognition. Psychological Review 76:165–78.

Ombrédane A (1951) L'aphasie et l'élaboration de la pensée explicite. Paris: PUF.

Parisse C, Rosenthal V, Andreewsky E (1987) An approach to machine recognition of handwritten texts. In Rose J (Ed): Cybernetics and Systems: Present and Future. 1:185–88.

Pierce RS, Beekman L (1977) Effects of linguistic and extralinguistic context on semantic and syntactic processing in aphasia, in Journal of Speech and Hearing Research 20:669–83.

Rumelhart DE, McClelland JL, the PDP Research Group (Eds) (1986) Parallel distributed Processing. Explorations in the Microstructure of Cognition. Cambridge, MA: MIT Press/Bradford Books.

Seron X (1979) Aphasie et Neuropsychologie: Approches Thérapeutiques. Brussels: Mardaga.

Seron X, Deloche G (1989) Cognitive Approaches in Neuropsychological Rehabilitation. Hillsdale NJ: Lawrence Erlbaum Associates.

Shallice T (1988) From Neuropsychology to Mental Structure, Boston, MA: Cambridge University Press.

Sharkey N (1993) Connexionist Natural Language Processing. Oxford: Intellect Books.

Skinner BF (1938) Verbal Behaviour. New York: Appleton–Century–Crofts.

Vygotsky LS (1986), Thought and Language. Translated by Hanfmann E, Vakar G, Cambridge MA: MIT Press, (First Russian edition, 1934).

Winograd T, Flores F (1986) Understanding Computers and Cognition: A New Foundation for Design. Norwood: Ablex.

Chapter 12
Writing Rehabilitation in Aphasic Patients

SERGIO CARLOMAGNO AND ALESSANDRO IAVARONE

Dysgraphic phenomena have been reported in the earliest literature on language disturbances in brain damaged people. However, writing disturbances in aphasic patients have usually been considered a secondary aspect of their communication disorder. This point of view was supported by the (quite general) assumption that writing is a mere graphemic translation of spoken language. Consequently, for a long time, retraining in writing for aphasic patients was assumed only as an additional treatment task for 'global stimulation' of language. However, the view that writing cannot be considered only graphemic transcoding of spoken language has gained acceptance among neuropsychologists and aphasia therapists. This hypothesis was acknowledged by Hatfield and Weddell (1976) where the main aims of retraining aphasics in writing were stated in detail and selective intervention methods were tested.

In the last decade a number of papers have aimed to describe dysgraphic disturbances in brain damaged people in the framework of information processing analysis (see Edmundson and McIntosh, Chapter 8, and Lesser, Chapter 9, this volume). Such a framework allows us to explain dysgraphic patterns in terms of impaired and intact components of the processing system. The information processing approach led therapists to develop cognitively oriented therapeutic programmes for dysgraphia (Hatfield, 1983; Behrmann, 1987; Carlomagno and Parlato, 1989). This provided theoretical insight into describing the nature of the deficit and interpreting the effects of the treatment. Furthermore, it was claimed that the nature of the dysgraphic impairment (identification of the locus of damage within the processing model) could predict the way in which the dysgraphia should be treated. This optimistic view has been recently mitigated by the observation that these rehabilitation programmes did not replicate from successfully treated cases to patients suffering from a comparable deficit (Hillis and Caramazza, 1994). However, treatment strategies have been tied to different views about mechanism(s) of functional recovery.

Briefly, in some cases the treatment plan was intended to restore functioning of the processing system as in the pre-lesional situation: the *functional restitution* or *re-establishment* approach. In other studies the treatment aimed to reorganize cognitive functioning by recourse to an alternative response strategy: the *functional substitution* or *reorganization* hypothesis. This dichotomy (see Weniger and Taylor Sarno, 1990, for a detailed discussion) has received less attention than relationships between putative locus of impairment and treatment. However, it might provide a basis for interpreting success or failure of treatment.

In this chapter we debate whether and which therapeutic interventions have been effective in improving aphasics' writing skills. We present a survey of the literature on writing rehabilitation and discuss aims, methods and results. However, in order to reach a conclusion for everyday therapeutic practice, our survey will take into account cognitive interpretations of dysgraphic impairments and hypotheses about the effect of therapeutic interventions on functional recovery. Finally, we discuss to what extent writing rehabilitation plays a role in improving the everyday communication skills of aphasic patients.

Effectiveness of Retraining in Writing for Aphasic Patients

Earliest Group Studies

In 1976 Hatfield and Weddell discussed writing retraining in severe aphasic patients using different methods. Three main objectives motivated their study. First, it was assumed that treating dysgraphia could contribute to recovery of speech. The second objective was to see if spelling retraining would be effective in reducing a significant handicap which hinders the occupational rehabilitation of patients or their communication capabilities in everyday life. The third question asked if improved writing skills could supplement defective spoken language in cases of disartria or severe Broca's aphasia. Despite the traditional view that written language is closely linked to spoken language, this asks if writing could improve without speech improving. The authors write 'the question is raised about the extent to which the written language system is tied to the spoken system ...' (p.77).

One of the treatments, the *visual-kinaesthetic* method, consisted of a step-by-step passage from simple copy to copy-from-memory and, finally, to writing from dictation. The therapy aimed to restore, by visual (and/or visuomotor) strategies, writing of words of practical importance in everyday life. Two patients suffering from severe expressive aphasia were treated. The results showed a significant improvement in one patient. When retested, one month after therapy completion, there was little retention of treated words but there was some learning of partial knowledge about spelling (e.g. of initial letter, approximate word length and consonant-vowel structure).

In the second treatment, *global stimulation*, the subject tried to write target words after he was repeatedly exposed to words presented in different contexts: copying the word, sentence completion task, reading and so on. One global aphasic patient (case S3) received two therapy sessions a week for two months. In each session, four words were trained, and on each occasion there was a pre-test and a post-test for treated words (writing from dictation). The post-session test scores showed that there was some learning across the session. However, a retest after one month showed that the improvement had not been maintained. A qualitative analysis showed that the best preserved spelling features were the approximate word length and the initial letter of the stimulus. The third method was based on the suggestion that writing involves a segmental transformation of phonological strings into their graphemic counterparts (Luria et al., 1969). That was regarded by Hatfield and Weddell as an effective method, since practising of phoneme-grapheme correspondence rules in some words could be generalized to untreated words. The authors treated two patients by practising auditory phonemic analysis of words, i.e. *moon* → /m/ + /u/ + /n/, and some phoneme-grapheme correspondences, i.e. pairing a single phoneme with the first phoneme of a familiar word, /m/ → *mother,* and writing the corresponding letter. The first patient (case S4) progressed on phonemic analysis but she was unable to set up phoneme-grapheme correspondences. For instance, attempting to write letter M of nonsense syllable *lem* she repeated /m/ several time and she wrote down ER. Note that she had been trained to pair the phoneme /m/ with the first letter of the word *mother* in order to cue the letter M. In the same way, when writing the letter M of the word *lamb*, she repeated /m/ but she wrote down the letter B. According to Hatfield and Weddell writing ER, the final letters of the word mother, or B, which is the silent final letter in *lamb*, could suggest persistence of visual images of words which interfered with the phoneme-grapheme procedure. The second patient (case S5) appeared to be more sensitive to this training. Unfortunately, since she was Austrian, intrusions of German phoneme-grapheme correspondences prevented the authors from showing significant recovery.

Results of the study by Hatfield and Weddell (1976) failed to show any stable effects of the methods used in the study. It is likely, however, that, since the study involved severe aphasic patients, failure to find maintained performance could be due to the gravity of aphasic disturbances. From the theoretical point of view, we should note that the global stimulation approach to dysgraphic disturbance was defined as an *umbrella approach* which 'weakens consolidation of any theory' (p.77). Thus, the authors attempted to define two selective methods for retraining in writing aphasic patients and the two methods were structured to match the functional deficit.

Then it was stressed that spelling in normal adults, aside from translation of phonemes into graphemes, can reflect visually based procedures. It was thus suggested that visual strategies also, tied to writing procedures used by normal spellers, could be useful in patients with severely reduced spoken language. Visual memorizing of whole word forms was found to be ineffective. However, some visual features of written words (initial letter, approximate word length and consonant-vowel structure) were found to be preserved in patients who had received visual treatment. Furthermore, a particular writing behaviour was observed in spontaneous responses of patients S3 and S4. For instance, attempting to write the word *thin,* patient S3 wrote first the N, then the I, then the T and last the H, achieving the correct spelling. Such writing in non-linear order and the preserved visual features of words were suggested to be linked to spontaneous visual strategies which could be exploited in future treatment programmes.

On the other hand, practising phonemic analysis and phoneme-grapheme correspondences could result in improved writing for patients with partially preserved spoken language. That was the case for patient S5, although the improvement was confined to the German language. Finally, it was also suggested that the nature of dysgraphia could be taken into account in dealing with the one or the other therapeutic programme. However, this particular point was not further discussed, perhaps because of lack of a theoretically driven classification of dysgraphic disturbances. The choice of treatment indeed was based only on clinical criteria.

Another investigation of the treatment of writing disorders in aphasic patients was carried out by Seron, *et al.,* 1980, using a computer-aided technique. The method, which aimed at retraining patients by typewriting from dictation, provided them with visual cues: the number of letters in the target; the relative position of the letter in the string, and so on. Progression was assured by fading out cues and by increasing the orthographic complexity of the stimuli. Furthermore, in order to test for learning transfer, in the testing sessions a separate list of stimuli was used and patients were requested to use handwriting.

A first post-test showed a significant improvement in all subjects for percentage of words correctly written, for total number of errors and for similarity between responses and target items. At the second post-test, six weeks later, no retention of the improvement was found except in the case of one patient whose improvement, according to the authors, could have been due to spontaneous recovery.

Again Seron and coworkers' results suggest that writing rehabilitation in aphasic patients does not seem useful. However, the results pointed out that spontaneous compensatory strategies should be taken into account to explain failure to find positive results. As a matter of fact, analysis of writing errors showed that most patients were writing by phoneme-grapheme correspondences since the majority of errors were plausible phonemic errors: i.e., /o/ → o instead of → au or → eau which in French sound alike. Furthermore, the orthographic complexity of the target was found to be an important source of errors since performance on words with as many letters as phonemes was significantly better than on words containing more graphemes than phonemes, i.e., /lavabo/ → lavabo vs /manto/ → manteau. Such errors indicated a spontaneous tendency for patients to write by phoneme-grapheme correspondence which was in conflict with the technique which stimulated visual strategies. We discuss the relevance of these compensatory strategies later.

Single Case Studies

A further contribution in dysgraphic rehabilitation was supplied by Hatfield (1983) using information processing models. Such models of writing have been put forward by Morton (1980); Shallice (1981); Ellis (1984). Typical information processing models of writing function can be summarized as follows (see Figure 12.1). Writing, like reading, involves two primary routes. The first entails the direct retrieval of word spelling which is stored in the orthographic output lexicon (lexical route). The second route involves segmental translation from phonology to orthography (phonological route or phoneme-grapheme conversion). According to these dual route models, acquired dysgraphia can be explained in terms of damage of one or more components of the processing system. Thus, dysgraphia may be classified into *surface* or *lexical*, where the lexical route is impaired, while phoneme-grapheme conversion is spared (Beauvois and Dérouesnè, 1981). In *phonological* dysgraphia, the reverse occurs (Shallice, 1981), and in *deep dysgraphia*, phoneme-grapheme conversion is unavailable and the lexical route may also be damaged at different levels of processing (Bub and Kertesz, 1982, Ellis, 1984).

Hatfield conducted a detailed investigation of four patients aimed at classifying them according to the proposed model. Three patients were shown to exhibit the writing pattern of deep dysgraphia, i.e., pronounceable nonsense letter strings could not be written, because of defective non-lexical procedures, and partial damage of the lexical route prevented them from writing abstract and function words. The fourth exhibited the pattern of surface dysgraphia. In this case, since the lexical route was impaired, the patient made many errors in writing

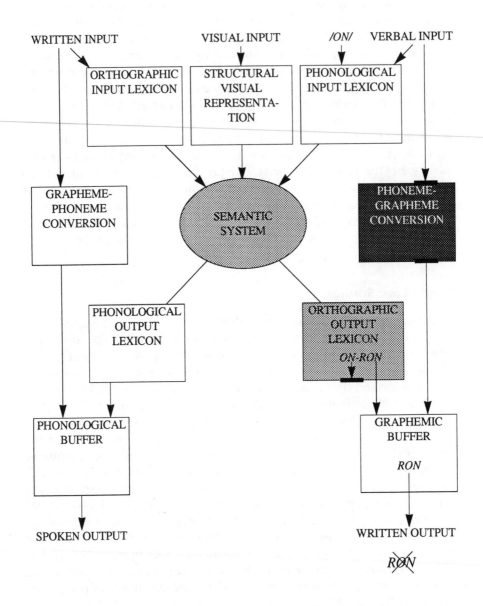

Figure 12.1 A model for the processing of writing and reading. In the schema the therapeutic hypothesis for treatment of the deep dysgraphic patient BB (Hatfield, 1983) is schematically represented.

irregular words, i.e. those words where phoneme-grapheme conversion procedures alone do not produce correct spelling, for example, the word *yacht* in English. Hatfield proposed to *reorganize* the writing function using the better preserved of the two routes: i.e., in the case of the deep dysgraphic patients, the partially spared lexical route. It was observed that one deep dysgraphic patient, BB, when attempting to write the function word *in*, spontaneously spelled the homophonic content word *inn*. The training method was linked to the spontaneous strategy exhibited by the patient. It involved instructing the patient to write, by means of the spared lexical route, a content word which was homophonic or quasi-homophonic with the target function word and then to correct the spelling. For example, to write the word *on* the patient was instructed to write the name *Ron* and then to delete the *R*. In this case the function of the word *Ron* was acknowledged to bypass the impaired access to the spelling of the word *on*, (see Figure 12.1). The therapeutic programme yielded positive results in the case of patient BB, since his score on function words rose from 34 per cent to 63.5 per cent.

Hatfield's study highlighted some theoretical implications for planning writing rehabilitation programmes. It was first assumed necessary to have a clear picture of the cognitive processes underlying writing function in normal literate adults. Second, malfunctioning and intact processes had to be identified with a theoretically driven testing procedure. Finally, it was suggested that writing could be reorganized by recourse to (partially) spared component(s) of the writing system.

Hatfield's study was pioneering in that it demonstrated the application of a processing model to therapy. In a further single case study, Behrmann (1987) presented a homophone retraining programme which was implemented with the surface dysgraphic patient CCM. In this case pre-therapy testing showed that the lexical route was impaired: CCM produced regularization errors when writing irregular words, i.e.: *shoes* → *shuse*, and non-homographic homophones, i.e., *no* versus *know*. The treatment was intended to pair a written homophone with its pictorial representation so that the orthography of the target item was linked to the corresponding meaning. Training activities included copying, matching words with their pictorial representation, writing from dictation, selecting the correct spelling in a multiple choice task and so on. There was significant improvement in writing treated homophones and untreated irregular words.

According to Behrmann, in the case of CCM, the cognitive processing model allowed the identification of a malfunctioning component of writing (the orthographic output lexicon) and the development of a therapeutic programme focused on the impaired aspect. However, with respect to Hatfield's 1983 study, there is an important difference when the nature of improvement is considered. Behrmann aimed to restore, by direct training, the activity of the damaged component of the processing system: i.e., the orthographic output lexicon. In contrast, Hatfield used residual processing abilities to achieve a functional recovery in an unusual way. Note that in Hatfield's study there was an explicit prediction about the behaviour underlying the improvement.

The last therapeutic strategy was developed by de Partz (1986) for a deep dyslexic[1] patient. This patient was unable to read nonwords aloud, had difficulties with function words and abstract words and made semantic paralexias. To improve his oral reading he was trained to apply grapheme-phoneme correspondence by means of a lexical relay code. In this approach, the patient, who was unable to sound out letters, had to pair graphemes with the initial phonemes of familiar words, i.e., *m* → /m-aman/. This one-to-one conversion strategy allowed him to retrieve the correct phonological output of the target item. After nine months of treatment his reading performance significantly improved both on words and nonwords. However, difficulties persisted on words where a sequence of graphemes corresponds to a single phoneme (see above *manteau*), and on words where the phonemic value of an ambiguous grapheme is context-related, i.e., *g* in *gateau* or in *genre*. Thus the post-therapy reading pattern was indeed that of a *surface* dyslexia. In other words, recovery was linked to acquisition of a reading strategy different from those reading procedures used in the pre-lesional state or in the pre-therapy period.

Returning to Hatfield's (1983) and Behrmann's (1987) studies, both authors claimed that their therapeutic programmes were explicitly based on a model describing the organization of cognitive processing underlying writing function. Such a conclusion, however, has been recently questioned by Hillis and Caramazza (1994). They have argued that while cognitive theory may offer a detailed description of the quality of surface symptoms suggesting a specific locus of damage, the diagnosis itself does not allow the conclusion that the damaged component can be remedied nor can it predict which factors might influence functional recovery.

To support their claim, Hillis and Caramazza (1990) described some rehabilitation studies carried out on individual patients suffering from deficits of lexical processing. For instance (see study 1) patient SJD, was suffering from severe impairments of phonological procedures and from partial damage to the orthographic output lexicon (deep dysgraphia). These deficits accounted for a high rate of omissions and semantic paragraphias when writing verbs. However, the phonological output lexicon was spared and she was taught to use intact oral naming and to convert the phonological form of verbs to the corresponding orthographic form. The treatment procedure entailed teaching SJD to associate a phoneme with a keyword she could spell. The keyword contained in the first position the grapheme corresponding to the first phoneme of the verb. Writing the first letter allowed SJD to cue the complete orthographic representation of the word. Phoneme-grapheme correspondences were successfully acquired by SJD and she could prevent semantic paragraphias or omissions when writing verbs.

SJD's positive therapy results were contrasted by Hillis and Caramazza (1994) with failure in the case of patient PM. This patient was also suffering from impaired phoneme-grapheme conversion and an impairment to the orthographic output lexicon, but a spared phonological output lexicon. Following treatment PM was unable to set up phoneme-grapheme correspondences and to use them when writing.

According to such results (see also other studies in the same paper), it is evident that the identification of locus of impairment with reference to a model of cognitive functioning does not predict the way in which an efficient therapeutic programme might be constructed. For the latter purpose, according to Hillis and Caramazza

> we would need not only a theory of the cognitive mechanisms which underlie a specific cognitive function, and how these may be affected by brain damage, but also, and more importantly, a theory of how a damaged system may be affected by specific therapeutic procedures. (Hillis and Caramazza, 1994: 450).

We would note, however, that the authors assumed that damage of component A (orthographic output lexicon) should have predicted the effectiveness of rehabilitation procedures focusing on the impaired component B (conversion of a phoneme into the corresponding grapheme). That seems unconvincing without assuming that therapeutic interventions must, *in any case*, restore functioning of the damaged component B (re-establishment hypothesis). Conversely, the effectiveness of treatments focusing on the component B could likely rely on residual processing of the component B and on effectiveness of cognitive skills which should enable the patient to use it (reorganization hypothesis). The last interpretation of the functional recovery might explain the difference between SJD and PM found by Hillis and Caramazza (1994). For instance, in the former case residual processing could be made available by means of an overt response strategy, i.e., matching the first phoneme with the appropriate keyword and writing the first grapheme. In contrast, in the case of PM, failure to set up sound-letter correspondences could have arisen from interfering lexical procedures (see, for instance, case S4 described by Hatfield and Weddell, (1976). Alternatively, residual skills did not allow the development of appropriate response strategies, i.e., unlike SJD, PM was unable to perform phonological segmentation of the stimulus.

Consistent with the reorganization hypothesis were results of a single case study by Carlomagno and Parlato (1989). The patient, OG, was found mildly dyslexic and severely dysgraphic when assessed over a period of 15 months. He exhibited a particular reading pattern. For instance, he regularized stress, i.e., *èsile* (thin) → *esìle* (nonword), and made confusion between non-homographic homophones, i.e., *l'una* (one o'clock) versus *luna* (moon) in Italian. These errors suggested that the lexical route was unavailable and that reading was supported by grapheme-phoneme conversion procedures, see Coltheart, *et al.,* 1983. However, whilst word reading was about 80 per cent correct he scored only 30 per cent correct on nonword reading. To explain such a dissociation (a reading pattern similar to that of phonological dyslexia but reading errors similar to those of surface dyslexia) it was suggested that also non-lexical reading procedures were also partially damaged. However, word reading was deemed to take advantage of a spontaneous lexical strategy which enabled OG to access orthographic phonological correspondences more efficiently. In other words OG's reading likely consisted in segmenting a letter string into syllabic or subsyllabic units. In this way phonological counterparts were obtained for each unit. Finally, the resulting phonological units were assembled by matching with the phonological structure of a real word (lexical relay) to produce an oral response. This hypothesis was supported by 80 per cent correct reading of nonwords homophonic with a word, i.e., *cuadro* (nonword) instead of *quadro* (painting). (See Dèrouesné and Beauvois (1979) for a description of a similar pattern).

The therapy programme was to instruct the patient to apply an analogous strategy of lexical relay (code-name) between phonological coded syllables and their graphemic forms. Briefly, the patient was trained to orally segment a dictated stimulus, to link each syllabic unit to a code-name and, finally, to write the syllabic unit. Upon completion of the treatment programme, OG scored 83 per cent correct on writing words and 80 per cent correct on nonwords (pre-therapy score 34 per cent and 10 per cent respectively, and the improvement generalized to nonword reading (post-therapy score 80 per cent). We emphasize that such a finding could not be predicted on the basis of the re-establishment hypothesis. If therapy had re-established syllabic graphemephoneme correspondences. We have reason to think that functional recovery of OGs writing was linked to the acquisition of a response strategy which allowed him to use residual phoneme-grapheme and grapheme-phoneme correspondences. That response developed as a substitute for defective processing abilities (re-organization hypothesis).

We will discuss two further single case studies which have provided support to the functional substitution (re-organization) hypothesis in approaching writing rehabilitation. Zesiger and de Partz (1991) described a therapy programme for a surface dysgraphic patient. This patient was found to produce mainly regularization errors (93 per cent) when writing irregular words. Furthermore, in a lexical decision task he showed a high rate of errors on irregular words and on nonwords homophonic with real words. The last finding suggested additional damage to the orthographic input lexicon which prevented him from using reading skills as a correction device for his writing deficit. Treatment involved pairing of the written irregular word with the corresponding pictorial representations as in Behrmann's (1987) study. However, the pictorial representation was embedded into an orthographic representation of the word. For instance, the two Ms of the word *flamme* (flame) were represented as tongue-shaped portions of fire. Following this procedure, memorizing the orthographic representation of the word was assumed to be cued by visual imagery. This hypothesis was supported by results since, at post-therapy testing, items treated by means of the imagery procedure were better than words treated by means of simple memorizing of whole word forms. Furthermore, the patient was shown to apply by himself the procedure of visual imagery and to retain what he had learned six months after therapy ended.

The second study was performed by Ferrand and Deloche (1991) on a patient suffering from severe Broca's aphasia. He exhibited a marked deficit of the phonological route of writing: he could not write nonwords, nonsense syllables or single letters. Furthermore, a marked effect of word length, i.e., monosyllabic words, were written correctly while polysyllabic words were not, suggested an additional deficit of the graphemic buffer (see Figure 12.1). The therapeutic strategy aimed to instruct the patient to segment dictated words into monosyllabic words, i.e., *boisson* (drink) → *bois* (wood) + *son* (sound) and to write them. Note that for the two words there are a few non-homographic homophonic words, i.e., *boit* (he drinks) or *sont* (they are), which could have biased the therapeutic programme. However, Ferrand and Deloche assumed that, since results from a lexical decision task indicated a spared orthographic input lexicon, the patient could use it as a correction device for the words to be written. Results agreed with the prediction, as the patient's score in writing polysyllabic words increased from 28 per cent to 85 per cent.

It should be stressed that, in both studies, there was an explicit prediction about the role of component(s) not belonging to the writing system in organizing the response strategy. Visual imagery was deemed to support learning the orthographic form of words in the case described by Zesiger and de Partz (1991), while the orthographic input lexicon, a component belonging to the reading system, was assumed to correct written responses in the case by Ferrand and Deloche (1991). Such an interpretation of functional recovery might be extended to those therapeutic attempts where functional recovery was deemed to be consistent with restoration of a damaged component.

Consider, for example, the writing improvement obtained by CCM (Behrmann, 1987). According to her hypothesis, the treatment restored functioning of the orthographic output lexicon so that CCM became able to retrieve orthographic representations of treated homophones and of irregular words. An alternative explanation is possible. At pre-therapy testing, CCM correctly read aloud irregular words and did not show confusion with non-homographic homophonic words, which would indicate that the orthographic input lexicon was spared. This module could offer the patient a visual check mechanism for monitoring the orthographic features of words she was writing. In other words functional recovery could be due not to re-establishment of the orthographic output lexicon but to acquisition of a new writing strategy involving knowledge of whole word forms stored in the orthographic input lexicon. On the other hand, we should note that patient BB (Hatfield, 1983) and patient OG (Carlomagno and Parlato, 1989), before starting their successful rehabilitation programmes, had been trained by practising letter-to-sound correspondences. However, in both cases there was no learning, i.e., restoration of phoneme-grapheme correspondences. On the contrary, in both cases, it was possible to obtain functional recovery by means of particular response strategies.

On the whole, results of single case studies support the hypothesis that writing rehabilitation is effective. However, the effectiveness of each programme appears to be constrained not only by the interpretation of dysgraphic disturbances but also by the interpretation of mechanisms subserving recovery. We will return in the conclusion to the relevance of these issues for therapeutic practice.

From Single Cases to Group Studies: Returning to Everyday Therapeutic Practice

The two treatment strategies, visual (visuo-lexical) and phonological, originally suggested by Hatfield and Weddell (1976), could be predicted by cognitive models where both lexical and phoneme-grapheme conversion routes are acknowledged to underlie writing function. However, contrary to almost all single case studies, group studies failed to demonstrate significant effects of these rehabilitation approaches.

A recent study by Carlomagno, et al., (1991a) support the hypothesis that in the study by Hatfield and Weddell (1976) failure to find positive effects for treatment was due to individual variability in organizing an effective response strategy. Six chronic aphasics patients were treated with two treatment programmes intended to stimulate writing by using either phoneme-grapheme conversion procedures or lexical strategies. A written naming task, structured as a crossword puzzle of increasing difficulty, was used to stimulate writing via the lexical route (visual-semantic treatment). Patients were given semantic information and visual cues about targets and these were faded out across sessions (see Table 12.1).

Table 12.1 The visual-semantic treatment used by Carlomagno et al. (1991b).

Task	Available cue
Step 1	
Copy and delayed copy semantic distracters.	The target is presented with phonological, visual and
Step 2	
Serial ordering of letters belonging to target	Prepositioning of the first letter or of a central letter. The number of letters belonging to the target is available. Additional treatment may involve the final letter.
Step 3	
As in step 2	The letters belonging to the target are given with 2 or 3 distracters. Other cues as in step 2.
Step 4	
Handwriting	The number of letters belonging to the target is available.

The treatment task is written naming arranged in a crossword puzzle. It involves 80 items (40 objects and 40 action) whose names are controlled for length (4–9 letters), frequency and orthographic complexity[2]. The items are arranged in groups of 10 which are alternated in each session in order to avoid overtraining on a few items. The treatment follows a progression rate through different steps. In each of them one or more visual cues are available as illustrated above. Usually, to move from one step to the next, patients have to obtain a score of 80 per cent correct responses. The programme has been implemented on a Macintosh computer. In this case the target figure is displayed on the screen with the available cues. The patient writes by keyboard and he or she can select, by means of the mouse, the position where he or she wants. Feedback is provided and the correct letter appears. The computer programme provides a listing of the patients responses and an analysis of errors. Finally, new target items can be easily introduced by means of an image scanner.

Conversely, nonword writing from dictation with phonological cues (keywords) was used to improve writing by non-lexical phoneme-grapheme correspondence (phonological treatment). This last treatment was similar to that used by Carlomagno and Parlato (1989) although it involved a single letter level. Writing assessment (pre- and post-therapy) included written naming and writing words and nonwords from dictation in order to control for pattern(s) of improvement, and, in order to control for learning transfer, practise lists contained items different from those used in assessment. The six patients received each of the two treatments in a cross-over ABCB time-series design, where B was a non-writing therapy and A and C were one of the two writing rehabilitation programmes.

Group results showed a significant improvement which appeared to be due to the two treatment programmes, since no writing improvement was observed following the non-writing therapy. Furthermore, patients retained what they had learned 40–50 days after completion of treatment (see Figure 12.2).

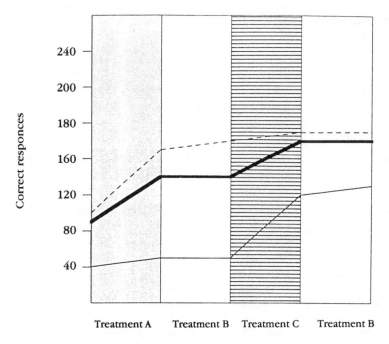

Figure 12.2 A schematic representation of major results obtained by Carlomagno, et al., 1991b. (——) Whole group, (———) Patient GI, (----) Patient ZG

Although overall results showed that both rehabilitation strategies had been effective, looking at single case results showed that in 3 out of the 6 patients phonological treatment was effective, whereas the visual-semantic was not. For instance, patient GI produced only 45 correct out of 240 stimuli (pre-therapy score = 41) after visual-semantic treatment. In contrast, after phonological treatment, 116 correct responses were recorded. The reverse pattern was observed in ZG who scored 167 correct responses after visual-semantic treatment (pre-therapy score = 95), whereas no improvement could be found after phonological treatment. For the remaining two patients we observed a strong effect for the visual-semantic treatment but an effect for the phonological was still present.

To explain these findings Carlomagno *et al.,* (1991a) have suggested that previous group studies did not take into account the variability of each patient in organizing an appropriate response strategy. For instance, patient 4 in the study of Hatfield and Weddell (1976) was trained to write by phoneme-grapheme correspondence but he was described as spontaneously applying visual strategies. Furthermore, the patients who participated in the study by Seron and coworkers (1980) were given visual cues. However, they were shown to use mostly phonological transcoding. In other words, spontaneous responses were found, in both cases, to rely upon residual writing procedures different from those the therapy programme was addressing. In contrast, each patient improved by means of one of the two therapeutic treatments, probably the one which was stimulating a spontaneous tendency to use residual lexical or non-lexical processing.

Further results from the study were consistent with this hypothesis. Patterns of improvement were found to be consistent with the writing procedure that each programme intended to stimulate. As a matter of fact only, written naming and word writing improved by the visual-semantic treatment (stimulating lexical procedure) whereas the effect of the phonological treatment produced better performance only on transparent[2] words and on nonwords (non-lexical procedure). This finding suggests that an effective treatment method should stimulate only one of the two writing procedures: i.e., avoid activating interfering strategies.

Note that the phonological treatment used nonword writing from dictation which was unlikely to allow patients to use lexical strategies. On the other hand, the visual-semantic treatment avoided activating phonological writing by means of a crossword puzzle task, i.e., the typi- cal task where normal subjects use visual and semantic information to cue whole word forms of target items. It should be stressed that the study by Carlomagno and coworkers involved unselected aphasic patients. Thus, it was assumed that in almost all patients both writing routes were damaged but residual knowledge of orthographic repre- sentations of words and/or residual phoneme to grapheme conversion procedures could be still present.

Residual knowledge of whole word forms was shown by Ellis (1982) in the erroneous responses of a deep dysgraphic patient. Hatfield (1985) made a similar observation describing the writing behaviour of another deep dysgraphic patient. This patient was consistently found to write letters of the target in non-linear order. The rate of correct letters was related to the temporal order in which they were written and not to the serial position within the word. Furthermore, erroneous responses respected length and shape of the target word. This suggested that the patient maintained some knowledge of the whole word form of the target stimulus and he could use it for accessing orthographic representations. We have already mentioned that similar behaviour had been previously described in patients S3 and S4 by Hatfield and Weddell (1976) and by Seron et al., (1980) in patients(s) of their cohort.

The visual-semantic treatment devised by Carlomagno et al., (1991a) trained patients to assist written naming through semantic and visual cues. The visual cues were not different from those partial responses which were found to underlie spontaneous compensatory strategies in the above mentioned studies (see Table 12.1). Following the visual-semantic treatment, patient ZG became able to spell correctly untreated items both in written naming and word writing from dictation. It was argued that the patient became able to access the whole word forms by using residual knowledge about word meaning and word spelling. On the other hand, in the case of phonological treatment, learning generalized across untreated items (there were seven untreated consonants). It was argued that patient GI, following the treatment, became able to apply phonemic analysis and to generate keywords for the seven untreated consonants, (see generalization of learning to untreated syllables in the case of OG (Carlomagno and Parlato, 1989)).

Further support for the hypothesis that the visual-semantic treatment stimulated residual knowledge about whole word forms was provided in a more recent study (Carlomagno, et al.,1991b). In this study, two chronic aphasic patients, respectively suffering from Wernicke's (TG) and moderate global aphasia (AR), received the visual-semantic treatment. The choice of this treatment was because the two patients were unable to consistently perform phonological segmentation of dictated nonsense syllables. That was particularly evident when they attempted to do it on stimuli containing consonant clusters. For AR, a further reason was that he sometimes exhibited visual strategies when writing. For instance, when asked to write the word *cintura* (belt) he wrote first NT, then added the segment URA on the right, and finally completed the word on the left. TG did not show such behaviour but during therapy sessions he did write in non-linear order. Each of the two patients received 22 one-hour sessions following the programme outlined in Table 12.1. Results supported the hypothesis that treatment stimulated the lexical writing route (see Table 12.2). We found, indeed, significant improvement in word writing and slightly better performance in written naming. However, improvement could not be found in nonword writing.

We should stress that the choice of visual-semantic treatment could be suggested in the case of AR by his tendency to write in non-linear order. According to Hatfield's study (1985) this behaviour might suggest residual knowledge about whole word forms and (complete)

Table 12.2 Results of the study by Carlomagno et al., 1991b. Number of correct responses produced by patients TG and AR before and after 22 sessions of visual semantic treatment. Pre-test 1 was given four months before the pre-test 2 (pre-therapy assessment). Post test 2 was given one month after therapy stopped.

	Pre-test 1	Pre-test 2	Pre-test 1	Pre-test 2
Patient TG				
Written naming (80)	13	18	45*	37
Word writing (198)	35	53	114	128
Non-word (80)	4	10	18	17
Patient AR				
Written naming (80)	24	31	47*	43
Word writing (198)	27	34	102	135
Non-word (80)	5	4	3	17

*Five uncorrect responses by TG and seven uncorrect responses by AR were correctly written semantic paragraphias (see text).

inability to use a phonological writing procedure. According to the study by Hatfield and Weddell (1976) the same behaviour might entail poor response when the patient is trained to write by phoneme-grapheme correspondences. Both hypotheses appear to be confirmed by results.

On the other hand, poor performance of AR and TG in nonword writing at pre-therapy testing (inability to use phoneme-grapheme conversion) could suggest that phonological treatment would have been ineffective. However, we should note that patient GI (Carlomagno *el al.*, 1991 and patient SJD, (Hillis and Caramazza, 1990) were found unable to write nonwords from dictation at pre-therapy testing but they were shown to be improved by phonological treatments. We must conclude that current evidence does not allow us to judge whether therapy via lexical or non-lexical writing procedures is more effective; i.e., we cannot properly assess the effectiveness of residual processing of the two writing routes using word versus nonword writing performances. Additionally, difficulty in choosing the effective treatment might be due to the fact that simple evaluation of the two writing routes does not take into account the status of cognitive component(s) not belonging to the writing system, which might be involved in organizing substitute response strategies.

Microcomputer Technology in Writing Rehabilitation

In recent years researchers have tried to use the Personal Computer in neuropsychological rehabilitation in order to provide patients with a prosthetic device or to provide therapy. In order to improve patient's acceptance, treatment tasks can be programmed in gamelike format and allow clinicians to modify modality of presentation, type of feedback and number of cues. Furthermore, the Personal Computer can provide collection and analysis of patient's responses that might be used in regulating feedback or in determining content of subsequent therapy sessions. (See Katz, Chapter 14 and Crerar and Ellis, Chapter 13). As far as writing rehabilitation is concerned we have already mentioned the study by Seron et al., (1980) which used writing from dictation. Moreover, treatments focusing on written naming can be easily arranged: the stimulus is displayed on the screen and patient's responses are written by means of the keyboard. Furthermore, cues can be built in: letters belonging to the target can be presented in an anagram format, the first letter or target to be copied can be provided and so on.

A similar treatment programme running on an Apple II computer has been recently provided by Deloche (1991). In each session the subject was requested to type the name of 16 objects displayed on the screen one at a time. In some treatment conditions patients could be provided with visual or lexical cues. Furthermore, when the patient typed an incorrect letter, the wrong letter did not appear but acoustic feedback signalled the error. If a further error was produced, the correct letter appeared guiding the patient to complete the word.

Eighteen chronic aphasics each received 25 treatment sessions. Pre- and post-therapy testing used practice (80 items) and control (40 untreated items) lists and involved oral and written naming. Group results showed a significant improvement (from 40 per cent to 54 per cent correct responses) which generalized to untreated items and to oral naming. Single case results showed that the scores of 16 patients increased by at least 5 per cent correct responses on treated items, and for 12 of them improvement generalized to untreated items. Furthermore, ten out of 18 patients showed a significant improvement on oral naming. A further qualitative analysis concerned relationships between oral and written language. The patterns of improvement (oral versus written naming) and writing errors (plausible phonemic errors, effect of the orthographic complexity of stimuli and so on) at the pre- and post-therapy assessment were studied. It was found that in nine cases written naming was tied to spoken language at the pre-therapy evaluation: i.e., written naming probably resulted from a sound to letter conversion of self dictated names. In seven of these patients improvement in written naming reflected improved oral naming at the post-therapy evaluation.

However, for two of them written naming improved without a parallel improvement of oral naming. That was true for four other patients who, at the pre-therapy evaluation, showed better performance in written naming than oral naming. Although the study does not mention whether improvement generalizes to other writing tasks, the last two findings are consistent with a view that (visuo-lexical) treatment of written naming disturbances may induce writing improvement without effecting spoken language.

Towards a Pragmatic Conclusion on Writing Rehabilitation in Aphasic Patients

It was beyond the scope of this chapter to discuss relationships between cognitive theory and therapeutic practice or neurological mechanisms subserving functional recovery. Our aim was to offer a practical survey of therapy for writing disturbances in aphasia. However, from the practical point of view, most of the single case studies showed that cognitively-oriented rehabilitation programmes had an effect on the writing performance of aphasic patients. In these cases cognitive theory provided a detailed description of dysgraphic disturbances (identification of target symptoms). That, in turn, could provide a rationale for therapy and pattern of improvement. Also, cognitive theory could offer insights for interpreting the effect of (phonological or visuo-lexical) therapies on groups of unselected aphasic patients (Carlomagno et al., 1991 a,b).

However, identification of locus (i) of impairment alone did not provide guidance for the choice of an effective treatment technique. That choice would face not only the interpretation of the cognitive deficit but also putative mechanisms underlying functional recovery (Hillis and Caramazza, 1994). With reference to.this, although the re-establishment hypothesis requires further testing, most available data provide support for the reorganization strategy for planning a writing rehabilitation programme. However, re-organization strategy would face difficulties in evaluating the role of residual processing abillities and of the non-writing cognitive skills which might be involved.

Residual processing abilities sometimes turn into overt spontaneous compensatory behaviour which might suggest the appropriate therapeutic strategy; i.e., patient BB spelled a homophonic content word instead of a function word (Hatfield, 1983) and patient AR was writing in non-linear order. In both cases effective therapeutic attempts reflected patient's spontaneous strategies. However, observing such behaviours is rare and far from providing appropriate diagnostic instruments. For instance, in the case of OG (Carlomagno and Parlato, 1989), residual phonological abilities (segmenting dictated stimuli and matching dictated nonsense syllables with written names of Italian towns) could not be predicted by the pre-therapy writing pattern. In this case, indeed, the therapeutic approach was constructed by analogy to the reading strategy. On the other hand, in the case of OG, it was not possible to evaluate the exact role of residual reading abilities (syllabic grapheme-phoneme correspondences) in producing functional recovery.

A further study provided evidence that reading abilities play a role in supporting writing improvement (Ferrand and Deloche, 1991). Similarly, cognitive skills not belonging to (spoken and written) language could support functional recovery of writing (Zesiger and de Partz, 1991). Interaction between writing and non-writing skills in functional recovery of writing could not be predicted by cognitive theory. We agree with Wilson and Patterson (1990) who suggest, as many have before them, that successful therapy attempts were (and are) more a matter of intuition by therapists than direct consequence of a theoretically driven approach. Nevertheless, recourse to efficient non-writing components(s) did help in many cases and further therapeutic attempts will take advantage of this possibility.

As a final consideration we will discuss the impact of writing rehabilitation on communicative skills of aphasic patients. A study by Basso, Capitani and Zanobio (1982) attempted to analyze the relationship between recovery in oral and written comprehension and production in rehabilitated and non-rehabilitated patients. Improvements of all pairs of modalities were found to be significantly associated in the 250 patients who had received global language stimulation for at least six months. According to these data it might be questioned whether selective writing rehabilitation plays a role in improving aphasics' communicative skills. Likely, if a global stimulation approach is sufficient to obtain improvement in writing skills, we have no reasons to propose highly detailed rehabilitation strategies for aphasics' writing disturbances.

However, successful rehabilitation attempts by Carlomagno et al., (1991 a and b) concerned unselected aphasic patients who, in spite of global stimulation therapy, did not show further writing improvement. In these studies specific writing therapies were found effective and patients maintained improved performance. Thus, it seems more interesting to raise the issue of whether writing improvement was of benefit in the patients' daily life. With reference to that question, it should be noted that writing disturbances may be a considerable handicap in occupation or everyday life even for those patients who maintain sufficient oral skills. Following writing retraining programmes, three out of the six patients of the first study by Carlomagno and coworkers were found to practise writing by themselves: two patients were keeping a diary and the third regained partial activity in managing his business (Carlomagno et al., 1990). Patient TG, who participated in the second study, could practise his hobby: crossword puzzles (Carlomagno et al., 1991b). Thus, we found evidence that writing improvement generalized, at least in these four cases, to everyday activity.

On the other hand, increasing interest in functional communication in recent years points to the possibility that residual writing abilities might supplement and/or replace oral language. Fawcus and Fawcus (1990), for instance, described strategies of patients suffering from severe apraxia of speech in sending messages. Two of them were found to use written messages although these messages contained spelling errors. Patient RG (Carlomagno et al., 1991b), upon completion of a visual-semantic treatment, had better written naming than oral naming and used writing when oral messages were unavailable. We feel justified in proposing writing therapy for those patients whose oral language is severely impaired. Such impairment might be supplemented by means of written messages.

Notes

1. The classification of acquired dyslexias in the cognitive approach is analogous to that of dysgraphias since reading, as well as writing, involves lexical and non-lexical routes which may be damaged independently. In the case of *surface dyslexia* (damaged of the lexical route) reading by grapheme-phoneme correspondence results in difficulties assigning the correct phonemic value to an ambiguous grapheme. (See also Andreewsky and Cochu, Chapter 11).
2. Transparent languages are those written languages where one-to-one sound to letter correspondences apply. Most Italian words respond to this rule. Other words contain one or more phonemes which correspond to a multiple (2 or 3) letter strings depending on the syllabic context. Obviously, on the latter words, phoneme to grapheme conversion alone does not allow correct spelling.

Acknowledgements

This study has been supported by a grant of Consiglio Nazionale delle Ricerche (Italy) and of Centro Ricerche Clinica Santa Lucia (Italy).

References

Basso A, Capitan E, Zanobio ME (1982) Patterns of recovery of oral and written expression and comprehension in aphasic patients. Behavioral Brain Research 6:115–28.

Beauvois MF, Dèrouesné J (1981) Lexical or orthographic agraphia. Brain 104:21–49.

Behrmann M (1987) The rites of righting writing: homophone remediation in acquired dysgraphia. Cognitive Neuropsychology 4:365–84.

Bub D, Kertesz A, (1982) Deep agraphia. Brain and Language 17: 146–65.

Carlomagno S, Parlato V (1989) Writing rehabilitation in brain damaged adult patients: a cognitive approach. In Seron X, Deloche G (Eds) Cognitive approaches in neuropsychological rehabilitation. Hillsdale NJ: Lawrence Erlbaum Assoc.

Carlomagno S, Iavarone A, Colombo A, (1994) Cognitive approaches to writing rehabilitation: from single case to group studies. In Humphrey G, and Riddoch J (Eds) Cognitive Neuropsychology and Cognitive Rehabilitation. Hillsdale NJ: Lawrence Erlbaum.

Carlomagno S, Colombo A, Emanuelli S, Casadio P, Razzano C (1991a) Cognitive approaches to writing rehabilitation in aphasics: evaluation of two treatment strategies. Aphasiology 5:355–60.

Carlomagno S, Faccioli F, Losanno N, Iavarone A, Colombo A, (1991b) Strategies visuo-lexicales pour la rééducation des troubles de l'écriture chez les adultes aphasiques. Paper presented at Réunion de la Société de Neuropsychologie de Langue Française, Paris.

Coltheart M, Masterson J, Byng S, Prior M, Riddoch J, (1983) Surface dyslexia. Quarterly Journal of Experimental Psychology 35A:469–95.

Deloche G (1991) Rééducation des troubles de la denomination d'images assistée par ordinateur. In de Partz MP, Leclercq M (Eds) La rééducation neuropsychologique de l'adulte. (Editions de la Societé Neuropsychologique de Langue Française, Paris).

de Partz MP (1986) Reeducation of a deep dyslexic patient: rationale of the method and results. Cognitive Neuropsychology 3: 149–77.

Dèrouesné J, Beauvois MF (1979) Phonological processing in reading: data from alexia. Journal of Neurology, Neurosurgery and Psychiatry 42: 1125–32.

Ellis AW (1984) Reading, writing and dyslexia: a cognitive analysis. Hillsdale NJ: Lawrence Erlbaum Assoc.

Fawcus M, Fawcus R, (1990) Information transfer in four cases of severe articulatory dyspraxia. Aphasiology 4:207–12.

Ferrand I, Deloche G (1991) Thérapie éxperimentale de l'écriture dans un cas d'atteinte de la voie phonologique avec préservation de la production des monosyllabiques. Paper presented at Réunion de la Société de Neuropsychologie de Langue Française, Paris.

Hatfield MF, Weddell R, (1976) Re-training in writing in severe aphasia. In Lebrun Y, Hoops R (Eds) Recovery in Aphasics. Amsterdam: Swets and Zeitlinger.

Hatfield MF (1983) Aspect of acquired dysgraphia and implication for re-education. In Code C, Müller DJ (Eds) Aphasia Therapy. London Edward Arnold.

Hatfield MF (1985) Visual and phonological factors in acquired dysgraphia. Neuropsychologia 23 (1):13–29.

Hillis AE, Caramazza A (1994) Theories of lexical processing and rehabilitation of lexical deficits. In Humphrey G, Riddoch J (Eds) Cognitive Neuropsychology and Cognitive Rehabilitation. Hillsdale NJ, Lawrence Erlbaum.

Luria AR, Naydin VL, Tsveskova LS, Virnaskaya EN (1969) Restoration of higher cortical function following local brain damage. In Vinken P, Bruyn GN (Eds) Handbook of Clinical Neurology vol 3. Amsterdam: North Holland.

Morton J (1980) The logogen model and the orthographic structure. In Frith U (Ed) Cognitive processes in spelling. London: Academic Press.

Seron X, Deloche G, Moulard G, Rousselle M (1980) A computer-based therapy for the treatment of aphasic subjects with writing disorders. Journal of Speech and Hearing Disorders 45: 45–58.

Shallice T (1981) Phonological agraphia and the lexical route in writing. Brain 104:413–29.

Weniger D, Taylor Sarno M (1990) The future of aphasia therapy: more than just new wine in old bottles? Aphasiology 4:301–6.

Wilson B, Patterson K (1990) Rehabilitation for cognitive impairment: does cognitive psychology apply. Applied Cognitive Psychology 4:247–60.

Zesiger P, de Partz M P (1991) Rééducation cognitives des troubles de l'orthographie et/ou de l'écriture. In de Partz M P, Leclercq M (Eds) La rééducation neuropsychologique de l'adulte. (Editions de la Societé Neuropsychologique de Langue Française, Paris).

Chapter 13
Computer-based Therapy for Aphasia: Towards Second Generation Clinical Tools

M. ALISON CRERAR AND ANDREW ELLIS

Introduction

In the United Kingdom the use of computers in mainstream language therapy, i.e., by clinicians on the ground rather than by the research community, is still very much the exception rather than the rule. While information technology has transformed the face of business and commerce, and has been embraced by most academic disciplines even in the humanities, it has had relatively little impact on the assessment and treatment of language disorders. The primitive state of computer provision in clinical settings no doubt has a lot to do with this, but there are other contributory factors. Key among these is the surprising dearth of methodologically sound efficacy studies of computer-based treatment. The lack of research exploring the clinical application of computers is puzzling because the general-purpose nature of these machines would seem to offer considerable potential as instruments of therapy, research and clinical management. Deadlock exists at present: progress in this non-acute, non-profit environment depends on skilled software support, but investment in computing equipment and personnel is not justified unless scientific studies demonstrate that there are clear therapeutic and/or economic benefits to be gained. In this chapter we discuss some promising findings which begin to offer such a justification.

The chapter is divided into three sections. The first briefly summarizes previous microcomputer usage in aphasia therapy, mentioning representative work and drawing on a published review summarizing the state-of-the-art as our research began (1990). This *background* section provides an insight into the limitations that motivated our own work. The middle section called *the microworld project,* presents an account of a treatment study combining cognitive neuropsychological principles

223

and computer technology which took place in Edinburgh during 1990 and 1991. We report improvements in the understanding of written sentences in a group of long-term aphasic subjects with previously stable impairments of verb and preposition processing. The final section, *the computer as a clinical tool*, reviews the range of advantages that computerisation brought to this project. We try to convey the psychological benefits shown by patients and the diagnostic edge afforded to clinicians in an environment which promoted genuine partnership in therapy. We recommend that at the present state of knowledge, the most promising direction beyond first generation drill and practice programs is towards interactive environments involving a dynamic client-clinician-computer triad in which the traditional assessment/treatment boundary may be blurred in favour of a diagnosis-within-treatment approach. This is not to deny the essential role of assessment in the evaluation of efficacy, but to promote the idea that in all but the simplest single-word therapies, treatment will necessarily be heavily diagnostic. This is because conventional assessment tests reveal *what* a patient cannot do, but not *why* – finding out why (in a cognitive neuropsychological sense) is important in targeting remediation. Far from de-skilling clinicians, we feel that second generation environments present unprecedented opportunities for the clinician to exercise on-line diagnostic logic and ingenuity. The reader is referred to Katz, Chapter 14 in this volume.

Background

In the past, the whole enterprise of speech-language therapy has suffered from a shortage of systematic efficacy evaluations (Howard and Hatfield, 1987). The situation is steadily improving with the publication of a number of well-designed, theoretically motivated treatment studies (Byng, 1988), but methodological inadequacies continue to undermine claims of effectiveness in many cases. It is hardly surprising, then, that the sub-field of computer-based therapy should also manifest procedural weaknesses. A timely review of computerized cognitive rehabilitation was uncompromising in its conclusions:

> No computer cognitive rehabilitation procedures have been shown to generalise to real life and there is no existing empirical basis for the sale or distribution of any computerized cognitive rehabilitation programmes for non-research purposes. (Robertson, 1990: 381).

Robertson (1990) observed that many computer therapies lacked theor-etical underpinning, that the quality of the software was often poor and that the design criteria seemed simply to be that the systems were within the technical competence of their authors and within the capacities of their machines. Robertson also highlighted the lack of publications relating to computer-based treatment studies in major refereed journals and the tendency for the experimental designs used to be inadequate to establish specific treatment effects because simple A-B designs were found to predominate. The problem with simple before-after designs is that:

> (they do not) control for non-specific therapeutic effects, effects of repeat testing, spontaneous remission or similar threats to external validity...Hence many of the presumed training effects reported in the less rigorous literature may simply reflect the practice effects of tests administered by pleasant and supportive psychologists (Robertson, 1990: 383).

Robertson further noted that most applications were entrenched in the drill and practice mould, whereby a small number of domain-specific (generally single-word) tasks are repeated with the computer as presentation medium.[1] In this category he cited the early picture-matching and confrontation-naming programs of Katz and colleagues (e.g. Katz and Nagy, 1984; 1985; Katz, et al., 1989). While acknowledging the pioneering nature of this work, Robertson observed that the experimental methods employed did not permit detection of generalization effects of treatment to items other than those seen in therapy.

A series of studies examining typing to dictation, all using the same basic method, sought to detect generalization effects to untreated words in handwriting to dictation mode (Deloche, et al., 1976; Deloche, et al., 1978; Seron, et al., 1980). The therapist provided the spoken stimulus and the computer provided interactive feedback during the typing exercises by means of highlighting the position of the next letter to be typed and indicating correctness or otherwise of letters. All three studies reported benefits (which in the most recent study were across three measures of performance and maintained in four out of five patients six weeks after cessation of treatment); however, in none of the cases can improvement be unequivocally attributed to the treatment since a simple A-B design was used.

Another single-word cueing application was the study of Bruce and Howard (1987). They selected five subjects who had naming difficulties, but who knew the first letters of the words they sought and could respond to phonemic cues from a clinician. The subjects were trained on an Apple IIe computer with voice synthesizer. Fifty line drawings were presented and the patients, by depressing the key corresponding to the first letter of the object, could activate the appropriate synthesized phoneme. The ensuing study looked at performance over 50 treated and 50 untreated words, both with and without computer-cueing. Performance benefited from cueing and some generalization to untreated items was observed. The authors reported that one patient managed to internalize the cueing strategy, thus overcoming dependence on the prosthesis.

There have been some attempts to distinguish the performance effects of varying delivery and feedback mechanisms. In a study by Katz et al., (1990), 22 aphasic subjects were randomly allocated to a computerized reading program, a computer stimulation program of the arcade game type, or to a no-treatment group. The two treatment groups received three hours exposure per week for 13 weeks. Unfortunately, as Robertson (1990) notes, conclusions were drawn from the raw data without statistical analysis and the claims that improvement on the computerized reading led to improvement in conventional reading, and that the benefit was attributable to the language content of the treatment software, were not supported by the data.

Two studies by Loverso and colleagues (Loverso, et al., 1985; Loverso, Prescott and Selinger, 1988, based on earlier work on the elicitation of verbs (Loverso, Selinger and Prescott, 1979), set out to compare alternative treatment deliveries in bringing patients to predetermined performance levels. In the earlier study Loverso, et al., (1985) found that 67 computer sessions were needed, compared with 36 therapist sessions, to achieve the required levels of performance on six tasks, and a comparable improvement on the Porch Index of Communicative Ability (Porch, 1971). The 1988 study reported results for 20 aphasic subjects. The conclusions here were that the unsupervised computer sessions were not as effective as the computer-assisted therapist sessions, and that the benefit of a clinician was apparent for both fluent and non-fluent aphasics in the moderate to marked ranges of severity.

Kinsey (1990) conducted a study to compare the effects of delivery and feedback mechanisms on patient performance. Twelve aphasic patients were subjected to three experimental treatment environments; conventional, computer delivery and feedback, and computer delivery with conventional feedback. The stimuli were a series of multiple-choice linguistic and non-linguistic tasks. In the conventional situation the therapist administered the tests manually using score sheets and stop watch. However, conventional feedback must have been very difficult to administer spontaneously, as a complicated protocol was laid down based on percentages of positive, intrinsic, nonverbal, no response, inappropriate, etc. feedbacks, derived from clinical interaction data. Computer delivery and data recording was entirely automatic. Computer feedback was comprised of a high pitched sound with textual reinforcer for correct responses and a low pitched sound with continued display of the task for incorrect responses. Nothing significant emerged in the analysis of the non-linguistic tasks, which caused no difficulty for the group in any environment. However, Kinsey discovered that feedback type, rather than delivery type, was the salient factor in improving performance on linguistic tasks, the computer feedback being the better form. Thus the consistent computer-generated feedback proved superior to the conventional therapist-delivered variety. However, as Kinsey explained in her paper, the study was compromised by using the same subjects in the different test conditions, providing opportunities for unwanted interference or carry-over effects.

In 1987, the clinical forum section of the journal *Aphasiology* (vol 1/2), was given over to a leading article by Katz (1987) on the efficacy of aphasia treatment using microcomputers, and to several responses. *Drill and practice* was unquestionably the dominant paradigm and the major benefit of computers was seen as the increased amount of drill that patients could be given. The responding papers raised a number of key issues. On methodology, Loverso (1987) pointed out that experimental designs used so far had failed to demonstrate efficacy, and that software had not progressed beyond drill level. Wolfe (1987) complained that software developers failed to incorporate models of rehabilitation in their designs, and Seron (1987) was concerned that software embodied only the transference of techniques that could equally well be applied by a clinician. He argued the futility of efficacy studies that compared the clinician and computer on similar tasks and called for the development of 'programs that are beyond the capacities of the clinician and thus not comparable with current practice'. (Seron, 1987: 162). This statement encapsulates a fundamental problem with the therapeutic use of micro-computers to date. In the same collection, Enderby (1987) stressed the neglect of the computer's role in assessment, pointing out the potential for increasing accuracy, greatly assisting data analysis and decreasing inter-observer error. She also made the important point that computeri-zation could erode the artificial separation of assessment and treatment by permitting monitoring during treatment.

At the end of his paper, Katz looked forward to hardware and soft-ware developments that might benefit aphasiology, claiming, 'By utiliz-ing artificial intelligence functions, treatment programs can make decisions about whether or not an intervention is needed, and if so, what cue should be selected.' (Katz, 1987: 148), though Seron (1987) queried whether, in the current state of knowledge, there was any possibility of offering an expert system in neuropsychology. This exchange is of interest in view of the subsequent appearance in the clinical forum section of the same journal of a leading article by Guyard, Masson and Quiniou (1990), reporting preliminary progress in applying artificial intelligence (AI) techniques clinically. Their system was the product of collaboration between linguist-clinicians and AI workers and represents a level of complexity beyond the simple, computerized exercises mentioned so far. The project was very ambi-tious, but at the time of publication had delivered only limited modules on nominal gender in French. While the spirit of the investigative processes described was sensitive and insightful, there must be some doubt as to whether the goals were realistic and whether the proposed system would prove clinically viable. In particular, the intention to scale down eventually from the development environment (a SUN workstation running Prolog) to an Apple Macintosh seems impracticable without reducing the specification.[2] We also wonder whether by relying only on patients' written responses, the authors have perhaps underestimated the diagnostic importance of such things as gesture, subvocalization, and eye movement, which at present cannot be adequately captured and interpreted automatically.

This brief survey of relevant work indicates that on the whole the clinical application of microcomputers has failed to keep pace with technological developments, with theoretical developments (such as models of rehabilitation and of cognitive functioning), and with the methodological requirements of sound experimental design and analysis. It seems that the initial phase of exploratory, anecdotal and pro-missory articles which appeared in the early 1980s has not been superseded by studies of greater depth and sophistication. The main reason for this is the continuing lack of opportunity for clinicians to collaborate with interested professionals; a situation that stems in large part from the limited resourcing of paramedical services to which we alluded above. The tendency has been to automate previous techniques, rather than to design new and different computer-inspired ones. (For further detailed discussion see Katz, this volume.) In the next section we describe a study which aimed to address the key issues raised in the literature review and to move towards a new generation of clinical software in which the complementary strengths of computer and clinician would be more fully exploited.

The Microworld Project

The acute shortage of sound efficacy studies of computer-based language therapy and the limited scope of existing treatment software prompted us to design an experiment which we hoped would satisfy a number of theoretical and practical objectives. Apart from wishing to fulfil methodological conditions such that the results of therapy could be interpreted confidently (Byng and Coltheart, 1986; Howard and Patterson, 1989) and to advance beyond drill and practice in the treatment paradigm, we were also keen to capitalize on the benefits of computing for assessment purposes and to combine assessment and treatment in a single investigative rationale. Work within the cognitive neuropsychological tradition (Ellis and Young, 1988; Edmundson and McIntosh, this volume) provided an overarching framework for the study, guiding the contents of the assessment tests, the experimental design and the highly analytical approach to treatment.

The focus of the research was difficulties of written sentence comprehension in aphasic subjects with good single-word understanding. In this chapter we present overviews of the experimental design, of the nature of the software[3] and of what happened during therapy. The aim is to explain informally how the combination of investigative method and software tools allowed us a) to answer a number of specific questions, for example, about the dissociability of language functions and about function-specific and item-specific effects of treatment; and b) to demonstrate beyond doubt that any benefits observed were attributable to the interventions applied. A comprehensive account of this work can be found in Crerar (1991) and Crerar, Ellis and Dean (forthcoming).

Within the general area of sentence processing deficits, two functions of special interest were isolated, namely the processing of verbs and the processing of locative prepositions. These two grammatical categories were chosen because they had been, singly or together, the focus of a number of previous studies which had produced interesting results and raised questions for further investigation. In particular, the work of Caplan, Baker and Dehaut (1985); Schwartz, Saffran and Marin (1980); and Byng (1988) influenced our thinking. Caplan, et al.,. (1985) conducted three studies testing 56, 37 and 49 aphasic subjects respectively with nine different sentence types involving the mapping of thematic roles. Sample stimuli were *It was the elephant that the monkey hit* and *The elephant that the monkey hit hugged the rabbit.* The subjects were required to demonstrate the thematic roles by acting out the sentences with toy animals. Caplan and colleagues found that sentences with canonical word order consistently proved easier than their non-canonical counterparts. Verb argument structure also affected performance and sentences with two verbs were harder than those with one. Sentence length was therefore not, of itself, a determinant of complexity; the salient features appeared to be non-canonical word order, a three-argument verb or a second verb.

Schwartz, Saffran and Marin (1980) investigated the aural comprehension of five Broca's aphasics using simple active declarative sentences, passive sentences and locative prepositional sentences, all in reversible form, in a series of picture-matching experiments. The locative prepositional sentences were introduced to eliminate possible lexical variability (the nouns used, *square* and *circle* being pre-tested for recognition). This idea was later extended to verb sentences, where the authors created stick characters called *circle* and *square*, with heads of the appropriate shape, for use as protagonists. Noun-prep-noun (N-P-N) and noun-verb-noun (N-V-N) constructions were considered equivalent in this work. Patients were then compared in their ability to handle active verb sentences versus locatives. Schwartz and colleagues concluded that, 'these agrammatic subjects have a syntactic mapping defect such that they are unable to utilize a fixed and principled set of procedures to recover the relational structure of spoken sentences' (Schwartz et al., 1980: 261).

Byng (1988) reported a treatment study which applied cognitive neuropsychological principles and the mapping deficit hypothesis of

Schwartz, Linebarger and Saffran (1985) to the investigation of expressive and receptive verb and preposition processing problems in two single cases. Following a short amount of therapy on written locative sentences (devised so that the patient could self-administer at home), patient BRB performed flawlessly in auditory and written modes. His improvements generalized to reversible active declarative sentences in both modalities (though these were not seriously impaired to start with), to Byng's own verb video test (which tests mapping without parsing by using video film sequences of verb pairs such as *buy/sell*), and to spontaneous speech. The benefits reported were attributable to the intervention applied and strongly supportive of the notion of a general mapping deficit underlying all tasks.

The Microworld

Previous research (Caramazza and Zurif, 1976) has shown that agrammatic subjects can make use of contextual cues in natural English to interpret sentences where the meaning is clear from the semantics of the component words alone (e.g., *The apple that the boy is eating is red*), but where parsing is essential to recover the correct meaning (e.g., in reversible or improbable sentences) their performance may decline to chance. Reversible sentences are those where subjects and objects (or agents and themes) can be plausibly interchanged (e.g., *The cow chased the dog/The dog chased the cow*). They have become standard material for assessing syntax processing, but fully reversible sentences are notoriously difficult to devise – in the above example one could argue that dogs are more likely to chase cows than cows are to chase dogs. On the other hand, deliberate use of improbable sentences (such as *The man bites the dog*) to trap lexico-pragmatic reliance invites undesirable interferences effects a) because aphasics have been reported to object that improbable scenarios do not make sense (Schwartz et al., 1980) and b) because some subjects might begin to operate successful compensatory heuristics, such as 'the silly interpretation is right'.

In order to eliminate both these potential difficulties, a computer-based microworld was devised after the fashion of Schwartz, et al's (1980) cartoon characters *circle* and *square*. Those authors had used line drawings to depict their protagonists in sentence/picture-matching tasks, where, by virtue of the artificiality, the scenarios were fully reversible. A typical target sentence from their work is *The circle shoots the square*, where subjects were offered two candidate pictures to choose from, the correct one and a reverse role distractor in which a square character was depicted shooting a circle character. We adapted this idea by creating three stick characters called *ball*, *box* and *star* (match-stick figures with appropriately shaped heads realised in colour computer graphics) and extended it by allowing these characters to be either animate or inanimate – thus we had a microworld of only three objects/nouns. We also pruned other aspects of vocabulary to the bare minimum necessary for the experimental design, having only five verbs *(paints, draws, gives, holds, thinks)* and six prepositions *(in, under, behind, above, between, beside)*. Allowable sentence structures were likewise confined to a small number of contrastive types outlined under *efficacy study* below. Thus typical microworld sentences were *The star paints a box* and *The ball is under the box and the star*. Figures 13.1 and 13.2 show specimen computer screens presented to patients for each of these stimuli. The purpose of minimizing the vocabulary was that patients' understanding of the single lexical items could be tested in isolation before combining the elements to assess sentence-level impairments. By controlling the vocabulary in this way confounding factors were reduced and syntax processing deficits were easier to identify than in unrestricted English.

Selection and Baseline Phase

Of 22 aphasic subjects referred for assessment, 14 subjects who exhibited deficits in the processing of verbs and prepositions as measured by a computer-based sentence/picture-matching Syntax Screening Test (Crerar, 1990) were selected as candidates for treatment.[4] The 14 candidates chosen ranged in age from 27 to 74 (the mean age was 52.4) and were between 6 months and 11 years post-onset (mean time post-onset was 4 years and 4 months). Before being admitted to the treatment phase of the research each subject was assessed on three

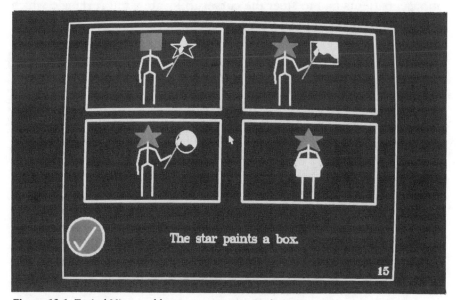

Figure 13.1. Typical Microworld assessment screen (verbs). (screen as at onset of task)

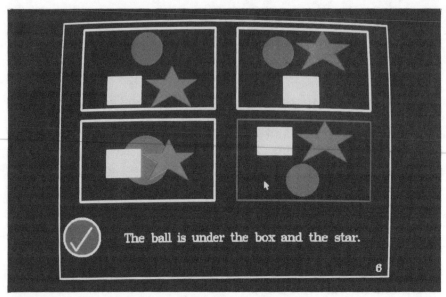

The ball is under the box and the star.

Figure 13.2. Typical Microworld assessment screen (prepositions). (Here the correct window has been selected using the mouse)

occasions, with a minimum of 4 weeks and a maximum of 16 weeks between consecutive test sessions. On each occasion three computer-based tests (Crerar, 1990) were administered; each test used the assessment interface shown in Figures 13.1 and 13.2. The first, the Interface Test, measured the patients' ability to operate the computer-based assessment environment independent of a linguistic task. Using a mouse, patients had to steer the cursor to locate a red rectangle which had been randomly placed in one of four windows on the screen; once inside the correct window a single mouse click registered their choice. Twenty stimuli were presented. The second test, the Lexical Test, used the same format, but this time a single word (such as *box* or *holds*) appeared beneath the four windows and subjects had to distinguish the matching picture from three distractors. The final test, the Syntax Screening Test, used the same program shell, but this time a full sentence appeared beneath the four windows (as in Figures 13.1 and 13.2) and subjects had to read the sentence and identify the corresponding picture. The Syntax Screening Test comprised 42 target sentences, seven in each of the following categories – verbs, prepositions, pronouns, adjectives, scope and quantification and morphology. In this way a preliminary profile could be gained of the relative impairment and preservation patterns of these various functions and the stability of performance could be ascertained over a period of months before the onset of treatment.

Before using new diagnostic tools with aphasic subjects we tested the software with normal subjects. Forty-five normal subjects, mostly college employees, were recruited to validate the Syntax Screening Test. The sample comprised 15 subjects in each of the age bands 25 to 39, 40 to 54, and 55 to 69. Within each age band there were males and females in three educational classes[5] (but not necessarily equal numbers of these two subgroups in each age band), thus the subjects ranged from heads of departments to kitchen staff with no post-school education. The normal subjects attended for one session only, during which they were presented with the Interface Test, Lexical Test and finally the Syntax Screening Test. The comparison of the normal and aphasic subjects across these three preliminary test yielded a great deal of valuable data; we have space here merely to give readers an impression of the level of impairment of the aphasic subjects prior to intervention. In summary, no subgroup of the normal subjects attained less than 90 per cent accuracy on the Syntax Screening Test.[6] The aphasic subjects as a group, returned mean scores of 54 per cent, 57 per cent and 56 per cent respectively on the three baseline administrations of the Syntax Screening Test – thus (as a group) they were both stable over time and significantly poorer than the normal subjects. Their degree of impairment was also evident from timing data. The test completion times for the normal subjects ranged from 4 minutes to 11 minutes, whereas, with the exception of one who operated at normal speed, the aphasics took between 19 minutes and 50 minutes to complete the Syntax Screening Test.

The 14 aphasic subjects reported here were selected for verb and preposition treatment on the basis of the results of this screening test. Figure 13.3 illustrates the performance of the normal subjects and the aphasic subjects across the six modules of the Syntax Screening Test. While the aphasics as a group were impaired in all the functions tested, Figure 13.3 confirms that they found particular difficulty with verbs and prepositions and also with morphology, which was therefore chosen as a control function. It should be noted that by the end of the baseline phase of the study just described, the aphasic subjects were accustomed to self-administration of computer-based assessments of the type used subsequently to detect treatment effects.

Efficacy Study

In order to be able to measure function-specific effects of therapy, to explore the dissociability of the two functions (verbs and prepositions) and to investigate the effects of treatment orderings, the 14 subjects (known as P1 ... P14) were divided into two groups of seven. Group A received verb therapy followed by preposition therapy and Group B received the treatments in the opposite order. A cross-over treatment design was implemented. This comprised two treatment blocks each of six hours duration (two separate hours per week for three weeks),

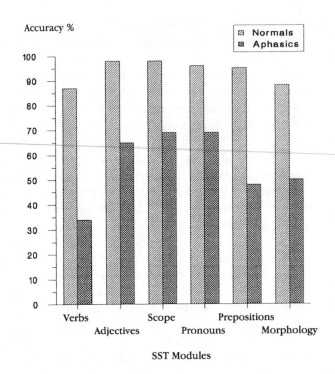

Figure 13.3 Comparison of aphasic and normal performances over the six Syntax Screening Test modules. (14 aphasics, 3 trials each; 45 normals, 1 trial each)

preceded, separated and followed by a block of assessments (two separate hours per week for two weeks). The treatment study therefore extended over a period of 12 weeks).

Each set of assessments consisted of the same four tests: Verb Test, Preposition Test, Morphology Test and Real World Test (Crerar, 1990). The first three were computer-based using the now familiar assessment shell (see Figures 13.1 and 13.2) while the Real World Test was paper-based. The Verb Test and Preposition Test both contained 40 sentences, 20 of these were treated during therapy, and the remaining 20 were never seen in therapy. The treated sentences were subdivided into small sets of homogeneous sentence structures so that comparative performance across different sentence types could be studied before and after therapy. The treated side of the Verb Test had four sentence types, exemplars of which are: *The ball points a box; A box is held by the ball; The ball gives a star to the box;* and *The ball paints the box that the star holds.* There were three treated structures in the Preposition Test (since there is no locative equivalent of a passive), matched with the verb items for complexity, e.g, *The ball is in the box; The box is under the ball and the star;* and *The ball is behind the star that is under the box.* Only the verbs *paints, holds* and *gives* and the prepositions *in, under* and *behind* were treated. The untreated items were constructed so as to be able to measure generalization of treatment effects to unseen sentences containing treated verbs/prepositions in both treated sentence structures and untreated sentence structures, and to untreated verbs/propositions again in treated and untreated sentence structures.

The Morphology Test was included as a control function, performance on which was not expected to change as result of treating either verbs or prepositions. As morphology was not treated, this was a 20-sentence test with no subdivision into treated and untreated items. The Morphology Test contained stimuli to test recognition of such things as plural, past tense, comparative and possessive markers, e.g. *The box's ball is red; The ball is smaller than the box.*

The final test given to patients pre-therapy, after therapy on the first function treated, and again after completion of the second therapy block, was the Real World Test. This was designed to provide an indicator of whether as a result of treating verbs, prepositions and grammatical structures in the microworld, improvement would transfer to reading tasks based on real world scenarios independent of the computer environment. For this purpose a paper-based sentence/picture-matching test was devised, as similar in format as possible to the screen layout, but using a much wider, everyday vocabulary (20 nouns). The Real World Test consisted of line-drawings laid out as for the computer-based assessments and containing 20 verb sentences and 20 preposition sentences. Each set of 20 included both treated and untreated sentence structures and both treated and untreated verbs or prepositions. For example, *The clown gives a flower to the girl* is a treated structure with a treated verb, *A clown is drawn by the boy* is a treated structure with an untreated verb and *The dog in the window is above the cat* contains an untreated preposition in an untreated sentence structure.

The computer-based assessment tests were always self-administered by patients with no interference from the observing clinician. Data collection was automatic. On completion of a test, a summary of performance was displayed on the computer screen, could be printed out and was stored on hard disc for later statistical analysis. The data recorded was

1. identification of the patient;
2. date;
3. total number of correct responses;
4. total time taken for test completion including any pauses;
5. the number and length of pauses taken;
6. the identification of each picture selected (these were numbered 1 to 4, with the correct picture being number 1 and the other distractors

being consistently numbered so that response patterns to specific sentence structures provided meaningful information;

7. the window number where the chosen picture had been displayed (since pictures were randomly allocated to windows by the software, this facility would alert us to any patient who had visual neglect of a quadrant or hemifield);

8. response latency in hundredths of a second to every stimulus presented.

Where tests were subdivided into treated and untreated items, a score out of 20 for each side of the test was given and the mean reaction time to each half was calculated.

The Real World Test was scored by hand. Since picture positions were fixed on the page, it was necessary only to record the window chosen by the patient. The total time taken for each half of the test (verb items and preposition items) was recorded. A purpose-designed score sheet was provided for this test, with correct response numbers pre-printed, so that manual scoring could be completed quickly by the clinician.

The Treatment Software and its Use

Having administered the foregoing tests for the first time we had considerable insight into what an individual patient could do accurately and where he or she was having problems. Because 14 patients were involved simultaneously, we also had a feel for the relative levels of impairments between subjects, both in terms of speed and accuracy. However, although the test data was more informative for our purposes than could have been obtained from previous assessments, it is important to realize that we still only knew *what* each subject could and could not do (and how long it took); we did not, with any certainty, know *why* they were experiencing the problems they were. This point is essential to appreciate the treatment approach.

On the basis of pre-therapy performances, individual goals for therapy were drawn up for each patient. Attention was paid to error patterns in formulating hypotheses to explore during treatment sessions. Often, errors were confined to particular sentence structures and very commonly within a sentence set one error type would predominate. Thus passive sentences elicited mostly reversal errors, whereas errors on active dative sentences almost always involved reversal of the object and indirect object. However, the reasons for these errors turned out to vary between patients. It was considered crucial in therapy to try to discover why errors were arising; this was thought to be the key to targeting remediation more effectively. For each subject, therapy was concentrated on those items which had been incorrect in assessment.

To assist with this heavily diagnostic approach to treatment, remediation programs were built to handle the 20 treated items contained in the Verb Test and Preposition Test. The assessment software had used a sentence/picture-matching format and had required no direct participation by the clinician. In contrast, the remediation programs were quite different in format and relied critically on a three-way interaction between client, clinician and computer. In order to explode the subtasks of sentence comprehension and help the therapist to determine the point and cause of breakdown, the treatment software offered two modes of operation: picture-building mode and sentence-building mode; these are illustrated in Figures 13.4 and 13.5 respectively.

In picture-building mode, the patient, confronted with a target sentence, was required to construct an appropriate picture element by element. The software partitioned the target sentence into major semantic units (e.g. [the ball] [paints] [a box]) and constrained the patient to completing these in left-to-right order. Three candidate images were offered for each bracketed portion. In this way the understanding of the lexical components could be checked.[7] Sentence-building mode presented the converse task, i.e., the generation of a sentence to describe a given picture. Again, the patient was offered three choices for every sentence component. The sentence partitioning was the same as for the picture-building tasks, and again, left-to-right working was enforced. In this way, each subtask was externalized for

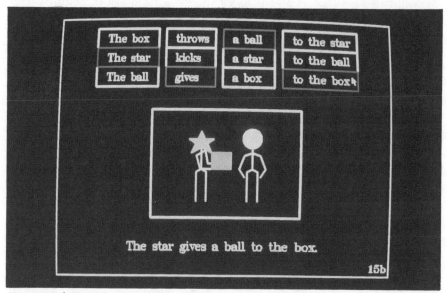

Figure 13.4. Typical picture-building treatment task underway (prepositions). (The bracketed elements have been tackled in left-to-right order, selecting on each occasion an appropriate picture from three candidates at the top to build up an image in the large central window. The final sentence component is now activated – selection of the blue box will complete the task.

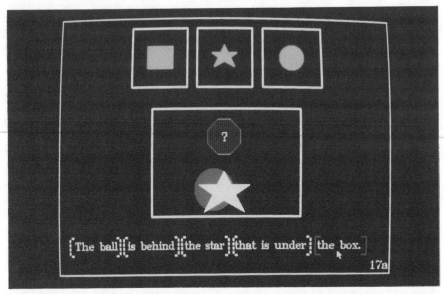

Figure 13.5. Typical sentence-building treatment task underway (verbs). The picture is given and the subject must build a sentence to describe it from the lexical components at the top. Here an error has been made in selections for the object and indirect object.

observation and discussion. The software was versatile in allowing the sentences to be tackled in any order and modes to be switched at will. It could also be used as a vehicle for the exploration of difficulties (e.g., teasing apart problems of meaning from problems of syntax) and for confirming progress (e.g., by perhaps constructing an incorrect sentence to a picture target and asking the patient to fix it, or interleaving different sentence types to check that grammatical constructions were secure outwith their homogeneous sentence sets).

Therapy sessions can therefore be characterized as heavily constrained by subject matter (i.e., the 20 treated sentences) and by software design (i.e., the fixed number of choices for any component, the left-to-right completion ordering and the two task modes). However, it is important to realize that despite this disciplined framework, what went on in each therapy session was in fact highly non-deterministic. Individual therapy goals were prepared for each patient on the basis of assessment results, but more than this, the interactive nature of treatment was based on an explorative partnership between patient and clinician, in which the dialogue between them, its form and direction, unfolded unpredictably in a dynamic way. The therapist presented task sequences designed both to advance his or her own understanding of the patient's problems and to improve his or her competence. Diagnostic insights were discussed with clients as they arose and patients were actively encouraged to consider their difficulties at a conscious level, to advance hypotheses where they were capable of doing so, and to participate in guiding the course of the interaction.

In attempting to disentangle the sometimes highly complicated inter-actions between language processing subsystems, a cognitive neuropsy-chological framework was used. Because the software externalized for the clinician the particular subtask the patient was attempting at any time, it was often possible to observe pathological processes in progress and to be fairly specific about the locus, or loci, of impairment within a functional model of language processing. Interestingly, even inside the confines of the Microworld, where opportunities for anomia were mini-mized, and where, in view of the written mode, one might have expected spoken language difficulties to be relatively unimportant, we observed many problems over and above the purely grammatical ones we had set out to study. It was clear that most subjects needed to stimulate the semantic system by verbalizing the lexical elements (orthography alone was insufficient – this applied to older and less well educated normal subjects too); however, phonological output problems could interfere in bizarre ways. For example, one of our patients, P10, had severe phono-logical problems. Unable to achieve a distinct phonetic contrast between *ball* and *box,* he renamed them *round* and *square.* However, his spoken attempts at *square* approximated more nearly to *star* than to his target, with the result that confronted with the word *box* P10 intermittently selected a picture of a star. Patients confronted with pictures often had difficulty retrieving the spoken word-forms for *ball* and *box* because they began with the same initial phoneme. These examples are given to indi-cate the sort of confounding factors that can occur even in a Microworld of three nouns. The also indicate that diagnostic insights that can be gained by a combination of the software tool, a controlled linguistic envir-onment and the clinician's on-line invocation of a model of normal lan-guage processing.

Summary of the Results

The accuracy results of the two aphasic groups are summarized in Figures 13.6a, 13.6b 13.7a, and 13.7b. From these graphs it is immediately appar-ent that the outcomes were dissimilar: Group A returned a classic cross-over profile, while Group B did not (c.f. Figures 13.6a and 13.7a). Statistical analysis showed that Group A, who received verb therapy first, improved significantly on verb items between test sessions 1 and 2 as a consequence of verb treatment. Accuracy on preposition items was unchanged following verb therapy. The session 3 results obtained after preposition therapy also showed significant function-specific effects of treatment, with maintenance of the improvement on verb items. A com-parison of treated and untreated items was not significant, showing that generalization of treatment had taken place to untreated microworld tasks. The Real World Test results (see Figure 13.6b) showed a similar function-specific response pattern, with significant effects of treatment after each therapy block. Moreover, improvement was not confined to real world items containing verbs/prepositions treated in the microworld. Finally, performance on the Morphology Test was static throughout, providing further evidence of the specificity of the treatments and ruling out any suggestion of coincidental remission or general stimulation effects.

Figures 13.7a and 13.7b show the results for Group B who received preposition therapy first. There was a significant improvement between sessions 1 and 2, after preposition therapy, but not between sessions 2 and 3 after verb therapy. It can be seen from Figure 13.7a that the group responded to treated preposition items after therapy (there was very little effect on untreated items), but that the improvement fell off sharply once therapy was withdrawn. However, there was also some improvement on verb items after preposition therapy (statistically, the size of improvement on the two functions was not distinguishable, so in this case the treatment was not shown to be function-specific). Although some further improvement occurred in treated and untreated verb items following verb therapy, the overall change between sessions 2 and 3 failed to reach significance. The Real World Test results for this group were disappointing: a significant treatment effect was found between sessions 1 and 2 but not between sessions 2 and 3. Like Group A, this group showed no effects of either treatment on their Morphology Test results.

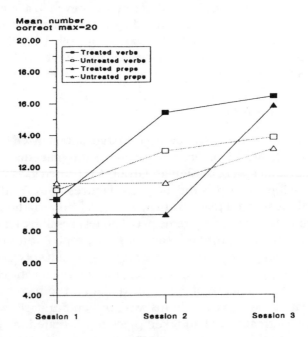

Figure 13.6a. Verb and preposition treatment results for Group A. Verb therapy was given between test sessions 1 and 2. Preposition therapy was given between sessions 2 and 3.

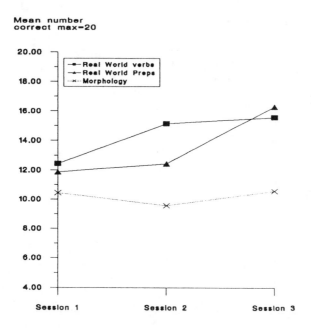

Figure 13.6b. Morphology and Real World Test results for Group A. Verb therapy was given between test sessions 1 and 2. Preposition therapy was given between sessions 2 and 3.

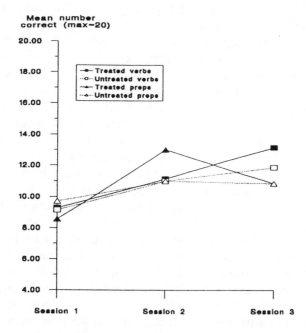

Figure 13.7a. Verb and preposition treatment results Group B. Preposition therapy was given between sessions 1 and 2. Verb therapy was given between test sessions 2 and 3.

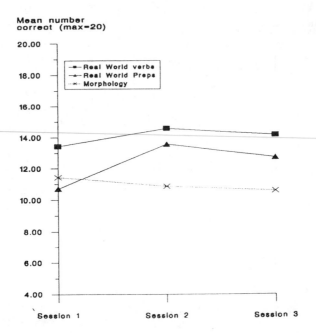

Figure 13.7b. Morphology and Real World Test results Group B. Preposition therapy was given between sessions 1 and 2. Verb therapy was given between test sessions 2 and 3.

Unfortunately, on the basis of this single study we cannot be sure how far the differences in outcome between the two groups were due to the treatment orderings; nor can the administering clinician be eliminated as a contributory factor. Moreover, although the groups had appeared well-matched in terms of their mean scores on a number of pre-therapy tests (not reported here), in fact the range of scores in Group B was much wider. In other words, Group A was a more homogeneous group. From a consideration of individual results and the outcome of a second treatment phase, we suspect that the poorer results of Group B were due mainly to the inability of particular individuals in that group to show generalization effects from treated to untreated items and to maintain item-specific treatment effects.

In order to test the durability of treatment effects in the more successful patients, six members of Group A and one member of Group B were recalled for reassessment after five months with no further treatment. Statistical analysis of the results of the Verb Test and Preposition Test for this group of subjects showed significant effects of treatment between session 1 (pre-treatment) and session 3 (after completion of both blocks of treatment), but no significant change between session 3 and session 4 (after five months no-treatment). That is, the beneficial effects of treatment were retained over a 5-month interval during which no further treatment was given. No significant difference was found between verb items and preposition items or between treated and untreated items, showing that both functions had benefited equally from treatment and that generalization to untreated items had been sustained. A similarly durable performance pattern was obtained on the Real World Test.

The response pattern of Group A allowed us to establish that performance on verb items (such as *The ball paints a box*) and preposition items of similar construction (such as *The ball is under the box*) is dissociable. This result is not just a group artefact, it was seen very clearly, for example, in the results of patient P1 (see Figure 13.8). It is interesting to note that the striking dissociation in this subject was created by the verb therapy. Thus the experimental design led to a finding which was not present at first assessment. At session 2, P1 was accurate on verb items and could be shown to understand all the lexical elements in the preposition sentences, including the preposition meanings which he could gesture. His deficit therefore lay neither in the appreciation of word meanings nor of the grammatical significance of S-V-O (or S-P-O) word order. In fact he was found to be relying on a compensatory strategy based on visual perceptual saliency (Levelt, 1989), to substitute for his loss of grammatical knowledge about the function of locatives. The dissociation found in Group A's results coupled with the function-specific effects of treatment led us to suspect that there may be an inherent advantage to treating verbs first. It may be that reinforcing S-V-O ordering, lexical selection and the mapping of relations on verb items first is logical, since these skills appear to be necessary but not sufficient to handling the locatives.

Running an experiment with 14 subjects simultaneously allowed us to evaluate the data both by groups and as individual cases. The *case series* approach arguably combines the advantages of single case and groups studies while avoiding the pitfalls of drawing conclusions from single cases or from group averages which do not do justice to clinical reality (c.f. Newcombe and Marshall, 1988).

Finally, questionnaires were sent to patients and separately to their carers at the end of the treatment study. These suggested wider functional generalization of therapy. The main areas where participants or their associates reported improvement was in spontaneous speech, in reading for pleasure, in alertness and concentration span and in a general sense of confidence, well-being and interest in life. The following selection of quotations gives an indication of the sort of comments received.[8]

> Modest but unmistakable improvement. Able to call upon a wider vocabulary of individual words, and increased frequency of use of short phrases. More interest in communicating. (P14's son – 6 years post onset).

> A very big improvement. I can make out what H says now. It is great. Long may it continue to improve. (P10's friend – 3 years post onset).

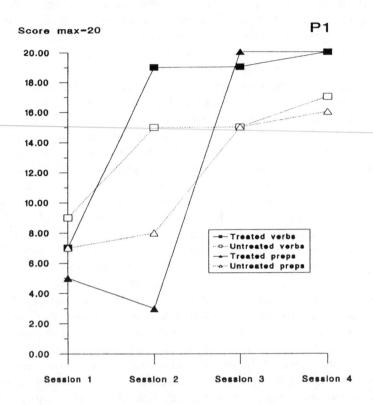

Figure 13.8: Verb and preposition treatment results for patient P1. Verb therapy was given between test sessions 1 and 2. Preposition therapy was given between sessions 3 and 4. No therapy was given between sessions 3 and 4.

There really has been a marked improvement since you started this study...S reads in phrases now and has started to read on her own. (P7's mother – 11 years post onset).

You will be happy to know that B has started to try to read books again – very slowly, but with a good deal of success. (P1's wife, personal note, Dec 1991 – 6 years post onset).

[Attention span has] greatly improved...friends see change for the better. (P12's wife – 1 year post onset).

Think he will persevere better at a task than before. (P6's therapist – 1 year post onset).

He moves around the town more on his own now, seems confident of making himself understood in the shops. To me, this is a wonderful improvement but he seems so casual about it! Maybe this is the true sign of success – the improvement has come, has been totally absorbed and is now 'normal' and useful. No need to think about it any more! (P1's wife – 5 years post onset).

Has made a tremendous difference. J had not ventured outside the house on his own since his stroke. Now he can go for a short walk and also, when I go shopping I can leave him to browse on his own. (P5's wife – 6 years post onset).

Confidence has certainly dramatically improved and with this followed a better sense of well being and increased interest in things around him. (P9's carer – 7 years post onset).

Microworld therapy proved very popular with this pilot group of patients despite the fact that treatment sessions involved working relentlessly for an hour at the limits of patients' abilities. Almost all the subjects would recommend this form of therapy to others and most would have liked extended therapy.

The Computer as a Clinical Tool

Microcomputer technology was indispensable to this study, but, the benefits it brought to assessment and treatment were rather different. The assessments all took the form of sentence/picture-matching tasks. These were self-administered by patients with the clinician as observer, thus providing a replicable assessment environment, free from any suggestion of clinician bias. Unlike with paper-based tests, it was possible to randomize the window positions of the images to guard against possible familiarity effects. Computerization permitted automatic data collection, removing the possibility of errors in scoring and in calculating summary statistics. It also enabled the recording of response latencies in a non-intrusive way and to an accuracy not otherwise possible. Assessment results were displayed immediately on completion of a test, could be printed for inclusion in the subject's file and were stored on hard disc in a form suitable for further analysis without re-keying.

The patients seemed to like the honesty of the feedback they received. They perceived the VDU display of results to be objective, which of course it was, and appreciated being able to get an instant, no-nonsense appraisal as soon as the test was over. Subjects took a great interest not just in their overall accuracy scores, but in their timing relative to previous performances, and to the significance of their error patterns, which were always discussed in a constructive way. Having a poor score was not necessarily demotivating in an environment where we were more interested in understanding the implications of the error patterns than in dwelling on absolute attainment. Indeed, patients were reassured by feeling that some order was seen in the apparent chaos of their responses. Error patterns were available on the screen directly after each test and many subjects were able to understand something of the importance of these – with suitable explanation.

Apart from being psychologically beneficial to the patients, enabling subjects to conduct their own assessments freed the clinician from her usual clerical role in assessment. Thus it was possible to make detailed observations (based on such things as eye gaze, mouse movement and subvocalizations) which were for the most part elicited by this particular environment and would anyway have almost certainly been missed had the clinician been presenting stimulus materials, scoring responses and perhaps also attempting to operate a stop watch.

In contrast, during therapy sessions no data was recorded automatically and no scoring took place. Observation sheets were used to record what had been tackled, any diagnostic insights that had been made and notes to guide the next therapy session. The remediation software provided an exploratory environment to facilitate investigation of the reasons why errors had been made in assessments, and through a better understanding of the difficulties, to try to intervene effectively. The remediation software does not treat the patient *per se*, it relies critically on the quality of the human clinical input. The factors that can contribute to sentence processing breakdowns are many and diverse. In addition, in any individual patient the occurrence of at least some of them can be probabilistic rather than constant. The experience of this study is that aphasic subjects would make little, if any, progress if exposed to this software without expert clinical help. However, it is possible that some more able subjects might benefit from unsupervised sessions providing that they first undergo therapist-directed therapy and can understand their own treatment goals. It is entirely feasible that a version of the system could be used by patients at home to supplement clinical sessions, given willing and suitably trained carers.

To conclude, we have described a computer system and a study to assess its efficacy in the treatment of sentence processing impairments. The combination of experimental design and theoretical basis allowed us not only to demonstrate unequivocal effects of treatment, but also to address specific issues of interest to cognitive neuropsychology. The most important finding was that it is possible to effect statistically significant and durable improvements in the cognitive functioning of some individuals who are many years post-stroke and who have stable language processing deficits – and that this can be achieved with a short input of treatment. We cannot be certain whether the results obtained here were due to reactivation of normal mechanisms or to the training of successful compensation strategies. Of the 13 subjects who were much slower than normal at first assessment, though some impressive reductions in time taken were made, none was restored to normal speed. So while accuracy-based scores indicate highly successful outcomes for some subjects, their slowness still constitutes a major functional handicap and probably points to a residual (general) computational deficit that may well be untreatable.

There are a number of current developments in information technology which have great clinical potential, for example, voice recognition and voice synthesis for personal computers are improving in quality and decreasing in price such that widespread use of automated auditory/verbal assessments and therapy will soon be feasible. The advent of optical disc storage and more powerful microcomputers offers the possibility of harnessing sophisticated computer graphics and moving film sequences for therapeutic use. The nascent field of virtual reality offers exciting opportunities for patients to be immersed in multi-modal assessment and treatment environments. The emergence of co-operative workgroup technology opens up the possibility of therapist and patient interacting simultaneously with shared screen objects and shared sound from separate geographical locations. These are just a few developments that await therapeutic exploitation. However, if more advanced technologies are ever to find their way into clinical settings, evidence must first be produced that computers can unquestionably contribute to better research and more effective patient care. The study we have described uses entry-level equipment and begins to make that case.

Notes
1. *Drill and practice* was a term coined to describe early computer-assisted learning programs which presented exercises (e.g. mathematical calculations requiring a simple answer) and provided limited (right/wrong) feedback.
2. Prolog is notoriously greedy with respect to processing overheads and the hardware necessitated is beyond clinic budgets (even in France!)
3. The software described here runs on any IBM PC AT compatible microcomputer (from a 286 machine with 64K RAM upwards). It requires a VGA colour monitor, a Microsoft compatible mouse and two megabytes of hard disc storage. The software was written in Borland's Turbo Pascal and runs under DOS.
4. Referring therapists knew the aims of the study, so we were selecting from likely candidates. Much wider use of the system is necessary to establish the proportion of aphasic individuals who would qualify for sentence-level therapy in these particular functions.
5. The basic subjects had no further education since leaving school, the intermediate ones had sub-degree level qualifications ranging from secretarial to Higher National Certificate and the advanced subjects had at least one degree.
6. A mean score of 90 per cent was achieved both by the subgroup aged 55 to 69 and by the subgroup with basic educational attainment. The highest mean score (97 per cent) was returned by the advanced education subgroup.
7. Although individual lexical items had been prechecked using the Lexical Test, we anticipated that errors might occur at sentence-level given the increased cognitive load.
8. The majority of the subjects were having regular speech-language therapy up to the commencement of this study and had experienced many different therapies since their strokes. Thus their favourable comments (and those of their carers) were not the result of a therapy/no therapy contrast.

Acknowledgements

This research was funded by grant no. K/MRS/50/C1320 from the Scottish Office Home and Health Department awarded to Elizabeth Dean and Alison Crerar. We are grateful to Elspet Ewing, Alison Paton and Jean Thomson who referred patients to the study. Special thanks are due to Elizabeth Dean for her substantial clinical and organizational inputs. The aphasic subjects who participated in the research program taught us a great deal.

References

Bruce C, Howard D (1987) Computer-generated phonemic cues: An effective aid for naming in aphasia. British Journal of Disorders of Communication 22; 191–201.

Byng S (1988) Sentence processing deficits: theory and therapy. Cognitive Neuropsychology 5/6:629–76.

Byng S, Coltheart M (1986) Aphasia therapy research: methodological requirements and illustrative results. In Hjelmquist E, Nilsson L B (Eds) Communication and Handicap. Amsterdam: North-Holland, Elsevier.

Caplan D, Baker C, Dehaut F (1985) Syntactic determinants of sentence comprehension in aphasia. Cognition 21:117–75.

Caramazza A, Zurif E B (1976) Dissociation of algorithmic and heuristic processes in language comprehension: evidence from aphasia. Brain and Language 3:572–82.

Crerar M A (1990) Interface Test, Lexical Test, Syntax Screening Test, Verb Test, Preposition Test, Morphology Test, Verb Remediation Program, Preposition Remediation Program, Digit-span Recall Test. Unpublished software, copyright 1990. Real World Test. Unpublished aphasia test, copyright 1990. Edinburgh Dept. of Computer Studies, Craiglockhart Campus, Napier University.

Crerar M A (1991) A computer-based microworld for the assessment and remediation of sentence processing deficits in aphasia. Unpublished PhD thesis. Edinburgh: Napier University.

Crerar M A, Ellis A W, Dean E C (forthcoming) Remediation of sentence processing deficits in aphasia using a computer-based microworld. Paper to appearb in Brain and Language.

Deloche G, Seron X, Sallient B, Moulard G, Chassin G (1976) Re-education programme d'un cas d'agraphie. Acta Neurologica Belgica 76:201–11.

Deloche G, Seron X, Rousselle M, Moulard G, Seron X (1978) Re-education assistee par ordinateur de certaines dysorthographies. Re-education Orthographique 16:9–24.

Ellis A W, Young A W (1988) Human Cognitive Neuropsychology. London: Lawrence Erlbaum Associates Ltd.

Enderby P (1987) Microcomputers in assessment, rehabilitation and recreation. Aphasiology 1/2:151–6.

Guyard H, Masson V, Quiniou R (1990) Computer-based aphasia treatment meets artificial intelligence. Aphasiology 4/6:599–613.

Howard D, Hatfield F M (1987) Aphasia Therapy: Historical and Contemporary Issues. London: Lawrence Erlbaum Associates Ltd.

Howard D, Patterson K (1989) Methodological issues in neuropsychological research. In Seron X, Deloche G (Ed). Cognitive Approaches in Neuropsychological Rehabilitation. London: Lawrence Erlbaum Associates Ltd.

Katz R C (1987) Efficacy of aphasia treatment using microcomputers. Aphasiology 1/2:141–9.

Katz R, Nagy V (1984) An intelligent computer-based spelling task for chronic aphasic patients. In Brookshire R (Ed) Clinical Aphasiology: Conference Proceedings. Minneapolis MN: BRK Publishers.

Katz R, Nagy V T (1985) A self-modifying computerised reading program for severely-impaired aphasic adults. In Brookshire R (Ed), Clinical Aphasiology: Conference Proceedings. Minneapolis MN: BRK Publishers.

Katz R, Wertz R, Davidoff M, Shubitowski Y, Devitt E (1989) A computer program to improve written confrontation naming in aphasia. In Prescott T (Ed), Clinical Aphasiology 1988: Conference Proceedings. Boston MA: Little, Brown & Co.

Katz R, Wertz R, Lewis S, Esparza C, Goldojarb M (1990) A comparison of computerised reading treatment, computer stimulation and no treatment for aphasia. In Prescott T (Ed) Clinical Aphasiology 1989: Conference Proceedings: Boston MA: Little, Brown & Co.

Kinsey C (1990) Analysis of dysphasics' behaviour in computer and conventional therapy environments. Aphasiology 4/3:281–91.

Levelt W J M (1989) Speaking: From Intention to Articulation. Cambridge, MA: MIT Press.

Loverso F L (1987) Unfounded expectations: computers in rehabilitation. Aphasiology 1/2:157–9.

Loverso F L, Prescott T E, Selinger M (1988) Cueing verbs: a treatment strategy for aphasic adults (CVT). Journal of Rehabilitation Research and Development 25/2:47–60.

Loverso F, Prescott T, Selinger M, Wheeler K, Smith R (1985) The application of microcomputers for the treatment of aphasic adults. In Brookshire R H (Ed) Clinical Aphasiology. Minneapolis MN: BRK Publishers.

Loverso F, Selinger M, Prescott T (1979) Application of verbing strategies to aphasia treatment. In Brookshire R H (Ed) Clinical Aphasiology Conference Proceedings. Minneapolis MN: BRK Publishers.

Newcombe F, Marshall J C (1988) Idealisation meets psychometrics: the case for the right groups and the right individuals. Cognitive Neuropsychology 5/5:549–64.

Porch B E (1971) Porch Index of Communicative Ability. Palo Alto, CA: Consulting Psychologists Press.

Robertson I (1990) Does computerized cognitive rehabilitation work? A review. Aphasiology 4/4:381–405.

Seron X, (1987) Cognition first, microprocessor second. Aphasiology 1/2:161–3.

Seron X, Deloche G, Moulard G, Rousselle M (1980) A computer-based therapy for the treatment of aphasic subjects with writing disorders. Journal of Speech and Hearing Disorders 45:45–58.

Schwartz M F, Linebarger M C, Saffran E M (1985) The status of the syntactic deficit theory of agrammatism. In Kean M L (Ed) Agrammatism. New York: Academic Press.

Schwartz M F, Saffran E M, Marin O S M (1980) The word order problem in agrammatism: I. Comprehension. Brain and Language 10:249–62.

Wolfe G (1987) Microcomputers and the treatment of aphasia. Aphasiology
    1/2:165–70.

Part IV: Efficacy and Effectiveness

The chapters in this final section provide a critical overview of issues relating to the efficacy and effectiveness of the treatment of aphasia. The first chapter by **Richard Katz** leads on from the previous chapter and reviews in some detail the contribution computer technology can make to the treatment of aphasia. This extensive review of the literature argues for the central role of the aphasia therapist in the effective utilization of computer technology. The chapter demonstrates the value of the use of computers in the treatment and rehabilitation of reading and writing skills and more generally in supporting the broader therapeutic process, including the tabulation of test data and the production of diagnostic reports. Possible developments through the use of expert systems are noted. In line with the argument implicit throughout this collection of papers, he highlights the difficulty in applying the broad principles of computer technology without first understanding the need of individuals with aphasia.

The penultimate chapter by **Klaus Willmes** offers an invaluable introduction to the use of statistical methods as applied in single case treatment. The increased attention and use of single case design in evaluating aphasia treatment is considered. It is also noted that many of the tasks available to assess speech and language often lack reliability and validity which present difficulties in objectively evaluating treatment. The chapter illustrates a number of important issues by reference to statistical techniques which are critical for research clinicians seeking to improve and evaluate treatment techniques for aphasia. He shows the need for aphasia therapists to be aware of the principles of research design and statistical analysis, especially when working within the paradigm which focuses on single case methodology. In passing, Klaus also notes that a great deal of the analysis can be carried out by therapists with personal computers.

The final chapter by **Robert T. Wertz** fittingly provides an overview of the efficacy of treatment for aphasia. This chapter is of critical importance to aphasia therapists, who, within the broader context of changing approaches to the provision of health care, are constantly being required to justify expenditure on treatment. In a clear exposition of the evidence currently available the chapter attempts to answer the question whether treatment for aphasia really works. The conclusions he draws are pertinent for aphasia therapists seeking to offer the most effective and beneficial treatment regimes. He strongly advocates the need for clinicians to act as if they were researchers, primarily to support the long term needs of people with aphasia. It is clinicians, he argues, who are best placed to provide day-to-day information of the effectiveness of treatment, and it might be argued, should be morally obliged to do so. For the student, the practising clinician, teachers and researchers in aphasia and related areas, the need to evaluate the effectiveness of their own contribution to the treatment of aphasia is paramount.

Chapter 14
Aphasia Treatment and Computer Technology

RICHARD C. KATZ

Aphasia rehabilitation has always utilized technological advances available to society. Portable cassette tape recorders, video-tape recorders, and other devices commercially developed and marketed for the general public are familiar additions to the aphasiologist's collection of clinical tools. Occasionally, special devices are developed by adapting existing technology to the needs of clinicians, for example, the use of analog tape recording technology in the development of the Bell and Howell Language Master (Keenan, 1967). When personal microcomputers were first introduced and successfully marketed in the 1970s, it was expected that this new electronic tool would follow the same course of adaptation to rehabilitation. What has happened over the past 15 years is both less and more than anticipated. The computer has not replaced the clinician in spite of its impressive speed, power, flexibility and promises of artificial intelligence. It has been the catalyst for much more than that. The introduction of computers to aphasia rehabilitation has caused considerable controversy, culminating in questioning efficacy of treatment, the role of the clinician and value of aphasia therapy itself. (See Chapter 13.) Clinicians are guided by training, objective measure, research literature, and clinical experience when administering treatment. There are few universally accepted rules of aphasia treatment (e.g., Rosenbek, 1979), but some general approaches to aphasia treatment are accepted by most clinicians. Newly designed clinical tools require a rationale that is consistent with that which is known or believed to be known.

Limits of Aphasia Treatment and Computer Programming

Aphasiologists do not expect treatment software to be effective just because the clinician-provided treatment on which it is based has been shown to be efficacious. Four characteristics of computer programming described by Bolter (1984) emphasize the limitations of the application of computers to aphasia treatment. Computers are *discrete* (i.e., digital), making description of qualitative features difficult. Events must first be separated into distinct, unconnected elements before they can be acted upon by a computer. Computers are *conventional*, that is, they apply predetermined rules to symbols that have no effect on the rules. Regardless of the value of the symbols or the outcome of the program, the rules never change. Computers are *finite;* their rules and symbols are limited to those defined within the program. Unforeseen problems and associations do not result in creation of new rules and symbols. Finally, computers are *isolated*, that is, problems and solutions exist within the computer's own parameters, apart from the real world. Problems are stated in terms of structure so that symbols can be manipulated and solved by following a specific strategy. The strategy behind the solution is called an *algorithm*, a finite series of steps described with adequate detail to guide the program (or anyone else) to answer the questions. Computers, therefore, can only consider problems in which all the variables and rules are known ahead of time, and can be solved in a step-by-step procedure with a finite number of steps, like a game of chess.

Clinicians know that aphasia treatment is very different from a game of chess. Treatment is recognized as a multi-level, interactive behavioral exchange. Not all behaviors have been identified; those that have may vary in importance between patients and situations. In addition, while clinicians recognize some fundamental approaches to aphasia treatment, all the rules are not known and those that are may not always be right (Rosenbek, 1979), although considerable effort has been made to quantify and measure the influence of salient aphasic behaviors (e.g., Porch, 1981) and events during treatment (e.g., Boone and Prescott, 1972).

The applications of linguistic theory to aphasia treatment and to computers serve to illustrate this point. Researchers involved in *computational linguistics* believe that language can be reduced to a mathematic procedure in which algorithms can be developed to reveal the formal structure of natural language processing (Fenstad, 1988). Their work eventually could allow people to interact with computers using natural human language. Researchers construct computer programs based on linguistic and neuropsychological models of language behavior for the purpose of better understanding normal and disordered use of language (e.g., Gigley and Duffy, 1982; Wallich, 1991). The challenge to use linguistic rules to construct software to identify and treat aphasic language behavior is appealing (e.g., Guyard, Masson and Quiniou, 1990) and can ultimately teach us much about language and aphasia, but some authors (e.g., Kotten, 1989; Katz, 1990) feel that the pathological language behavior of aphasic people is influenced just as importantly by other factors, including elements that are cognitive (e.g., attention, vigilance, memory, resource allocation); cybernetic (e.g., slow rise time, noise build-up, intermittent inperception); behavioral (e.g., discriminatory stimuli, chaining, extinction); pragmatic (e.g., functionality, social status); and emotional (e.g., interest, relevance, novelty, enjoyment).

If all the intervening variables were known, the value of treatment would be the same whether delivered by clinician or computer. However, treatment has a diagnostic, evaluative quality. Clinicians can not anticipate all possible patient behaviors, researchers can not identify all therapeutic variables, and programmers can code only a limited number of contingencies. Viewing the clinician's behavior as a model, how many symbols and algorithms do we need to represent aphasia therapy? A program that truly represents clinician-provided treatment will quickly exceed the capacity of modern computers. With expensive and skilful programming and by reducing the scope of the problem to a size manageable for the computer, treatment software can be squeezed and shaped to imitate cognitive and language therapy in small, trivial and predominantly symbolic activities. Rather than emphasize state-of-the-art aphasia treatment, the resultant computerized activity highlights the technical limitations of the computer medium.

Odor (1988) referred to this problem when he wrote that computer-assisted learning defers decisions to programmers who are not physically present during the session, but must gather and send information only through the computer medium, plan in advance how to handle the learning interaction, and then encode these steps into a computer program. Consequently, the scope of treatment software is limited because computer programs are not powerful enough to represent every potentially relevant nuance of interaction during therapy. Odor concluded that computer-assisted instruction is often based on convergent rather than divergent theories of learning. Most computer treatment studies reported in the aphasia research literature describe convergent activities, particularly drills, in which specific responses are learned. Dean (1987) stated that the inability to incorporate divergent strategies in computer programs severely limits their value and application to treatment of aphasic patients, particularly chronic aphasic patients, for whom such treatment appears promising (Chapey, Rigrodsky and Morrison, 1976). The adaptation of divergent therapy to computer-provided treatment remains a challenge for contemporary software developers.

Computers in Aphasia Rehabilitation

Advantages of computers are well-know to clinicians and have been described in detail elsewhere (e.g., Petheram, 1992; Schwartz, 1984;

Crerar and Ellis, Chapter 13). Decreasing price and increasing availability and support have made computers a desirable option in rehabilitation. Speed, accuracy, reliability and ease-of-use are characteristics valued wherever personal computers are used, but the power of computers is not simply the result of faster microprocessors or larger storage devices. Computers are used by clinicians to present stimuli, evaluate responses and store performance for later review. Patients can control some important aspects of their therapy, such as content, duration and frequency. Schuell, Jenkins and Jiménez-Pabón (1964) stated that principles of aphasia treatment should be utilized through our increasing repertoire of clinical techniques. As the technology improves, the role of computers will change. There are many areas in which computers have the potential for becoming significant tools for treating aphasia.

Supplementary Treatment

The concept of homework is hardly new; supplementary treatment in the form of workbooks and other activities has always been an option for clinicians (e.g., Eisenson, 1973). Patients can work longer and more often on a variety of activities designed to stabilize, maintain or generalize newly acquired skills. Contemporary commercial treatment and educational software provides clinicians with the opportunity to extend controlled treatment-related language and cognitive activities beyond the confines of the treatment session. The computer can present many different stimuli in any order at any time and still provide the patient at least some level of feedback, all with minimal supervision and intervention from a clinician. The computerized tasks are presented in a structured setting that incorporate important therapeutic principles and factors, such as control of both stimulus characteristics and response requirements and recording of session performance over time for later analysis. Programs can vary along a continuum according to structure and content, ranging in complexity from simple repetitive drills to interactive tasks that not only evaluate individual responses, but measure overall performance and adjust the type and degree of intervention provided (e.g., Katz and Wertz, 1992).

Modality Considerations

Face-to-face conversation, i.e., talking and listening, is our primary mode of communication. Management of auditory and verbal skills are central to the concept of aphasia rehabilitation (Schuell, Jenkins and Jiménez-Pavón, 1964). Listening and talking are the communicative behaviors used to classify most types of aphasia (Goodglass and Kaplan, 1983; Kertesz, 1982), and are the focus of most aphasia therapy.

Listening and talking, more than other language modalities, affect the likelihood of an aphasic person's successful re-integration into the community, the final demonstration of the success of therapy. For most patients, their families, friends and physicians, the perception of recovery and treatment success is measured by improvement in listening and talking.

Computers offer little assistance to clinicians treating aphasic speaking and listening problems that occur during conversation. Contemporary treatment software seems to have little direct influence in these areas. The contribution of computers to aphasia treatment appears to be in reading and writing. Computers are basically visual-motor graphic machines. Information from the user is normally entered by typing on a keyboard; the output of the computer displayed on the monitor screen and read by the user. This makes the computer well-suited for presenting reading tasks and, through typing, writing tasks. Reading and writing skills appear to be an appropriate focus for computerized aphasia treatment for several reasons. Most aphasic patients have problems in reading (Rosenbek, LaPointe and Wertz, 1989) and writing (Geschwind, 1973). Reading requires minimal response from the patient. Programs for treating reading can run on standard personal computers, without expensive modification or specialized peripheral devices. Typing on the keyboard can be used to examine many aspects central to writing (Selinger, Prescott and Katz, 1987), with the obvious exception of the mechanics of handwriting. Also, reading and writing as communicative acts are usually done alone; having greater interpersonal distance, they are in many ways less direct and responsive than speaking and listening. As such, reading and writing may be appropriate therapeutic activities for aphasic people. Computerized reading and writing treatment tasks can free up valuable treatment time so that face-to-face, individual therapy can emphasize auditory comprehension and verbal output skills. While the computer can provide valuable reading and writing activities (e.g., Scott and Byng, 1989), additional non-computerized, clinician-provided reading and writing therapy could be provided when indicated by changes in patient performance.

Treatment Efficacy

Measuring whether a specific task reduces the effects of aphasia is an essential part of any treatment regime. (See Wertz, Chapter 16, for detailed discussion of efficacy.) Speech-language pathologists assess the influences of various linguistic, physical, and psychological variables on communication and task performance in order to evaluate the effectiveness of a treatment approach or activity. The computer can provide treatment in a standard manner and routinely store performance data for later descriptive and statistical analysis of task effectiveness, thus addressing Darley's (1972) efficacy questions. Perhaps in the near future we will be able to say with confidence that a 55-year-old Broca's aphasic adult who one-year post onset is at the 50th percentile on the *Porch Index of Communicative Ability (PICA)* and should need between 125 and 150 trials to learn to write or print 10 words at the third-grade level (LaPointe, 1977). This benchmark of prognostic resolution would serve as an invaluable clinical yardstick against which the success of treatment could be measured (Matthews and LaPointe, 1981; 1983).

Generalization

The value of aphasia treatment may be determined by the degree skills acquired in treatment are observed in real-life situations. The computer can administer some aspects of treatment without the familiar presence and constant control of the clinician. Treatment activities practised away from the conscious and unconscious effects of the clinician may facilitate generalization. The computer provides immediate feedback during the activity; the clinician reviews performance and provides further intervention if indicated at a later time. Rosenbek, LaPointe and Wertz (1989) recommended a series of clinical activities to increase the likelihood of generalization. Several of the recommendations appear ideal for the computer:

1. expose each patient to numerous repetitions;
2. train a large number of items in a given category;
3. extend treatment outside of the clinic; and
4. organize treatment to maximize independence so patients learn to use treated responses when they want to rather than when told to by the clinician.

Independence

To foster independence and exploit availability of treatment-related activities, the patient should be able to run treatment software with minimal assistance. The required skills include selecting the treatment disk, securing the disk in the disk drive and turning on the computer. Aphasic patients can then determine when and how often they participate in supplementary language activities. This is consistent with Wertz's (1981) comment that we should allow patients to maintain as much independence as possible and that a long-term goal of aphasia treatment is to have patients become their own best therapists. The insight patients have into their problems and strengths can be utilized instead of ignored, and in this way, patients can take a more active role in their treatment.

Emotional Factors

In addition to addressing the language needs of aphasic people, other factors, such as motivation, dependency and quality of life, are concerns that may become increasingly important as recovery slows and the degree of disability and its subsequent effect on life becomes more apparent to the patient and family. Under conditions of perceived helplessness and hopelessness, people frequently become depressed (Seligman, 1975) and have greater difficulty coping with and adapting to changes and problems (Coelho; Hamburg and Adams, 1974). Bengston (1973); Langer and Rodin (1976); Schulz (1976) and others have shown that giving some options and responsibilities to persons in otherwise dependent situations, for example, the institutionalized elderly, can have a strong positive effect on their satisfaction and physical well-being. Decision-making and expression of personal preferences by each patient should be a basic part of patient management and treatment whenever possible.

Diagnostic Activities

Testing and treatment can be stressful for many patients. A good therapist can communicate empathy, honesty, and genuine concern to patients when needed; a computer has none to share. Also, computers measure only what they have been coded to measure. Using semi-autonomous computers for direct patient testing is similar to using technicians or assistants who have limited or no experience with aphasic patients. We can tell them what to expect, but we cannot tell them everything. The inability of software to deal with unpredictable events coupled with lack of empathy severely limits the role of computers as a diagnostician, especially for acute patients (i.e., patients who are rapidly changing and new to the medical setting). Computers are very useful for analyzing speech and voice (e.g., Conway and Niederjohn, 1988) or measuring the degree of aspiration in dysphagia (Mills, 1991). An appropriate diagnostic application for computers with aphasic patients is in routine, periodic monitoring of specific activities (e.g., attention, reading comprehension) for patients already involved in treatment, as they will be more familiar with the computer, its operation, and computer programs. In addition, computers are being used to help clinicians collect test data, calculate scores, print tables, draw graphs, write narrative descriptions, and finally, put all elements together to generate the diagnostic report.

Administrative Activities

Currently, computers are assisting clinicians in the performance of administrative and clinical duties, and in all likelihood will continue to do more in the near future. However, few speech pathologists complain about having too much free time. As computers do more for clinicians, clinicians can do more for their patients and the hospital administration. As is the case for many other professions, general purpose programs have many useful applications for clinicians working with aphasic patients, for example, report and letter writing (wordprocessing programs); organizing, recording and recalling information (database programs); and organizing, recording and recalling information (database programs); and organizing, calculating and projecting values (spread sheet programs). Recent innovations in word processing include the use of voice recognition to increase the speed of generating reports (Tonkovich, et al., 1991). In contrast, only a few programs are written specifically for the administrative needs of aphasia clinicians due primarily to the expense of developing software for a relatively small market. However, many general purpose programs now have features which allow the user to modify the way the program looks and operates, thus meeting the needs of the clinician. Programs incorporating a Graphic User Interface (GUI) make use of word processing, database and authoring programs easier for new and experienced users due to intuitive procedures and standard features (e.g., *point and click*, menu bar) and to use of familiar concepts, and metaphors (e.g., desktop, folders, trash can). For example, information (such as patient information) that was, in the past, organized and stored on index cards can be effectively processed using a GUI multi-purpose program that uses a file card metaphor, such as HyperCard (Apple Computer Inc., 1987–1991).

Recreational Activities

Many commercial recreational programs (such as arcade and adventure games) are finding a limited but useful role in treatment (Lynch, 1983). Enderby (1987) discussed the possibility of computers providing a path toward social and intellectual stimulation for aphasic patients. Stumbo (1995) described how computers, in addition to other resources such as board games, can be used to provide patients with social skill training. While recreation therapy can be a valuable service for patients, our involvement is not urgent or necessary. However, computer game activities offer the patient a diversion and a way of occupying their time in a novel, distracting, entertaining and sometimes intellectually stimulating manner.

Task Structure

There are many elements that are common to the structure of all treatment activities regardless of the underlying principles or mode of deliv-

GOAL

STEPS

INSTRUCTIONS

STIMULI

TARGET RESPONSES

RESPONSE REQUIREMENTS

GENERAL AND SPECIFIC FEEDBACK

INTERVENTION

CRITERIA

RECORD PERFORMANCE

Figure 14.1. Common treatment task components.

ery (Figure 14.1) some are obvious, none are trivial. An understanding of these task components is useful for describing, developing and evaluating treatment activities for the computer. All tasks have a goal, which is usually an intermediate step towards a major or long term goal. The patient should be aware of the goal of the task, and should also be aware of the logical order or steps within the task that advance toward the goal. The clinician should provide the patient with *instructions* so that the patient knows from the beginning what is expected. The *stimuli* used and the desired *responses* should be consistent with the purpose of the task. Responses should be described and quantified using a multidimensional *scoring system* (LaPointe, 1977; Porch, 1981) whenever possible to identify and measure the occurrence of salient behaviors within the task (Figure 14.2). Care should be taken

Score	Description of Response
3	Accurate and complete without prompt
2	Accurate and complete after prompt
1	Partially accurate after prompt
0	Inaccurate after prompt

Figure 14.2. Example of a multidimensional scoring system for a PACE-type task.

that the patient is not burdened with additional, unnecessary *response requirements* that could confound performance. Responses should be as simple as possible to reflect accurately the performance of the target behavior. *General feedback* (Stoicheff, 1960) to encourage the patient and *specific feedback* to describe the most recent response should be readily provided. The clinician should provide an *intervention* (strategy or cue) to improve performance as needed. Teaching specific responses may be the goal of some tasks; commonly, a more valuable goal is to develop a task to help the patient learn an intervention (e.g., self-cue or compensatory strategy) to improve communication during actual, functional situations (e.g., Christinaz, personal communication, re: Colby, et al., 1981). Criteria for *termination* of the task should be specified to provide a target against which the patient can measure progress. Responses and performance *scores should be stored* for later review and analysis. At that time, both the patient's performance and the intervention can be *evaluated* using various techniques (Prescott and McNeil, 1973; LaPointe, 1977; McReynolds and Kearns, 1983; Matthews and LaPointe, 1981; Matthews and LaPointe, 1983).

The following four major types of treatment activities are appropriate for presentation on the computer. The types are not exhaustive nor mutually exclusive; a treatment activity may have several purposes and demonstrate characteristics of more than one type, stimulation and drill and practice (e,g., Seron, et al., 1980).

Stimulation

As described by Schuell and her colleagues (1964), stimulation activities offer the patient numerous opportunities to respond quickly and usually correctly over a relatively long period of time for the purpose of maintaining and stabilizing the underlying processes or skills, rather than simply learning a new set of responses. The process, therefore, is the focus of the task. Stimuli are not selected primarily for informational content (e.g., interest and relevance), but for salient stimulus characteristics (e.g., length, number of critical elements, complexity and presentation rate). Computer programs can easily be designed that contain a large database of stimuli and control these variables as a function of the patient's response accuracy. Overall accuracy and other salient response characteristics (e.g., latency) are usually displayed at the end of the task. An early example of a computer stimulation task is the auditory comprehension task described by Mills (1982).

Drill and Practice

The goal of drill and practice exercises is to teach specific information so that the patient is able to (or appears able to) function more independently. Stimuli are selected for a particular patient and goal, and so an authoring or editing mode is needed to modify stimuli and target responses. A limited number of stimuli are presented and are replaced when criterion is reached. Since response accuracy is the focus of the task, the program should present an intervention or cues to help shape the patient's response toward the target response. Drill and practice exercises, therefore, are convergent tasks because the accurate response must match exactly the target response. Results are displayed or stored on disk and show the effectiveness of the intervention. An example presented in the research literature of a drill and practice exercise is the typing (writing) program described by Seron, et al., (1980); Katz and Nagy (1984); and Katz et al., (1989).

Simulation

Also called micro-worlds, simulations are programs that present the patient with a structured environment in which a problem or problems are presented and possible solutions are offered (See Crerar and Ellis, Chapter 13, for detailed discussion of micro-worlds). Simulations may be simple, such as presenting a series of paragraphs describing stages of a problem and listing possible solutions. Complex programs more closely simulate a real-life situation by using pictures and sound. The term *virtual reality* (Rheingold, 1991) describes a totally simulated environment created through the interaction of computer and human along verbal and nonverbal channels. Simulations have been used in fields such as chemistry, geology, meteorology and astrophysics to test conditions impossible to experience or to train people in situations that would otherwise be too dangerous to experience first hand. Simulations provide the opportunity to design divergent treatment tasks that could more fully address real life problem-solving strategies than those addressed by more traditional, convergent computer tasks, for example, by including several alternative but equally correct solutions to a problem, such as during *PACE* therapy (Davis and Wilcox, 1985). The question of whether simulations can improve generalization of the new behavior to real-life settings remains to be tested.

Tutorial

Research does not appear to support the notion that prepared tutorial material offers aphasic patients any direct benefit. However, some authors (e.g., Eisenson, 1973) have suggested that aphasic patients be best served by modifying their communication environment. In that respect, tutorials can offer valuable information to facilitate communication and influence quality of life for the family, friends and others who help shape the aphasic patient's world. For example, the computer tutorial could present information found in patient information pamphlets in an interactive format, with additional models provided when needed or requested. The tutorial program could be combined with an expert system program to function as a source of information for family members in the future when new problems and questions arise.

Efficacy of Aphasia Treatment Software

The computer can be a powerful clinical tool. It can administer activities designed by a clinician or programmer and, just as importantly, can measure patient performance on the tasks. Sophisticated programs can modify stimulus and response characteristics, provide cues, or change tasks altogether, all in response to patient performance. The computer used this way can increase the amount of time patients are involved in supervised activity. However, Loverso (1987) noted most computer advocates focus on appealing features of computers, such as cost effectiveness and operational efficiency, while the real issue that demands attention from clinicians is treatment effectiveness; treatment activities must be effective before they can be efficient.

Ineffective treatment programs would be damaging to the overall quality of treatment provided aphasic patients. Treatment provided by computers must undergo the same scientific scrunity and systematic modification as do all other aspects of treatment; otherwise, treatment software will not continue to develop and improve. Each computer treatment study reported in the aphasia literature measures not only the applicability of the computer medium, but a number of other factors, such as the underlying treatment model, its appropriateness for the types of patients tested, its realization as software, and how the computerized treatment program merges with the rest of the treatment regime. The efficacy of a particular software program will not indicate the appropriateness of computerized rehabilitation in general for all aphasic patients. That question can only be answered one program at a time.

A computer, however, is only as good as its software. Software can not reproduce every process and variable that occurs during treatment and so computerized treatment in this sense will never be as efficacious as clinician-provided treatment. One way clinicians increase the likelihood that software is efficacious is to develop and test their own treatment programs. Mills (1988) suggested that clinicians who program with only limited programming skills tend to produce limited programs. Experience has also demonstrated that programmers who program with only limited understanding of treatment principles tend to produce treatment software that is limited in its effectiveness.

How do computer treatment studies reported in the aphasia research literature measure up to what is known about treatment?

Dean (1987) wrote that existing computer treatment programs 'are not firmly grounded in a theoretical rationale for remediation' (p. 267), thus limiting their potential. To Katz (1984) and Loverso, et al., (1988), most contemporary treatment software consists of drills with no explicitly stated intervention goals; their use should be conservative and practical. Others (e.g., Lucas, 1977; Bracy, 1983; Skilbeck, 1984) have advocated the computer rather than the clinician as the primary treatment medium, while a few (e.g., Rushakoff, 1984) described the development of clinician-independent, autonomous computerized aphasia treatment programs. Robinson (1990) argued that the research evidence is simply not yet available to support the use of computers for the vast bulk of language and cognitive problems, and suggested that some researchers have obscured the basic issue by asking what works, with whom, under what conditions (see Darley, 1972). Robinson concluded that because computers are prematurely promoted in clinical work, their routine clinical use may be causing patients more harm than good. Certainly, there is no substitute for carefully controlled, randomized studies, the documentation of which has become the scientific foundation of aphasiology. Holland (1970) said it well when she wrote that the scientific community has a right to ask for our data, not our word. Katz and his colleagues over a ten-year period incorporated increasingly sophisticated designs and greater numbers of subjects to assess efficacy of computerized aphasia treatment, from simple A-B-A designs (Katz and Nagy 1982; 1983; 1984; 1985) to large, randomly-assigned group studies incorporating several conditions (Katz and Wertz, 1992). Perhaps one of the best examples of the process of demonstrating efficacy in a computerized treatment program involves 13 years of published research by Loverso and his colleagues, who have published a series of data based reports describing the development and testing of a model-driven clinician-provided treatment approach, the 'verb as core', from its origins as a 'clinician-delivered therapy' (Loverso, Selinger and Prescott, 1979; Loverso, Prescott and Selinger, 1988) to its encoding as a computer/clinician-assisted program (Loverso, *et al.*, 1985; Loverso, *et al.*, 1988; Loverso, Prescott and Selinger, 1992).

As important as documented research is to the development of our field, responsible aphasia clinicians are not blindly following some simple, step-by-step plan when providing treatment. The course of recovery for aphasic patients involves many levels of change (e.g., physiologic, cognitive, communicative, emotional, social). Clinicians base contemporary aphasia treatment on theory and experience and routinely measure patient response as a guide to maximize the effect of that treatment. By measuring and documenting performance, each clinician learns what works and what does not for different patients and for different types and severities of aphasia. If treatment works, the process is continued; if it does not, something different is attempted. The procedure is guided by theory, clinical experience, objective measurement and the objective to maximize improvement in the patient. Although clinicians can not guarantee success, a patient is rarely, if ever, in danger of being harmed or even wasting his or her time. This approach is accepted by many professions for providing treatment to patients in need. For example, the effectiveness of aspirin for headaches has never been tested in a controlled study, but physicians continue to prescribe it. Many physicians prescribe therapy to reduce stress in the belief stress predisposes people to a number of illnesses, although research to date frequently produces conflicting results (Blois, 1988). Medical textbooks (e.g., Geiringer, Kincaid and Rechtien, 1988) recommend trial use of cervical traction to relieve neck pain, even though the approach has never been tested, there is no medical basis for it, and some patients report an increase in pain, in which case physicians stop the treatment and try something else. Perhaps the most dramatic example of whether to withhold treatment revolves around the drug, azidothymidine (AZT). While randomized clinical tests were underway, the U S Federal Drug Administration permitted physicians, at their discretion, to prescribe the drug for asymptomatic HIV-positive patient in the hope of delaying the onset of symptoms (Young, 1988). When the research studies were completed (e.g., Parks, et al., 1988), AZT was shown to be efficacious in delaying symptoms for some patients, and just as importantly, in the interim the lives of many patients had been extended.

Research

The computer can become a very powerful clinical tool by incorporating what we know about aphasia, treatment and computer programming. The studies cited briefly below are part of a growing body of research which describes the efforts of researchers to measure and document the effectiveness of various computerized treatment programs for aphasic adults. (For a more extensive review, refer to Katz, 1986; 1987; Robinson, 1990.) Those that are concerned that researchers are advocating computers in place of clinicians are missing the point. In all computer aphasia treatment studies, speech clinicians selected and tested the patients, designed the treatment plans, designed and modified the treatment tasks, trained the patients to use the computers, and measured treatment efficacy.

Computer Utilization

Early studies focused on whether aphasic patients would be capable of using computers in treatment. Katz and Nagy (1982) reported that their five chronic aphasic subjects learned to place the treatment disk in the drive, turn on the computer, and use the keyboard to select options from menus and run specially written treatment software, all with minimal supervision after three sessions. One aphasic subject, who suffered a right cerebral vascular accident (CVA) found the computer generated characters difficult to read on the monochrome computer screen. Mills (1982) described an aphasic patient using a joystick successfully on an auditory comprehension task that offered up to four choices, one in each corner of the screen. Petheram (1988) conducted the most extensive test of compatibility between aphasic subjects and computer equipment. He tested five different input devices (mouse, joystick, tracker ball, concept keyboard, touch screen) with nine aphasic and three control (elderly) subjects on tasks that simulated eight common exercise formats (e.g., choosing from a menu) and found the tracker ball best on success rate and patient preference. The author concluded that the tracker ball was preferred by the subjects over the mouse and joystick because it allowed them to divide the point and click procedure into two distinct components. Burton, Burton and Lucas (1988) supplied disks containing 14 general language stimulation programs and questionnaires to 23 centres treating aphasic subjects in an effort to solicit information on therapist and patient preferences and success. Questionnaires were returned after three months and provided and provided information on 99 subjects who completed a total of 281 sessions. Average number of tasks used per session was under four. The majority of aphasic patients responded well to computers and enjoyed using them. Therapists reported favourable comments regarding use of the software. As expected, elderly and more severely impaired patients required additional support from the therapists.

Auditory Comprehension

The patient's impaired ability to understand spoken speech is frequently the focus of aphasia treatment. When treating auditory problems, Schuell (1974) indicated the patient should be provided with the opportunity to respond accurately many times. All would agree speech used in auditory comprehension tasks should be natural sounding. Contemporary treatment programs, however, have only a limited ability to manipulate and produce speech, and the intelligibility and quality of artificial speech varies considerably due to difference designs in hardware and software.

There are two major types of computer controlled artificial speech. Synthesized speech is the most common form of computer speech found in educational software. Two types of synthesized speech exist. Phoneme-based synthesized speech produces recognizable speech from a large set of phonemes and other sound combinations stored on the synthesizer card. Speech is only moderately intelligible as many sounds are distorted. For example, the sounds for the letter *T* and the letter *S* usually differ only in duration. Also, speech is pieced together from phonemes creating severe disruption of coarticulation, prosody and rate, further adding to the artificial quality of the output. In *phrase-based* synthesized speech, digitized representations of entire words and phrases, rather than phonemes and sounds, are read from a disk and stored on memory chips on the synthesizer card. The prosody within words and phrases is preserved somewhat and the quality of speech is better than with phoneme-based synthesized speech. Synthesized speech is best utilized when the capacity to produce unlimited novel output is required. Treadwell, Warren, and Wilson (1985) compared two varieties of synthesized speech (phoneme-based and custom) to live speech. The nine aphasic subjects performed well on a computerized listening task when listening to custom speech; accuracy and response time were only slightly better when listening to live speech. Phoneme-based speech produced poorer performance.

Digitized speech uses an auditory digitizing device to measure the pitch (frequency) and loudness (intensity) of a sample of natural speech many thousand times each sound. The frequency and intensity values of the speech sample are then stored as numbers in a file on a disk. When the sample of speech is first played back, the digitizer, controlled by special software, reads the stored frequency and intensity values from disk and reproduces the speech sample with good clarity, prosody and rate. Faster sampling rates result in higher speech fidelity, but required greater amounts of disk space and computer memory. Computer response time can be noticeably delayed because the digitized values are read initially from a disk in a disk drive. Sample speech can be accessed by the program as many times and in any order required. The capacity to digitize sound provides researchers and clinicians with an excellent tool to record and study speech signals (e.g., Conway and Niederjohn, 1988). Because digitization produces the most realistic sounding speech, it is preferable for auditory comprehension tasks. Mills and Thomas (1983) compared intelligibility of different forms of artificial speech, specifically synthesized speech (phoneme-based), digitized speech (4K Hz sampling rate) and analog speech (tape-recorded). As a group, the six aphasic patients performed best with analog speech and worst with synthesized speech.

Mills and Thomas (1981) and Mills (1982) used a computer to provided auditory comprehension practice for an aphasic adult. Four line drawings of common objects were presented on the screen as one-, two-, and three-part pointing commands were audibly presented by the computer and a speech digitizer (4KHz sampling rate). The patient responded by pressing the key or keys (1–4) associated with the target picture and then pressing the return key or by moving a joystick and pressing the joystick button. Pressing the return key alone provided the patient with a repetition of the auditory stimulus. An error on the first attempt resulted in feedback and a repetition of th stimulus. If a second error was encountered, the correct item was highlighted and the next stimulus item presented. A correct response resulted in a positive verbal message followed by presentation of the next stimulus item. Twelve stimulus words per session were presented. Improvement over five months' time was observed in accuracy, response time (latency), and responsiveness (need for fewer repetitions) for an aphasic adult who began the computerized treatment program two months after suffering a left cerebral vascular accident. The influence of the program is questionable, however, due to the patient's recent time post onset.

Verbal Output

Because of a multitude of problems including technical limitations and costs, little use has been made of the computer when treating language output problems of aphasic adults. The ability to evaluate a patient's verbal (linguistic) production without transcription is currently beyond the limitations of existing commercially available equipment and treatment software. Computer and microprocessor-driven devices are widely used that help physically impaired patients compensate for speech output (motor and/or sensory) problems by producing artificial speech or by printing words on a screen or on paper. A considerable degree of linguistic ability is required to formulate and monitor the accuracy of messages, making these devices less appropriate for aphasic patients.

In spite of the many difficulties, some researchers have developed programs to compensate for aphasic verbal output problems. Colby made extensive use of computers and speech synthesizers in attempts to increase verbalization and communication in autistic and other non-speaking children (e.g., Colby and Kraemer, 1975; Colby and Smith, 1973). Later, Colby, et al., (1981) built and programmed a small, portable microcomputer carried by a dysnomic aphasic subject on a sling and shoulder strap combination, thus allowing the use of the device in actual communicative situations. When the subject experienced difficulty remembering a word, she pushed keys in response to prompts from the computer. On a small LCD screen, the computer printed a series of cues (posed as questions) designed to help the computer predict the forgotten word, e.g., 'Do you remember the first letter of the word', '... the last letter', '... any other letters', '... any other words that go with the forgotten word?' The subject's answers were applied according to an algorithm outlined in the program, and a list of possible words was produced and displayed across the computer screen beginning with the most probable words. When the patient recognized the forgotten word, she pressed a button and the word was produced via synthesized speech. (Most dysnomic patients usually can recognize the correct word and say it after a visual or auditory model (e.g., Benson, 1975).) The subject was cued successfully by the portable computer in real-life situations that were functional and communicatively stressful. Christinaz (personal communication, 1984) later reported that the cueing algorithm subsequently generalized to non-computer settings. His subject and other patients tested reported after several weeks of use that they no longer required the computer, instead asking themselves the same series of questions previously displayed by the computer. Christinaz reasoned that the subjects had apparently 'internalized the algorithm' and now cued themselves without the need of the external prompts. The implications of Christinaz' observation are certainly interesting, potentially significant and hopefully will be tested soon. Portable computers are widely used as dedicated compensatory communication devices; acquisition and generalization of functional communication behaviors may occur if these or similar devices modeled self-cueing strategies for patients during actual communicative situations.

Dysnomic aphasic patients, such as the subject in the Colby et al., 1981 study, are usually mildly aphasic (Brown and Cullinan, 1981). Globally aphasic patients are at the other end of the severity continuum. Steele, et al., 1987; and Weinrich, et al.,1989, developed and tested a graphically oriented computer-based alternate communication system called, *Computer-Aided Visual Communication* system, or *C-VIC* for chronic, global aphasic adults. *C-VIC* is an interactive pointing board that runs on a Macintosh computer and uses a picture-card design, or metaphor. Subjects use the mouse to select one of several pictures or icons, each of which represents a general category. The selected icon then opens up to reveal pictures of the items within the selected category. After selecting the desired item, the picture is added to a sequence of other selected pictures; this string of pictures represents the message. The message can be read via the sequence of icons, words printed below the sequence, or in some cases, heard through digitized speech. Much attention is given to the selection of icons. Weinrich, et al., (1989) reported that concrete icons were learned and generalized faster than abstract icons, but neither type of icon generalized well to new situations. Steel, et al., (1987) described that although improvement on expressive and receptive tasks for a globally impaired aphasic subject using *C-VIC* followed training, communication through more traditional modes of communication remain unchanged.

Reading Comprehension

Katz and Nagy (1982) described a program designed to test reading and also provide reading stimulation for aphasic patients. Five aphasic subjects ran the computer programs two-to-four times per week for eight-to-twelve weeks. Although several subjects demonstrated improved accuracy, decreased response latency and increased number of attempted items on some computer tasks, changes in pre- and post-treatment test performance were minimal. The following year, Katz and Nagy (1983) reported a computer program for improving word recognition in chronic aphasic patients. The program was designed to accomplish a task difficult to undertake for a clinician and utilized the advantages of a computer. The program presented 65 words and varied the rate of exposure as a function of accuracy of response. The goal of the program was to help increase and stabilize the subject's sight vocabulary, but no changes were observed on pre- and post-treatment measures for the five chronic aphasic subjects. Later, Katz and Nagy (1985) described a self-modifying computerized reading program for severely-impaired aphasic adults. The objective of the study was to improve functional reading, and a program was developed to teach subjects to read single words without intensive clinician involvement. The program also generated through a printer writing homework activities that corresponded to the subject's performance. Four of the five subjects demonstrated pre- to post-treatment changes on the treatment items that ranged from 16 per cent to 54 per cent.

Scott and Byng (1989) tested the effectiveness of a computer program designed to improve comprehension of homophones for a 24-year-old subject who suffered traumatic head injury and underwent left temporal lobe surgery. Eight months after the accident the subject continued to demonstrate aphasic symptoms as well as surface dyslexia and surface dysgraphia. Reading was slow and laboured; she was able to understand printed words by sounding them out, presenting particular problems with homophones. The computer program, based on an information processing model, was designed to focus on this one aspect of the subject's reading problem. The subject demonstrated steady improvement on the 136-item treatment program which was run 29 times over a ten-week period. The subject improved in recognition and comprehension of treated (p<.001) and untreated (p<.002) homophones used in sentences. Improvement was also demonstrated on recognition of isolated homophones that were treated (p<.05) and on defining isolated treated (p<.03) and untreated homophones (p<.02). Recognition of isolated untreated homophones and spelling of irregular words showed no improvement.

Writing: Typing and Spelling Words

Many reading comprehension activities are easily transferred to the computer. Writing activities, however, are less easily adapted. The most obvious problem is the inability of the common computer to evaluate handwriting and printing. The computerized writing treatment programs described in the literature substitute typing for writing during the intervention. In a comparison of writing and typing abilities of aphasic subjects, Selinger, Prescott, and Katz (1987) examined seven left-hemisphere damaged subjects in order to assess differences between *PICA* graphic scores on subtests *A* through *E* using standardized *PICA* graphics responses, and *PICA* responses typed on a computer. No differences were found between scores on the *PICA* subtests as generated with a pencil and paper and on a computer. These results suggest that the graphic language abilities of brain damaged adults are equally represented by the two output systems.

Several investigators have incorporated complex branching algorithms in computerized writing programs to provide multilevel intervention. Seron, et al., (1980) described a minicomputer/clinician combination that helped aphasic patients learning to type words to dictation. The clinician said the target word and the subject typed a response on the computer keyboard. (The clinician had to know in advance the order of the stimuli programmed in the computer.) Intervention consisted of three levels of feedback: the number of letters in the target word; whether the letter typed was in the word; and when the correct letter was typed, whether that letter was in the correct position. The five subjects completed the program in seven to 30 sessions. Pre- and post-treatment tests required the subjects to write a generalization set of single words to dictation. A decrease (p<.05) in the number of misspelled words and in the total number of errors made on the post-treatment test suggested that the computer program had improved spelling of words written by hand. Four of the five subjects maintained improved performance on a second post-treatment test administered six weeks later.

Katz and Nagy (1984) used complex branching steps to evaluate responses and provide patients with specific feedback in a computerized typing/handwriting confrontation/spelling task. A stimulus was randomly selected by the program and a drawing representing the stimulus was displayed on the computer screen. The subject responded by typing on the keyboard. Feedback consisted of auditory sounds and text printed on the screen. Single and multiple cues from a hierarchy of six were selected by the program in response to the number of errors made for each of ten stimuli. A seven-point multi-dimensional scoring system was used to describe performance and track the effectiveness of the various cues. (Figure 14.3). Additional feedback included repetition of the successful and most recently failed cues. At the end of the computer session, pencil-and-paper copying assignments automatically generated via the computer printer were completed by the subject. Pre- and post-writing tests revealed improved spelling of the target words for seven of the eight aphasic subjects (p<.01).

Attempt	Score If Correct	Cue If Error
1	7	Repeat stimulus picture only
2	6	Anagram without feedback
3	5	Copying words from memory
4	4	Anagram with selection feedback
5	3	Multiple choice cues
6	2	Copying from printed word
7	1	ERROR / score equals 0 / next word

Figure 14.3. Hierarchy of cues and corresponding scores (Katz and Nagy, 1984).

Glisky, Schlacter and Tulving (1986) reported the ability of four memory-impaired, nonaphasic subjects to type words in response to definitions displayed on the computer screen. Cues included displaying the number of letters in the word and displaying the first and subsequent letters in the word, one at a time, as needed. Cues continued until either the patient typed the word correctly or the program displayed the entire word. All patients improved in the ability to type the target words without cues. Patients maintained their gains after a six-week period of no treatment and demonstrated generalization to another typing task, although generalization to writing was not measured.

Katz, et al., (1989) developed and tested a computer program designed to improve written confrontation naming of animals for nine aphasic subjects with minimal assistance from a clinician. The treatment program required subjects to type the names of ten animals in response to pictures displayed on the computer monitor. If the name was typed correctly, feedback was provided and another picture was displayed. If an error was made, hierarchically-arranged cues were presented and response requirements were modified. Five of the nine subjects reached criterion within six treatment sessions and the performance of all nine subjects improved an average of 40 per cent on the computer task (p<.0001). In addition, improvement was measured on non-computerized written naming tasks, such as written confrontation naming of the treatment stimuli and written word fluency for animal names (p<.001). PICA Writing modality score improved by +4.1 percentile points (p<.05). Improvement did not extend to PICA Overall and Reading scores. Because the goal of the program was to teach subjects the ten names, improvement did not nor was it expected to generalize to written word fluency for an unrelated category. The lack of change in these latter language activities for these ten chronic aphasic subjects contrasts with their improved performance on treated words.

Katz and Wertz (1992) conducted a longitudinal group study to investigate the effects of computerized language activities and computer stimulation on language test scores for chronic aphasic adults. Forty-three chronic aphasic subjects who were no longer receiving speech-language therapy were randomly assigned to one of three conditions: 78-hours of computer Reading Treatment, 78-hours of Computer Stimulation (non-language activities), or No Treatment. The

MATCHING

Letters
  single
  pair
  three
Numbers
  single
  pair
  three
Mixed Letters & Numbers
  pair
  three
Words
  short
  long

COMPREHENSION

Match Upper & Lower Case Letters
Words
  function
  category
  synonym
  antonym
  spelling
Phrase
  function
  definition
  spelling
  grammar
Questions
  who/what
  what/where
  where/when
  when/why
  why/who
  who/what/where
  when/why/what
  all question words
Complex Reading
  yes/no questions
  orientation
  attributes/comparisons
  logic

Figure 14.4. Hierarchy of computer treatment tasks (Katz and Wertz, 1992).

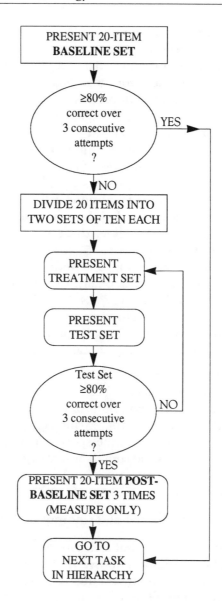

Figure 14.5. Flowchart for reading treatment software (Katz and Wertz, 1992).

Computer Reading Treatment software consisted of 29 activities, each containing eight levels of difficulty, totalling 232 different tasks (Figure 14.4). Treatment tasks required visual-matching and reading comprehension skills, displayed only text (no pictures), and utilized a standard, match-to-sample format with two-to-five multiple choices. Treatment software automatically adjusted task difficulty in response to

subject performance by incorporating traditional treatment procedures, such as hierarchically arranged tasks and measurement of performance on baseline and generalization stimulus sets, in conjunction
with complex branching algorithms (Figure 14.5). Software used in the
Computer Stimulation condition was a combination of cognitive rehabilitation software and computer games that used movement, shape,
and/or color to focus on reaction time, attention span, memory and
other skills that did not overtly require language or other communication abilities. Subjects in the two computer conditions worked on the
computer for three hours per week for 26 weeks. Clinician interaction
during the two computer conditions was minimal. Subjects from all
three conditions were tested with standardized measures (including
the *PICA* and *WAB*) at baseline, three months and six months, and
revealed improved scores (p<.05) for the Treatment group for the
PICA Overall, Reading, Writing, and Verbal modalities and for the *WAB*
Aphasia Quotient (AQ). Additionally, the Treatment group made more
improvement (p<.05) on the *PICA* Overall score than the other two
groups. No statistically significant differences in improvement were
demonstrated between the Stimulation and No Treatment groups on
any test measure. Results suggest that

1. computerized reading treatment can be administered with minimal
   assistance from a clinician;
2. improvement on the computerized treatment tasks generalizes to
   improvement on non-computer language performance;
3. improvement results from the specific language content of the software and not simply the stimulation provided by the computer; and
4. chronic aphasic patients can improve performance through computerized treatment.

Comparison of Traditional and Computer Medium

Comparing the effect of similar treatment activities provided by two
different mediums should improve understanding of the influence of
the medium and the relative effectiveness of the treatment. Many
researchers are attempting to simulate currently accepted testing and
treatment protocols on the computer. Some researchers feel that,
because of speed, reliability, and relative autonomy, computers are
ideally suited to administer tests to aphasic patients who can then work
at their own pace without embarrassment or fear of humiliation (e.g.,
Enderby, 1987). Odell, et al., (1985) developed two computerized
versions of the *Raven Coloured Progressive Matrices* (Raven, 1975) on
an IBM PC system.

The program used high-resolution graphics and a touch screen
input device to administer and analyze test performance quickly and
accurately with minimal supervision from a clinician. The authors

compared the two computerized versions of the *Raven's* test with a traditional, clinician-controlled, paper booklet administration of the test. The performances of 16 aphasic subjects were essentially equivalent under all three conditions, leading the authors to conclude that the computer testing conditions did not present greater visual or cognitive demands on the subjects.

Wolfe, Davidoff, and Katz (1987) compared the performance of non-brain damaged and aphasic adults on another nonverbal problem-solving task, *The Towers of Hanoi* puzzle, originally administered to aphasic subjects by Prescott, Loverso and Selinger (1984). The performance of 19 aphasic and 19 non-brain damaged subjects was compared using two different methods of presentation: two-dimensional color computer simulation of the puzzle versus the manipulation of the actual wooden model. Non-brain damaged subjects performed equally well under both conditions. Like the Odell, et al., (1985) study described earlier, aphasic subjects demonstrated similar performance on the task under both conditions. Aphasic subjects, however, required more time to complete the puzzle in the computer condition than when manipulating the actual wooden model. Also of interest was the fact that under the computer condition, aphasic subjects made more illegal moves, that is, attempted to move the pieces in a sequence not in accordance with the rules of the puzzle. The results suggest that while the computer medium did not affect the accuracy of performance for the aphasic subjects, task completion took longer and was less efficient under the computer condition.

Wertz. et al., (1987) compared the effectiveness of closed circuit television, computer-controlled video laserdisk, and traditional face-to-face interaction for providing appraisal and treatment to aphasic patients in remote settings. Results suggested no significant differences between the three conditions in the diagnoses assigned to the subjects using standard and modified tests. In addition, subjects in all three treatment conditions demonstrated clinically significant change (between 12 and 17 percentile points on the *PICA*). No significant differences in improvement among the three treatment groups was observed, indicating that aphasic patients can benefit from treatment provided in any of the three conditions. The results suggest that television and video laser disc over the telephone could be employed to provide services for patients who live where services do not exist.

Loverso, Selinger and Prescott (1979); Selinger et al., (1987) and Loverso, Prescott and Selinger (1988) developed and tested a treatment protocol for aphasic patients in which verbs were presented as starting points and paired with different wh-question words to provide cues to elicit sentences in an actor-action-object framework. Thirty verbs were used at each of six modules. The hierarchy was divided into two major levels, each consisting of an initial module and two sub-modules which provided additional cueing for subjects unable to achieve 60 per cent or better accuracy on the initial module. Level I presented stimulus verbs and the question words, *who* or *what*, to elicit an actor-action sentence. Level II elicited actor-action-object sentences by presenting stimulus verbs and the question words *who* or *what* for the actor and question words *how*, *when*, *where* and *why* for the object. Subjects responded verbally and graphically. Subjects were scheduled for treatment three-to-five times per week. During each session 30 stimulus verbs were presented for generation of sentences. Statistically significant improvement (p<.05) was demonstrated on the *PICA* following $3\frac{1}{2}$ months of treatment for each of the two aphasic subjects.

Later, Loverso, *et al.*, (1985) compared the effects of the same treatment approach when treatment was provided by a clinician and when it was provided by a computer and speech synthesizer assisted by a clinician. The aphasic subject responded in the clinician-only condition by speaking and writing and in the clinician/computer condition by speaking and typing. Stimulus presentation and feedback in the clinician/computer condition was normally provided only by the computer. The clinician only intervened if the patient's typed response was correct, but the spoken response was in error. The subject improved on the task under both conditions, but took longer to reach criteria under the computer and clinician-assisted condition. based on the subject's improvement, both on the treatment task and on clinically meaningful changes on successive administrations of the *PICA* (p<.01), the authors concluded that their listening, reading and typing activities under the clinician/computer condition had a positive influence on the patient's language performance. They suggested that, although still in the early stages of development, aphasia treatment administered by computers is practical and has the capacity for success. Loverso, *et al.*, (1988) replicated the Loverso, *et al.*, (1985) study with five fluent and five nonfluent aphasic subjects for the purpose of examining whether treatment provided under the computer/clinician condition was as effective as a clinician alone when treating various types and severities of aphasia utilizing their cueing-verb-treatment technique. The ten subjects required 28 per cent more sessions (p<.05) to reach criteria under the computer/clinician condition than under the clinician-alone condition. Fluent subjects required 24 percent and nonfluent subjects required 33 per cent more sessions under the computer/clinician conditions than the clinician-alone condition. Of the ten subjects, eight showed significant improvement (p<.05) on the *PICA* overall percentile measure, on the Verbal modality measure, and on the Graphic modality measure. All subjects maintained gains after a maintenance phase of one month post-treatment or longer. Similar results were reported following a replication of the study using 20 subjects (Loverso, Prescott and Selinger, 1992).

Summary

The true value of computers in the rehabilitation of aphasia continues to be studied. Just like the question of efficacy itself in aphasia rehabilitation (Howard, 1986; Fitz-Gibbon, 1986; Wertz, Chapter 16), the effectiveness of computer utilization in aphasia treatment cannot be answered with a simple *yes* or *no*. Much more work is needed. Treatment software may be an imperfect reflection of clinician-provided therapy, but by improving the software, clinicians and programmers will learn more about how and why treatment works.

Clinicians are responsible for treatment effectiveness, not the computer, software, programmer, publisher or researcher. As treatment cannot be effectively prescribed like medicine, software should be viewed as supplementary treatment with the clinician providing critical intervention as indicated by performance and other considerations. The role of computers and treatment software, like all tools, should extend the abilities of the clinician, allowing clinicians to intervene when skills, experience and flexibility are required. Rather than emphasize what computer can or cannot do better than clinicians, our focus should be on an intelligent division of labour between computers and clinicians, a combination that can do more than either alone. The real danger comes from a failure to appreciate the scope and depth of clinical work. An autonomous, robotic therapist, blindly following a set of rules supposedly representing the knowledge and experience of competent aphasia clinicians, is some fantasy dreamed up by those who focused too much on the costs of care and not enough on the efficacy of care. Until we can describe to others precisely how to treat specific problems in individual patients, it is unreasonable, unethical, and a misrepresentation of the complexity of aphasia therapy to assume that at this time a machine can perform the functions of a clinician.

While clinical perfection is beyond the scope of this chapter, a few steps in the general direction can be made to approach the goal. Better communication among the branches of rehabilitative services using computers will facilitate the process of improving the quality of care delivered to all patients. In the best tradition of scientific and rehabilitative efforts, aphasiologists can work together to shape computer technology for the development of their professions and the benefit of their patients.

References

Bengston VL (1973) Self-determination: A social-psychologic perspective on helping the aged. Geriatrics 28 (12):118–30.

Benson DF (1975) Disorders of verbal expression. In Benson DF, Blumer D (Eds)

Psychiatric Aspects of Neurologic Disease. New York: Grune & Stratton. (pp. 121–377).

Blois MS (1988) Medicine and the nature of vertical reasoning. The New England Journal of Medicine 318 (13):847–51.

Bolter JD (1984) Turing's Man: Western Culture in the Computer Age. Chapel Hill NC: the University of North Carolina Press.

Boone DR, Prescott TE (1972) Content and sequences of speech and hearing therapy. Asha 14:58–62.

Bracy OL (1983) Computer-based cognitive rehabilitation. Cognitive Rehabilitation 1(1):7–8, 18–19.

Brown CS, Cullinan WL (1981) Word-retrieval difficulty and dysfluent speech in adult anomic speakers. Journal of Speech and Hearing Research 24:358–65.

Burton E, Burton A, Lucas D (1988) The use of microcomputers with aphasic patients. Aphasiology 2(5):479–92.

Chapey R, Rigrodsky S, and Morrison E (1976) Divergent semantic behavior in aphasia. Journal of Speech and Hearing Research 19:664–77.

Coelho GV, Hamburg DA, Adams JE (1974) Coping and Adaptation. New York: Basic Books.

Colby KM, Kraemer HC (1975) An objective measurement of nonspeaking children's performance with a computer-controlled program for the stimulation of language behavior. Journal of Autism and Childhood Schizophrenia 5(2):139-46.

Colby KM, Smith DC (1973) Computers in the treatment of nonspeaking autistic children. In Masserman JH (Ed) Current Psychiatric Therapies (Vol 11). New York: Grune & Stratton, pp 1–17.

Colby KM, Christinaz D, Parkison RC, Graham S, Karpf C (1981) A word-finding computer program with a dynamic lexical-semantic memory for patients with anomia using an intelligent speech prosthesis. Brain and Language 14:272–81.

Conway RJ, Niederjohn RJ (1988) Generation of speech spectrograms using a general-purpose digital computer and a dot-matrix printer. Journal of Computer Users in Speech and Hearing 4(1):14–22.

Darley FL, (1972) The efficacy of language rehabilitation in aphasia. Journal of Speech and Hearing Research 37:3–21.

Davis GA, Wilcox MJ (1985) Adult Aphasia Rehabilitation: Applied Pragmatics. Austin TX: Pro-Ed.

Dean EC (1987) Microcomputers and aphasia. Aphasiology 1(3): 267–70.

Eisenson J (1973) Adult Aphasia. New York: Appleton-Century-Crofts.

Enderby P (1987) Microcomputers in assessment, rehabilitation and recreation. Aphasiology 1(2):151–6.

Fenstad JE (1988) Language and computations. In Herken R (Ed) The Universal Turing Machine: A Half-Century Survey. New York: Oxford University Press. pp 327–48.

Fitz-Gibbon CT (1986) In defence of randomised controlled trials, with suggestions about the possible use of meta-analysis. British Journal of Disorders of Communication 21: 117–24.

Geiringer SR, Kincaid CB, Rechtien JJ (1988) Traction, manipulation, and massage. In

DeLisa JA (Ed) Rehabilitation Medicine: Principles and Practice. Philadelphia PA: JB Lippincott. pp 276–9.

Geschwind N (1973) Writing and its Disorders. Paper presented at the Second Pan-American Congress of Audition and Language, Lima, Peru.

Gigley HM, Duffy JR (1982) The contribution of clinical intelligence and artificial aphasiology to clinical aphasiology and artificial intelligence. In Brookshire R H (Ed) Clinical Aphasiology: 1982 Conference Proceedings. Minneapolis MN: BRK Publishers. pp 170–7.

Glisky EL, Schlacter DL, Tulving E (1986) Learning and retention of computer-related vocabulary in memory-impaired patients: Method of vanishing cues. Journal of Clinical and Experimental Neuropsychology 8(3):292–312.

Goodglass H, Kaplan E (1983) Boston Diagnostic Aphasia Examination. Philadelphia PA: Lea & Febiger.

Guyard H, Masson V, Quiniou R (1990) Computer-based aphasia treatment meets artificial intelligence. Aphasiology 4(6): 599–613.

Holland AL (1970) Case studies in aphasia rehabilitation using programmed instruction. Journal of Speech and Hearing Disorders 35:377–90.

Howard D (1986) Beyond randomised controlled trials: the case for effective case studies of the effects of treatment in aphasia. British Journal of Disorders of Communication 21:89–102.

Katz RC (1984) Using microcomputers in the diagnosis and treatment of chronic aphasic adults. Seminars in Speech, Language and Hearing 5(1):11–22.

Katz RC (1986) Aphasia treatment and microcomputers. New York: Taylor & Francis.

Katz RC (1987) Efficacy of aphasia treatment using microcomputers. Aphasiology 1(2):141–50.

Katz RC (1990) Intelligent computerized treatment or artificial aphasia therapy? Aphasiology 4(6):621–4.

Katz RC, Nagy VT (1982) A computerized treatment system for chronic aphasic adults. In Brookshire RH (Ed) Clinical Aphasiology: 1982 Conference Proceedings. Minneapolis MN: BRK Publishers. pp 153–60.

Katz RC, Nagy VT (1983) A computerized approach for improving word recognition in chronic aphasic patients. In Brookshire RH (Ed) Clinical Aphasiology: 1983 Conference Proceedings. Minneapolis MN: BRK Publishers. pp 65–72.

Katz RC, Nagy V (1984) An intelligent computer-based task for chronic aphasic patients. In Brookshire RH (Ed) Clinical Aphasiology: 1984 Conference Proceedings. Minneapolis MN: BRK Publishers. pp 159–65.

Katz RC, Nagy VT (1985) A self-modifying computerized reading program for severely-impaired aphasic adults. In Brookshire R H (Ed) Clinical Aphasiology: 1985 Conference Proceedings. Minneapolis MN: BRK Publishers. pp 184–8.

Katz RC, Wertz RT (1992) Computerized hierarchical reading treatment in aphasia. Aphasiology 6(2):167–77.

Katz RC, LaPointe LL, Markel NN (1978) Coverbal behavior and aphasic speakers. In Brookshire RH (Ed) Clinical Aphasiology: 1978 Conference Proceedings. Minneapolis MN: BRK Publishers. pp 164–73.

Katz RC, Wertz RT, Davidoff M, Schubitowski YD, Devitt EW (989) A computer program to improve written confrontation naming in aphasia. In Prescott T E (Ed) Clinical Aphasiology: 1988 Conference Proceedings. Austin TX: Pro-Ed. pp 321–38.

Keenan JS (1967) A Language Rehabilitation Program – Aphasia. Chicago IL: Bell and Howell.

Kertesz A (1982) Western Aphasia Battery. New York: Grune & Stratton.

Kotten A (1989) Aphasia treatment: A multidimensional process. In Perecman E (Ed) Integrating Theory and Practice in Neuropsychology. Hillsdale, NJ: Lawrence Erlbaum. pp 293–315.

Kreindler A, Fradis A (1968) Performance in Aphasia: A Neurodynamical, Diagnostic and Psychological Study. Paris: Gauthier-Villars.

Langer EJ, Rodin J (1976) The effect of choice and enhanced personal responsibility for the aged: A field experiment in an institutional setting. Journal of Personality and Social Psychology 34:191–8.

LaPointe LL (1977) Base-10 programmed stimulation: task specification, scoring and plotting performance in aphasia therapy. Journal of Speech and Hearing Disorders 42:90–105.

Loverso FL (1986) Rehabilitation of language-related memory disorders in aphasia. In Chapey R (Ed) Language Intervention Strategies in Adult Aphasia (2nd Ed). Baltimore MD: Williams & Wilkins. pp 239–50.

Loverso FL (1987) Unfounded expectations: computers in rehabilitation. Aphasiology 1(2):157–60.

Loverso FL, Prescott TE (1981) The effect of alerting signals on left brain-damaged (aphasic) and normal subjects' accuracy and response time to visual stimuli. In Brookshire RH (Ed) Clinical Aphasiology: 1981 Conference Proceedings. Minneapolis MN: BRK Publishers. pp 55–67.

Loverso FL, Prescott TE, Selinger M (1988) Cueing verbs: a treatment strategy for aphasic adults. Journal of Rehabilitation Research and Development 25:47–60.

Loverso FL, Prescott TE, Selinger (1992) Microcomputer applications in aphasiology. Aphasiology 6(2):155–63.

Loverso FL, Selinger M, Prescott TE (1979) Application of verbing strategies to aphasia treatment. In Brookshire R H (Ed) Clinical Aphasiology: 1979 Conference Proceedings. Minneapolis MN: BRK Publishers. pp 229–38.

Loverso FL, Prescott TE, Selinger M, Riley L (1988) Comparison of two modes of aphasia treatment: clinician and computer-clinician assisted. In Prescott T E (Ed) Clinical Aphasiology (Vol. 18). Austin TX: Pro-Ed. pp 297–319.

Loverso FL, Prescott TE, Selinger M, Wheeler KM, Smith RD, (1985) The application of microcomputers for the treatment of aphasic adults. In Brookshire RH (Ed) Clinical 1985 Aphasiology: Conference Proceedings. Minneapolis MN: BRK Publishers. pp 189–95.

Lucas RW (1977) A study of patients' attitudes to computer interrogation. International Journal of Man-Machine Studies 9:69–86.

Lynch WJ (1983) Cognitive retraining using microcomputer games and commercially-available software. Cognitive Rehabilitation 1:19–22.

McReynolds LV, Kearns KP (1983) Single-Subject Experimental Designs in

Communicative Disorders. Baltimore MD: University Park Press.

Matthews BAJ, LaPointe LL (1981) Determining rate of change and predicting perform-ance levels in aphasia therapy. In Brookshire RH (Ed) Clinical Aphasiology: 1981 Conference Proceedings. Minneapolis MN: BRK Publishers. pp 17–25.

Matthews BAJ, LaPointe LL (1983) Slope and variability of performance on selected aphasia treatment tasks. In Brookshire RH (Ed) Clinical Aphasiology: 1983 Conference Proceedings. Minneapolis MN: BRK Publishers. pp 113–20.

Mehrabian A, Wiener M (1967) Decoding inconsistent communication. Journal of Personality and Social Psychology 6:108–14.

Mills RH (1982) Microcomputerized auditory comprehension training. In Brookshire RH (Ed) Clinical Aphasiology: 1982 Conference Proceedings. Minneapolis MN: BRK Publishers. pp 147–52.

Mills RH (1988) Book review (Aphasia treatment and microcomputers). Journal of Computer Users in Speech and Hearing 4(1):40–1.

Mills RH (1991) Machine vision technology: Quantification of videofluoroscopic swallowing data. Journal of Computer Users in Speech and Hearing 7(1):132–42.

Mills RH, Thomas RP (1981) Microcomputerized language therapy for the aphasic patient. IEEE Proceedings of the Johns Hopkins First Search for Personal Computing Aid to the Handicapped. pp 45–6.

Mills RH, Thomas RP (1983) The Talking Apple – Comparison of Three Microcomputerized Speech Production Methods. Paper presented at the American Speech-Language-Hearing Association National Convention, Cincinnati OH.

Odell K, Collins M, Dirkx T, Kelso D (1985) A computerized version of the Coloured Progressive Matrices. In Brookshire RH (Ed) Clinical Aphasiology: 1985 Conference Proceedings. Minneapolis MN: BRK Publishers. pp 47–56.

Odor JP (1988) Student models in machine-mediated learning. Journal of Mental Deficiency Research 32:247–56.

Parks WP, Parks ES, Fischl MA, Leuther MD, Allain JP, Nusinoff-Lehrman S, Barry DW, Makuch RW (1988) HIV-1 inhibition by azidothymidine in a concurrently random-ized placebo-controlled trial. Journal of Acquired Immune Deficiency Syndrome 1:125–30.

Petheram B (1988) Enabling stroke victims to interact with a minicomputer – a com-parison of input devices. International Disabilities Studies 10(2):73–80.

Petheram B (1992). A survey of therapists' attitudes to computers in the home-based treatment of aphasic adults. Aphasiology 6(2):207–12.

Porch BE (1981) Porch Index of Communicative Ability, Vol.1: Administration, Scoring and Interpretation. (3rd). Palo Alto CA: Consulting Psychologists Press.

Prescott TE, McNeil MR (1973) Measuring the effects of treatment of aphasia. Paper presented at the Third Conference on Clinical Aphasiology, Albuquerque NM.

Prescott TE, Loverso FL, and Selinger M (1984) Differences between normals and left brain damaged (aphasic) subjects on a nonverbal problem solving task. In Brookshire RH (Ed) Clinical Aphasiology: 1984 Conference Proceedings. Minneapolis MN: BRK Publishers. pp 235–40.

Raven JC (1975) Coloured Progressive Matrices. Los Angeles CA: Western Psychologic Services.

Rheingold H (1991) Virtual Reality. New York: Summit Books.

Ritchie D (1961) Stroke: A Study of Recovery. Garden City, NY: Doubleday.

Robinson I (1990) Does computerized cognitive rehabilitation work? A review. Aphasiology 4(4):381–405.

Rosenbek JC (1979) Wrinkled feet. In Brookshire RH (Ed) Clinical Aphasiology: 1979 Conference Proceedings. Minneapolis MN: BRK Publishers. pp 163–76.

Rosenbek JC, LaPointe LL , Wertz RT (1989) Aphasia: A Clinical Approach. Austin TX: Pro-Ed.

Rushakoff GE (1984) Clinical applications in communication disorders. In Schwartz A H (Ed) Handbook of Microcomputer applications in Communication Disorders. San Diego CA: College-Hill Press. pp 148–71.

Schuell H (1965) Differential Diagnosis of Aphasia. Minneapolis MN: University of Minnesota Press.

Schuell H (1974) Aphasia Theory and Therapy: Selected Lectures and Papers of Hildred Schuell. Baltimore MD: University Park Press.

Schuell H, Jenkins JJ, Jiménez-Pabón E (1964) Aphasia in adults. New York: Harper and Row.

Schulz R (1976) Effects of control and predictability on the physical well being of the institutionalized aged. Journal of Personality and Social Psychology 33:563–73.

Schwartz AH (1984) Introduction to microcomputers for specialists in communication disorders. In Schwartz AH (Ed) Handbook of Microcomputer Applications in Communication disorders. San Diego CA: College-Hill Press. pp 1–15.

Scott C, Byng S (1989) Computer-assisted remediation of a homophone comprehension disorder in surface dyslexia. Aphasiology 3(3):301–20.

Seligman M (1985) Helplessness: On Depression, Development and Death. San Francisco CA: Freeman.

Selinger M, Prescott TE, Katz RC (1987) Handwritten versus typed responses on PICA graphic subtests. In Brookshire RH (Ed) Clinical Aphasiology: 1987 Conference Proceedings. Minneapolis MN: BRK Publishers. pp 136–42.

Selinger M, Prescott TE, Loverso FL, Fuller K (1987) Below the 50th percentile: Application of the verb as core model. In Brookshire RH (Ed) Clinical Aphasiology: 1987 Conference Proceedings. Minneapolis MN: BRK Publishers. pp 55–63.

Seron X, Deloche G, Moulard G, Rouselle M (1980) A computer-based therapy for the treatment of aphasic subjects with writing disorders. Journal of Speech and Hearing Disorders 45:45–58.

Skilbeck C (1984) Computer assistance in the management of memory and cognitive impairment. In Wilson BA, Moffat N (Ed), Clinical Management of Memory Problems. Rockville, MD: Aspen Publication.

Steele RD, Weinrich M, Kleczewska MK, Wertz RT, and Carlson GS (1987) Evaluating performance of severely aphasic patients on a computer-aided visual communication system. In Brookshire RH (Ed) Clinical aphasiology: 1987 Conference Proceedings. Minneapolis MN: BRK Publishers. pp 46–54.

Stoicheff ML (1960) Motivating instructions and language performance of dysphasic subjects. Journal of Speech and Hearing Research 3:75–85.

Stumbo NJ (1995) Social skills instruction through commercially available resources. Therapeutic Recreation Journal 29: 30–55.

Tonkovich JD, Horowitz DM, Kawahigashi JN, Krainen GH, Kronick D (1991) An application of voice recognition technology for clinical documentation. Computer poster session presented at the 1991 American Speech-Language-Hearing Association Annual Convention, Atlanta, GA.

Treadwell JE, Warren LR, Wilson MS (1985) the influence of three types of speech production upon auditory comprehension in aphasia. In Brookshire R H (Ed) Clinical Aphasiology: 1985 Conference Proceedings. Minneapolis MN: BRK Publishers. pp 280–6.

Wallich P (1991) Digital dyslexia: Neural network mimics the effects of stroke. Scientific American, October p 36.

Weinrich M, Steele RD, Kleczewska M, Carlson GS, Baker E, Wertz RT (1989) Representation of verb's in a computerized visual communication system. Aphasiology 3(6):501–12.

Wertz RT (1981) Aphasia management: The speech pathologist's role. Seminars in Speech, Language and Hearing 2:315–31.

Wertz RT, Dronkers NF, Knight RT, Shenaut GK, Deal JL (1987) Rehabilitation of neurogenic communication disorders in remote settings. Journal of Rehabilitative Research and Development 25(1):432–3.

Wolfe GR, Davidoff M, Katz RC (1987) Nonverbal problem-solving in aphasic and non-aphasic subjects with computer presented and actual stimuli. In Brookshire R H (Ed) clinical Aphasiology: 1987 Conference Proceedings. Minneapolis MN: BRK Publishers. pp 243-8

Young FE (1988) The role of the FDA in the efforts against AIDS. Public Health Report 3:242-5.

Chapter 15
Aphasia Therapy Research: Some Psychometric Considerations and Statistical Methods of the Single-case Study Approach

KLAUS WILLMES

Introduction

Single-case experimental designs have gained growing attention for the evaluation of neuropsychological treatments in general. Wilson (1987; 1993) argues for the acceptance of such designs, which have originated mostly in behavioural psychology, in the efficacy evaluation of treatment of the individual patient. Objections against the usefulness of large-scale randomized controlled (clinical) trials for the investigation of specific aphasia therapy methods have been well summarized by Howard (1986), but see Schoonen (1991) and Wertz (1992; 1993) for arguments favouring group efficacy studies with an adequate research design including random assignment of patients and provisions for sufficient statistical power. Wertz points out that his arguments pertain in particular to answering the research question: 'Are various methods of therapy efficacious for various types of aphasic patients?' Kazdin (1992) is an excellent reader for classical and more recent papers on design considerations in clinical research in general.

Pring (1986) has given a current review of single-case methodology with reference to aphasia therapy concentrating on clinically applicable research designs and assessments. Along a similar line, Hesketh (1986) argues for the use of multiple baseline designs with visual inspection of the data in order to determine whether interventions were successful. McReynolds and Kearns (1983) provide an overview on single-subject experimental designs for research in the field of communication disorders. One example for a single-subject multiple baseline design across behaviours and subjects is given by Connell and Thompson (1986); an application of this type of design to evaluating the efficacy of treatment for sentence production deficits is by Thompson (1992).

Quite frequently, no inferential statistical procedures are employed when evaluating the changes in performance studied in a single-case experiment. It is sometimes argued that clinically relevant or clinically significant findings should be demonstrable without recourse to statistical testing procedures (Kearns, 1992). This has indeed been a reasonable argumentation for many treatment studies in behavioural psychology where (behavioural) measures could be obtained easily and frequently without obvious training effects induced by the assessment itself. In addition, effects of training were quite often easily reversible after withdrawal of the intervention.

As Pring (1986) has already argued, the typical situation in aphasia therapy is quite different. Treatment is not very likely to lead to rapid and extensive changes in performance, nor is this the case when treatment is removed. It may even be the case that due to (re)learning or the acquisition of new strategies improvements may tend to continue beyond the phase of actual treatment. A second consequence of the gradual type of improvement after treatment is a need to employ inferential statistical procedures to detect more subtle changes in the patient's level of competence. The presence of uncontrolled variability in the observed (dependent) variable(s) is another reason to resort to statistical tests of significance in order to draw inferences about the efficacy of treatment.

Psychometric considerations concerning the tasks and actual items used for assessment seem to be a rather neglected aspect in aphasia therapy research (Tompkins, 1992). As Coltheart (1983) has demonstrated, it will be rather unlikely that standardized tests for the specific treatable functions in a given patient already exist. Coltheart provides many examples of how to construct new assessment procedures to capture the nature of the deficit(s) hypothesized to be producing observed disorders. In the great majority of cases there is no information on the reliability and validity of these specifically tailored tasks available. Normative data are lacking as well. Although items contained in pre and post-treatment assessment often seem to have face validity, their relation to hypothesized underlying deficits within some processing model is usually not one-to-one.

Therefore, in the first part of this chapter a conceptual framework – borrowed from the criterion referenced test approached – for the generation of content valid items and the construction of tasks will be outlined. *Pre-treatment assessment* is important for several reasons. It is needed to determine (stable) baseline performance and to characterize pre-therapy patterns of impairment. A more precise identification of specific types of discrepancies in performance (dissociations) helps to delineate the localization of a functional lesion within some model of normal or impaired language processing. Evaluation of the effects of treatment will be demonstrated for the most basic type of single-case design with either one or two treatment periods. In particular, the crossover treatment design, as described by Coltheart (1983), will serve to illustrate statistical procedures for detecting differential changes in performance over some period of specific treatment. Most of the time it will be assumed that items have a pass/fail scoring. Randomization tests (Edgington, 1987) for items with graded responses or dependent variables with (quasi-) metric properties will be touched on more briefly.

The need for an adequate number of items to guarantee sufficient power of the statistical tests employed is often overlooked in therapy research (see Wertz, Chapter 16, for discussion of statistical power). It is argued that statistical power considerations should be incorporated in the planning of a single-case therapy study. Many of the procedures to be proposed could also be part of normal clinical work in line with Coltheart's plea to transform normal clinical work into methodologically acceptable research.

Pre-treatment Assessment

The generation of items used in assessment tasks is quite often taken for granted in language therapy evaluations. In exemplary applications of the cognitive neuropsychological approach to therapy (Behrmann and Herdan, 1987; Howard and Hatfield; Lesser, 1987; Seron and Deloche, 1988; see Edmundson and McIntosh, Chapter 8, for further discussion of the application of cognitive neuropsychology and aphasia therapy), as well as in single-case studies within other frameworks, the selection of items for assessment (as well as for treatment) has often been motivated on purely theoretical grounds. In the former case items get selected based on some model of normal language processing, which have been found useful in experimental studies or which have been assumed to tap pertinent properties of processing routes or components, intact or suspected of functional damage. Since even rather comprehensive standard test batteries are too heterogeneous within subtests or do not comprise the relevant sets of items, assessment tasks must often be specifically tailored to the requirements of the particular therapy study at hand. Assessment procedures like the PALPA (Kay, Lesser and Coltheart, 1990; and Lesser, Chapter 9) represent an intermediate step in that a large set of tasks comprised of sizeable sets of items are available for the study of aphasic language impairments according to explicit psycholinguistic theory. The collection of items is thus either theory-driven or sometimes simply *ad hoc*. This is inevitably so if those items on which a patient failed (consistently) in some baseline testing from a larger set are selected for further use (Behrmann and Herdan, 1987, Byng and Coltheart, 1986, Howard, et al., 1985). Even if tasks have been used in several studies, the adequacy of the items remains a matter of observational impression as far as empirical evidence for their reliability and, more important, validity are concerned.

The *criterion-referenced measurement* approach originating in educational psychology (Berk, 1980) offers a framework within which rules for item generation and task construction can be developed. These concepts make explicit many of the implicit notions usually employed when setting up assessment procedures in therapy research. Some basic concepts of this approach will be presented in the following section.

Criterion-referenced Measurement

Content validity is implicitly taken to be the major criterion for item generation and selection (Hambleton, 1980). A test is called *content valid* (Berk, 1980; Klauer, 1987) if it contains or represents a *universe* or *domain* of items, e.g., the universe of legal neologisms for a particular language or the universe of prepositions. Such a domain can be defined by complete enumeration of its members or, more frequently, by stating the properties which an item from the particular domain has to fulfil. Very often the domain of interest encompasses too many elements for all of them to be considered in a given assessment procedure; e.g., there is a very large number of legal neologisms that can be made up from words of a particular language according to some rules obeying the phonotactic or graphotactic restrictions in that language. Even if the domain is limited, not all elements will be employed most of the time. In general, the actual assessment task consists of a representative sample from the domain.

For a complete characterization of an item, a stimulus and a response component, i.e. an operation that must be performed on the stimulus, are combined to yield a specific item format, for example, one two-syllable word (or neologism) at a time written imprint is presented visually on a PC-screen for three seconds and the subject is required to make a lexical decision. This general framework is well established in educational psychology and associated with criterion-referenced measurement or mastery testing (Hambleton and Novick, 1973; Hambleton, et al., 1978; De Gruijter and van der Kamp, 1984) and has tacitly been employed in rudimentary form for therapy research as well. Two important aspects are the stratification of a domain into subsets (subdomains) and the formation of representative samples from each of them in order to draw inferences from the item sample to the word frequency intervals, number of syllables, concreteness/abstractness ratings, regular/irregular spelling, complexity of initial, middle, final consonant clusters, etc. Structuring the domain according to theoretically relevant aspects that potentially affect performance helps to reduce uncontrolled variation when analyzing subjects' responses.

In addition, the proportion of items from each stratum has to be taken care of. Representativeness can often be obtained by drawing a random sample of fixed size without replacement from each subdomain in accord with the proportion in the item universe itself. This approach to item generation and selection also provides a convenient way to obtain (data independent) *content valid parallel tests,* i.e., distinct representative samples from some domain. The notion of content valid parallel tests is implicit when a set of items is split, one subset being used in the therapy condition and the other part taken only for pre and post-treatment assessment. In general, a one-to-one relationship between a task domain and one component or route in some processing model is very unlikely. Several types of tasks or subdomains within one domain may be relevant and informative, e.g., not only lexical decision after auditory or visual presentation of words and neologisms but also writing to dictation or reading.

The degree of competence (ability) of a subject i for some domain can be defined as the probability p_i of solving items from a particular domain correctly (Klauer, 1987). Thus a probabilistic relationship between some (latent) competence represented by the (unknown) *universe score* and observable behaviour is assumed. Empirically, the level of competence must be estimated from a representative sample of items from that domain. The properties of the ability estimate depend on the particular test model employed, for example, the binomial model introduced below.

Besides characterizing a subject by computing a competence estimate, a (dichotomous) classification according to master/non-mastery with respect to a universe of items is often useful. Such a definition of mastery allows an operational definition and statistical check of types of dissociations in competence (see below). Second, the demonstration of mastery after a period of treatment can be taken as strong evidence for the effectiveness of therapy. Mastery thus can be taken as one criterion to decide whether to go on to more demanding tasks or to the treatment of a different function. Technically, *mastery* can be defined to hold, if the individual degree of competence p_i is no less than some high degree of competence, the so called *criterion probability p_c,* often chosen to be $p_c=0.90$ or 0.95 (90 or 95 per cent). The individual test performance is thus related to a certain level of competence, not to a distribution of scores across some reference population, as is done in a psychological test constructed according to the classical test theory model (Gulliksen, 1987) using percentile ranks or T-scores.

Fixing the particular p_c is arbitrary to some degree. As a rule it should not be set too close to 100 per cent for this amounts to needing very long tests or to subjecting a severely impaired patient to unreasonable goals. On the other hand p_c should, in general, not be set lower than 80 per cent as this would impoverish the concept of mastery. A relatively low criterion probability does make sense for a domain whose mastery is considered to be a prerequisite for proceeding to the treatment of some more complex problem. In educational psychology mastery levels of 90 or 95 per cent have generally been found adequate. In the following, one particular test model, the binomial model, is used extensively to characterize a subject's competence for some task domain.

The Binomial Model

The binomial model is used implicitly in all single-case studies in which the competence level for a set of pass/fail items is estimated by means of the relative frequency of correct responses. This model is treated in most introductory textbooks on statistics. It allows one to compute the probability of observing the number of one particular outcome from two alternatives (heads or tales when throwing a coin; pass or fail when responding to an item) in a number n of repeated independent trials of the same type. It is important to keep in mind that the probability p for one particular outcome of the two is taken to be constant across all, say n repetitions. As pointed out by Klauer (1987), three variants of the binomial model can be distinguished, which have also been described in Willmes (1990), but the *item sampling* variant of the binomial model rests on the least restrictive assumptions. It requires that for any (randomly selected) subject a new random sample without or with replacement is drawn from the infinite or finite item universe of interest with (possibly) different item difficulties.

Since language items tend to vary in their level of difficulty even for well defined domains irrespective of stratification, only the item sampling model seems to be feasible in most instances. It calls for a new random sample to be drawn from the respective domain for each new patient examined. Technically this would present no problems when using a microcomputer for item banking and item presentation. If random sampling is not employed, one has to assume that the set of items is not biased compared with the random sampling case.

One important assumption has to be met, however, by all variants of the binomial model: in theory, the responses to different items have to be statistically independent of each other. Unfortunately, the assumption of so-called *local stochastic independence* cannot be tested satisfactorily under reasonable conditions, particularly if items are used only for the assessment of one or some subjects. This assumption will be violated in particular if responses to preceding items affect the probability of passing subsequent items. Practice or learning effects as well as decreasing concentration or fatigue because of a long test are standard examples. More important, if answering a previous item correctly is a prerequisite for solving subsequent items, this independence will be violated. What one can do when allocating the items is to avoid circumstances that are known to violate statistical independence in any experimental setting. Quite often, randomization of the sequence of items will do.

Nevertheless, the problem of serial dependency should be taken seriously (Kratochwill and Levin, 1992). Data collected in a single-case study cannot be assumed to be statistically independent *per se*. But this assumption must hold for a valid application of many statistical tests such as the t-test or the analysis of variance. This problem has mostly been discussed in the context of studies, in which a larger number of assessments for a given subject exists (Cook and Campbell, 1979; Pring, 1986). Nevertheless, serial dependency cannot be ruled out even for the simple AB-design or for the comparison of performances in two (theoretically related) tasks observed on one occasion because it is the same patient who responds to the tasks.

Usually the performances, i.e., the number of correct and false responses, for both tasks are compared using the large-sample chi-square test or Fisher's exact test for a two-by-two contingency table (Siegel, 1956; Hays, 1963; Siegel and Castellan, 1988). For a valid application of either of the two tests one has to assume that the responses to all items are statistically independent, i.e., the response to a previous item or task does not influence the response to a later item or task at all – positively or negatively. If there is positive dependence between adjacent observations, the chi-square test rejects the true null hypothesis of no difference too often for a given type I error level (Moore, 1982; Tavaré and Altham, 1983). The actual type I error of falsely rejecting the null-hypothesis under scrutiny can easily become twice as large for rather small positive dependencies. This means that a numerical difference in performance level can incorrectly be declared significant by the researcher.

For the type of single-case data dealt with here there is no way of obtaining precise information on the type and size of dependencies. Therefore, all measures possible should be taken in the administration and sequencing of test items to counteract such effects. Only then can the use of the binomial model and related tests for two-by-two tables be justified. Marginally significant results should be interpreted with still more caution than in a group study context. In the following section the most basic inferential statistical problem of comparing the competence of one subject for two task domains is considered. This diagnostic question has to be answered in order to learn about the particular strengths and weaknesses of the patient under study. Mostly, more than two task performances have to be compared but this represents the most simple situation.

Comparison of the Performances in Two Tasks

The comparison of the performances in two (theoretically related) tasks A and B of an individual patient i with pass/fail items can be summarized as in Table 15.1 (Siegel and Castellan 1988: 104). There are n_A items for task A and n_B items for task B. The number of items passed for task A is denoted n_{A+} and that for task B n_{B+} respectively. The number of items failed then is the difference n_{A-} n_{A+} and $n_{B-}n_{B+}$ respectively. It is assumed that the numbers correct n_{A+} and n_{B+} follow two independent binomial distributions with competence probabilities p_A resp. p_B of passing items from task A or B. The relative frequencies n_{A+}/n_A and n_{B+}/n_B constitute estimates of the underlying degrees of competence p_A for task A and p_B for task B, respectively. The statistical null-hypothesis tested is that of identical competence; i.e., H: $p_A=p_B$ against a one- or two-sided alternative.

Table 15.1. Data scheme for the performance of one subject in two tasks with pass/fail scoring.

	Response		
	+	–	Total
Task A	n_{A+}	n_{A-} n_{B+}	n_A
Task B	n_{B+}	n_{B-} n_{B+}	n_R

The well known statistical tests suited to test this hypothesis are either the *exact Fisher (-Irwin) test* for two-by-two tables for small item numbers or the *chi-square test* with or without continuity correction for larger samples (Siegel and Castellan, 1988). Instead of having to perform the exact test by hand, published tables can be used (Finney, *et al.,*1963; Siegel and Castellan, 1988). A convenient alternative is the PC-program package *StatXact* (1989, version 2 in 1991), which can also do the (exact) test for large samples (Mehta and Patel, 1983). For rather small samples the difference in one-tailed or two-tailed p-values (i.e., the empirical significance level) can be considerable compared with the chi-square test. Since also comprehensive statistical computer packages like *BMDP* (Routine 4F), *SAS*, and *SPSS* as well as the tables cited enable one to perform the exact version of the test with great ease, they are recommended for standard use. As an example, consider pre-treatment data reported by Scott and Byng (1989) from a surface dyslexic patient. A random set of 68 homophones were selected for writing to dictation, 34 for treatment and 34 for control testing. The results are summarized in Table 15.2. *StatXact* provides the exact two-sided *p*-value of 0.6154. The *p*-value from the chi-square test is 0.4505, which becomes 0.6150 with Yates' correction for continuity.

Table 15.2. Pre-treatment data from a surface dyslexic patient in a writing homo-phones to dictation task (Scott and Byng, 1989); 68 homophone words split in two parts.

Task	Response +	–	Total
Treatment set A	23	11	34
Control set B	20	14	34

The test decision that there are no differences in task difficulty for the two sets of homophones is identical for all three statistical tests used, but the numerical difference between the *p*-values for the chi-square and the exact test is quite large.

Statistical Assessment of (double) Dissociations

In many areas of neuropsychology gross performance differences between certain tasks are taken to be indicative of selective impairment of some (specific) processing components like in cases of surface or deep dyslexia, to name one prominent example. Shallice (1988, Ch. 10) differentiates three types of dissociations between some task A and some task B under the condition that task B is performed better than task A. His suggestions have led to a more precise identification of specific types of discrepancies in performance and a characterization of pre- and post-therapy patterns of impairments. He offered no statistical procedures, however, to distinguish reliably between classical, strong and weak dissociations. Willmes (1990) has shown that the binomial model is well suited for this purpose. But it will also be argued that only additional normative data can help to address the problem of differences in task difficulty (Sergent, 1988).

For a *classical* dissociation, performance in task A must be below the normal range and must be much inferior to performance in task B, which in turn must fall within the normal range, possibly close to the premorbid level of competence. For a *strong* dissociation, both tasks must be performed below the normal range with task A being performed much worse that task B. A *trend* dissociation is character-ized by a significantly poorer performance on task A. Shallice also intro-duced a *robust* dissociation as a particular type of a strong dissociation in which performances on both tasks can be expressed as standardized scores obtained from non-brain-damaged subjects.

As Shallice points out, the operationalization in the latter case is particularly difficult if normal subjects have a competence of 1.0 (100 per cent) or very close to it; i.e., they respond correctly to (almost) all items. He also points out some of the pitfalls that task demands, resource capacities and resource artefacts or individual differences of reorganization after brain damage present when patterns of performance are taken to be indicative of (double) dissociations. In the following, statistical procedures that provide operational definitions of the different types of dissociation will be introduced.

A *trend dissociation* can be defined to hold if there is a significant difference in the degree of competence for two tasks as tested with Fisher's exact test. One could strengthen the criterion for a trend dissociation by requiring that there should be a prespecified minimum competence difference of $d = p_A - p_B > 0$. To test against this alternative, the statistical power of the chi-square test must be considered explicitly; i.e., the probability of deciding in favour of the alternative hypothesis if it actually holds. For a short exposition of the statistical power concept see Siegel and Castellan (1988: 9–1) or Cohen (1988, Chapter 1 and discussion by Wertz, Chapter 16). This explicit consideration of the power aspect also requires that a minimum number of items per task is computed, for which it is possible to detect a pre-specified d (i.e., difference) at fixed type I and type II error levels with a one-sided test. With decreasing size of d more items are needed. There are tables available (Hasemann, 1978) and a PC-program (PC-SIZE, Dallal, 1985a) to carry out the required sample size calculations; details are given in Willmes (1990). In subsequent statistical evaluation of the data a dissociation should be taken to hold only if there is a significant difference for the assumed type I error level *and* if the estimated effect size is at least as large as the effect size parameter value for which the sample size computations have been carried out.

For a valid demonstration of a *double dissociation* one must show two things: two complementary dissociations between tasks A and B for two different patients and a complementary and significant difference between both tasks for both patients (see Shallice, 1988: 234 for details). For an investigation of the complementary and significant difference between both tasks for both patients, two *one*-tailed Fisher's exact tests can be carried out for the comparison of performance on task A between patient 1 and 2 with, for example, patient 2 scoring higher than patient 1 and the same for task B with patient 1 performing better that patient 2.

Strong dissociation: In a task in which non-brain-damaged subjects show a ceiling effect in performance, one could require mastery at a competence level p_c somewhere between 80 per cent and 95 per cent if the task is assessing the (relatively) spared function, the competence level of the other task being set considerably lower at p_o. For multiple-choice items with m alternatives the probability of random guessing p_o $=1/m$ could be adopted as a low level p_o. For example, $n=32$ is the smallest item sample size for $p_c=90$ per cent and $p_o=1/4$ in four-choice items that allows separating mastery from guessing reliably. At least 25 out of 32 items need to be solved correctly in the task with greater proficiency and a maximum of 13 correct responses are allowed in the task assessing the more impaired function. Table II in Willmes (1990) gives the minimum sample size – under the condition that both tasks have the same number of items – that are required for several (p_o, p_c) combinations to be truly representing different competence levels. The minimum number of correct responses compatible with the respective p_c value is listed in parentheses. As can be seen from that table for items with only two response alternatives the number required is quite high because $p_o=50$ per cent is already a rather high competence attainable by pure guessing. With free response formats the choice of p_o is not so straightforward; one would have to choose a reasonable value for the type of assessment at hand. Alternatively, one could proceed as described for a trend dissociation with a larger difference d between p_c and p_o.

Classical dissociation: For a task solved well by normal controls, a very high mastery level must be adopted when using the binomial model ($p_c=99$ per cent or even higher if the task has a large enough number of items, e.g., more than 50). The procedures applicable are identical to the ones used with strong dissociations. For tasks with considerable variability of performance among normal controls, p_c may be fixed at some quantile of the distribution for normal controls, e.g., the 25th percentile, which is often taken to be the lower bound for average normal performance.

Robust dissociation: Shallice assumes that normative data from control subjects are available for this type of dissociation – at least information on the arithmetic mean and the standard deviation. The binomial model can only be applied adequately if it is reasonable to express the mean of normals as some pc and impaired competence as some p_o; e.g., the score that is equivalent to the mean minus two standard deviations in the reference group. One problem with this approach is that the distribution of scores in the normal group is often negatively skewed; i.e., a small proportion of normal subjects perform rather poorly. In such cases the standard deviation can be too large and the normal range found to extend too far down the range of competence. The choice of some quantile (e.g., the 10th percentile) as the value for p_o then might prove more adequate.

The valid interpretation of a dissociation crucially hinges on the assumption that the tasks used for assessment have identical inherent difficulty when considering the mental processing load required

(Blanken, 1988; Sergent, 1988; Shallice, 1988). This objective is particularly important in those instances in which performance is poorer on the more demanding task and the reverse pattern of performance has not been observed so far. Although cognitive neuropsychology and aphasiology seek to relate impaired performance to models of normal processing, data obtained from an average clinical sample of aphasic patients can be useful to inform us about the gradation of performances on different tasks in the absence of pertinent data from normal controls or if normal subjects exhibit ceiling effects on both tasks. To illustrate this argument, Willmes (1990) presented data from a supplement to the Aachen Aphasia Test assessing lexical discrimination abilities (Poeck and Göddenhenrich, 1988). However, such data are of no use when it is a matter of generating tasks specifically designed to examine one particular patient.

Number of Items Per Task

Significance should not be the only statistical criterion when using, for instance, the binomial model. The statistical power of the statistical tests must be taken into consideration, as well, in order to be able to also detect not so spectacular differences in performance. With poor statistical power it may always be the case that some relevant difference in competence might be overlooked just because too few items were used. Two cases are of particular interest in single-case therapy studies:

1. For a *mastery decision* it is important to prevent the identification of *mastery* as *no mastery* but also to identify reliably a subject with non-mastery competence. Several solutions have been proposed. A simple one consists of having the lower limit of the respective confidence interval for an individual competence p_i just covering p_c at the upper end and simultaneously being above some lower limit p_o. Table III in Willmes (1990) gives the minimum item sample size required for this approach, together with the minimum number of items to be scored correct. For example, in a two-choice lexical decision task at least 20 items are needed in order to demonstrate 90 per cent mastery, without covering the guessing probability of $p_o=0.5$. A total of 15 correct responses out of 20 is the minimum performance compatible with this requirement.
2. When comparing pre-therapy performance for a set of items, randomly split in two parts and one being used for treatment, or when trying to demonstrate *identical competence* for two tasks, it is not sufficient to show that there is no significant difference in competence. It might well be that due to a too small number of items the statistical test used has only poor power. There would be more confidence in the statistical decision if the null hypothesis could be proven to hold with reasonable accuracy (Westermann and Hager, 1986). Again, details can be found in Willmes (1990).

Evaluation of the Effects of Treatment

Only the most basic types of a single-case designs with either one or two therapy periods will be discussed. Howard (1986) has listed requirements that studies must fulfil in order to be adequate for distinguishing between effects of specific treatment, non-specific therapeutic intervention and spontaneous recovery when the efficacy of one specific treatment aimed at improving a specific linguistic function (e.g., writing isolated words to dictation) is to be evaluated. Coltheart (1983) has introduced the crossover treatment design as the most adequate and parsimonious design for that purpose. Byng (1988) also mentions the adequacy of this design for the comparison of two treatment methods for one function. It has also been applied with respect to two types of materials to be compared (Behrmann and Herdan, 1987). The latter case allows one to examine whether treatment effects have generalized to non-trained items from the same domain or a related domain. In educational psychology a distinction is made between retention or drill effects, trivial training effects and non-trivial training (learning, transfer) effects, depending on whether improvement pertains only to items used during therapy or extends to untreated items from the same domain or from a related domain involving a similar type of processing. Irrespective of the most appropriate design used to demonstrate one or several of these types of effects, three varieties of effects have to be evaluated statistically.

1. Increase of competence (improvement) for a treated linguistic function.
2. Differential improvement for treated and non-treated sets of items assessing the same or a related linguistic function.
3. Improvement for a treated function and no improvement for an unrelated non-treated function.

For all three types of changes in performance a further aspect concerns the final outcome level, i.e., the question of whether a numerical or statistically significant improvement has led to mastery competence. Only if a very low level of pre-treatment performance is followed by very dramatic improvements may inferential statistical procedures for the detection of changes in competence perhaps be neglected. But it is more likely that there is a need to detect reliably more subtle changes in impairment or differences in level of performance after treatment.

Improvement After Treatment

For a set of pass/fail items selected from some task universe and administered before and after a period of treatment, the results can conveniently be summarized in the two-by-two table shown in Table 15.3.

Table 15.3. Data scheme for the comparison of a subject's performances in the same task comprised of n items before and after treatment (probabilities corresponding to absolute counts per cell are given in brackets)

		Post-test		
		+	–	Total
Pre-test	+	n_{11} (P_{11})	n_{10} (P_{10})	$n_{1.}$ $(P_{1.})$
	–	n_{01} (P_{01})	n_{00} (P_{00})	$n_{0.}$ $(P_{.})$
		$n_{.1}$ $(P_{.1})$	$n_{.0}$ $(P_{.0})$	n (1.0)

The exact or the asymptotic version of the McNemar test for two related samples (Siegel and Castellan, 1988) are well known to serve as tests for significant improvement in the level of competence. The one-sided null hypothesis one wants to reject is H: competence post-treatment is not larger than before treatment. This is equivalent to assuming that the probability of responding correctly post-treatment to items failed pre-treatment is not larger than the probability of responding incorrectly post-treatment to items passed pre-treatment. This is again equivalent to assuming that there are no more changes to the positive side than the other way around.

There are tables available in the book by Siegel and Castellan of the exact one-tailed p-values for the latter hypothesis up to a total number of $N=25$ items with changes in performance ($N=n_{10}+n_{01}$) and in the paper by Willmes (1990, Table I of the appendix) for N, up to 70 for several conventional levels of significance. Cohen (1988, Table 5.3.1.) lists selected critical values up to $N=1000$ both for one-sided and two-sided alternatives. The exact test can also be carried out conveniently with the *StatXact* program package (1989). To give an example, data from pre- and post-treatment testing for some task with 60 items are shown in Table 15.4. Relative frequencies are given in brackets. Performance increases from 37 to 49 correct responses. As can be seen from the body of the table, there are $N=18$ items altogether with a change in performance from the pre- to the post-test. It is only the two cells with entries of 15 and 3 respectively, which represent change in level of competence.

Table D in Siegel and Castellan (1988) as well as the *StatXact* program give a one-side p-value of 0.004 for $N=15+3=18$ and $x=3$. When consulting Table I in Willmes (1990), one sees that a value of $n_{01}=15$ with $N=18$ reaches significance at the 0.005 level. Using Yates'

Table 15.4. Sample data for the data scheme from Table 15.3.

		Post-test		
		+	–	Total
	+	34	3	37
		(0.57)	(0.05)	(0.62)
Pre-test	–	15	8	23
		(0.25)	(0.13)	(0.38)
	Total	49	11	60
		(0.82)	(0.18)	(1.00)

continuity correction, the asymptotic chi-square test statistic value with 1 d.f. is 6.72 with a two-tailed $p=0.0095$. All tests thus indicate significant improvement in performance. Authors ought to report the full two-by-two table for assessment of change. Marginal frequencies or proportions provide no information about the amount of discordant responses for individual items in the pre-treatment and the post-treatment assessment. These 'fluctuations' in performance give valuable descriptive information about the degree of instabilities in competence.

Again, power considerations should be attended to when deciding on the number of items for a task that is to be evaluated for its therapeutic relevance. They are explained in Willmes (1990). As before, when testing for differences in competence, the number of items must be high for the detection of a small change in performance, in particular if a small pre-post difference in competence is accompanied by a high fluctuation rate. Only for very large treatment effects are item samples of about 20 items sufficient to back up a significant test result with a reasonably high power of 0.8 or more. Another obstacle for a sound demonstration of improvement lies in having pre-test competence too high so that further improvement may be hard to detect on the pertinent task.

A further measure for the efficacy of the administered treatment is the post-therapy level of competence achieved (outcome). The criteria for mastery introduced above are also applicable to the evaluation of outcome data. The post-treatment performance of $49/60=0.82$ in the example from Table 15.4 is just compatible with a criterion probability of $p_c=0.9$ (because the upper limit 0.9048 of the 95 per cent confidence interval is just above 0.9; Documenta Geigy, 1980).

It sometimes proves necessary to demonstrate the absence of a significant change in performance. For example, to obtain a strictly specific treatment effect with the crossover treatment design the non-treated function should remain unaffected (Coltheart, 1983). A first step is to fix a small maximum of improvement in competence that cannot be regarded as substantial improvement. But even with a liberal type I error level of 0.10 to 0.20 for a one-tailed test, large item samples of no less than 100 are needed to give the statistical test reasonable power. Such a large number of items often defies feasibility, so that the ensuing test for no effect tends to have low power, i.e., a notable difference in competence can fail to get recognized. Thus it is difficult to exclude the possibility of smaller generalized therapy effects or some spontaneous recovery making inferences less unequivocal. Other examples for this type of problem are the demonstration of a stable baseline or of stable treatment effects after a period of no treatment or no specific treatment. Anyway, it is recommended that the power estimate for the data at hand in a therapy study be obtained from the tables in Cohen (1988). The book contains several examples of how the computations are carried out.

The most compelling demonstration of modality or task specific effects using the crossover treatment design calls for the following pattern of performances (cf. Coltheart, 1983): significant improvement in task A but not in task B when the target treatment has been addressed with task A and the reverse pattern of performance when task B has been employed in the treatment. Willmes (1990) describes how to handle the related set of four statistical tests together with recommendations for the adjustment of type I and type II error probabilities because of multiple testing. Four exact (or asymptotic) McNemar tests have to be carried out in order to evaluate changes in performance from the pretest to the intermediate test after the first therapy period for the treatment of function A and then from the intermediate test to the post-test after the second therapy period for the treatment of function B. Willmes (1990) also indicates how one can test for differential improvement, i.e. a significant superiority of one treatment method over another across a treatment period, irrespective of whether one or both were effective.

Graded and (Quasi-)Metric Responses

All the considerations about defining a universe of tasks remain valid when a patient's responses are no longer scored dichotomously. For the statistical procedures to be described below, item scorings or other dependent variables may be either of the following types. Graded scores for item responses representing ordered categories for performances from 'very wrong' to 'very correct', total scores over a subset of pass/fail or graded response items, number of occurrences of a particular event (cf. the example in Wilson, 1987) or reaction times.

Conceptually, the research hypotheses are identical to the ones for dichotomous scores. Pre-treatment data have to be compared to identify patterns of performances. Pre- and post-therapy assessments for the (specific) treatment of one function have to be compared to identify changes in or stability of performances. Pre- and post-therapy data have to be compared for the identification of differential effects when treating two different functions or when comparing two treatment methods for one function. A basic distinction has to be made between the case in which the same items are used under two different pretest conditions or are contained in the pre- and the post-test compared to the case in which different items are taken for the comparison of two conditions are illustrated in Table 15.5.

Table 15.5. Two basic data schemata for single-case studies incorporating two assessments with different sets (left) or the same set of items (right)

Independent two-samples problem				Dependent (paired) two-samples problem		
Item	Task 1	Item	Task 2	Item	Pre-test	Post-test
1	y_{11}	1	y_{12}	1	y_{11}	y_{12}
2	y_{21}	2	y_{22}	2	y_{21}	y_{22}
3	y_{31}	3	y_{32}	3	y_{31}	y_{32}
–	–	–	–	–	–	–
–	–	–	–	–	–	–
–	–	–	–	–	–	–
n_1	$y_{n_1 1}$	–	–	–	–	–
		–	–	n	y_{n1}	y_{n2}
		n_2	$y_{n_2 2}$			

y_{ij} score (rating) for item i within task j; j = 1,2.	y_{ij}: score (rating) for the same item i at test time j; j = 1,2.

Different item sets sampled from the same domain may also be chosen for the comparison of pre and post-treatment competence. Whenever the same items are used for two assessments, statistical procedures taking into account this type of dependency should be applied. The (exact version of) the sign test or the Wilcoxon signed-ranks tests or the corresponding randomization test can be applied for the dependent two-samples problem. If different sets of items are employed, statistical procedures suited for the independent two-samples problem are adequate like the exact version of the Mann-Whitney U-test or the corresponding randomization test using the observations themselves and not just their ranks (Edgington, 1987; 1992).

To give an example for a not so obvious dependent-samples problem, consider a therapy study, in which the traditional and a modified PACE approach, incorporating linguistically structured therapy material, were compared (Springer, *et al.*, 1991). As a control test, a semantic classification task comprising 120 items from 10 semantic classes (12 items per class) was used to assess the lexical-semantic impairments. Item responses were scored on two different graded response scales, a naming score of

0–4 and the original PACE-score of 0–5. For an evaluation of individual patients' therapy effects across one period of therapy in an A–B–A–B design, score totals per semantic class with a maximum score of 48 respectively, 60 were computed. Since the same semantic classes with the same items were used in the pre- and the post-test, statistical procedures for the dependent two-samples problem were applied. Data for patient WB, with global aphasia are reported in Table 15.6. Only PACE-score totals for the 10 semantic classes will be considered.

This patient started with the modified PACE approach (Treatment B). With four therapy periods there are five control assessments such that there is a pre- and a post-therapy test for each treatment period. For each of the therapy periods the difference score (post-minus pre-) for each semantic field is also reported in Table 15.6. For both B-phases there is a

Table 15.6. Comparison of the efficacy of traditional PACE therapy (phase A) and modified PACE therapy (phase B) for patient WB; reported are the PACE score totals (max. 60) for the ten semantic fields assessed in the control test (120 items) for each of the five control testings before and after each therapy phase in the B-A-B-A design. In addition, exact one-sided p-values for the comparison of pre and post-test performances are given for the paired two samples randomization test as compared to the exact sign test, the exact Wilcoxon signed ranks test, and the paired samples t-test (results from the PC-program PITMAN, Dallal 1985b)

Therapy Phase		B		A		B		A	
Semantic Field	Test 1	Difference	Test 2	Difference	Test 3	Difference	Test 4	Difference	Test 5
1	22	18	40	-5	35	7	42	-2	40
2	30	14	44	-5	39	10	49	4	53
3	34	5	39	11	50	1	51	0	51
4	30	5	35	5	40	10	50	-5	45
5	33	10	43	1	44	5	49	-3	46
6	31	10	41	8	49	1	50	7	57
7	20	17	37	3	40	6	46	0	46
8	41	9	50	-8	42	12	54	-2	52
9	45	2	47	-1	46	11	57	-1	56
10	25	14	39	3	42	5	47	6	53
Mean	31.1	10.4	41.5	1.2	42.7	6.8	49.5	0.4	49.9
Standard deviation	7.8	5.4	4.6	6.1	4.6	3.9	4.1	4.0	5 5
Comparison of consecutive control tests		p-value one-tailed		p-value one-tailed		p-value one-tailed		p-value one tailed	
Randomization test		.0010		.2852		.0010		.4063	
Sign test		.0010		.3770		.0010		.3633	
Wilcoxon test		.0010		.3096		.0010		.3985	
Paired t-test		.0001		.2731		.0002		.3789	

consistent increase in performance across all semantic fields, whereas for both A-phases positive and negative differences tend to level out.

Possible (positive) serial dependence of responses within and across conditions again poses a potential problem for a valid interpretation of statistical test results. As for the chi-square test before, anticonservative decisions are the rule for all the well-known two-sample test statistics such as the independent and paired samples t-test, the Mann-Whitney U-test and the Wilcoxon signed ranks test.

The exact versions of the U-test and the Wilcoxon-test as well as the two-sample randomization test, which allow for an evaluation of total scores for dichotomous or graded items or reaction time data themselves and not only their ranks, can conveniently be carried out within the *StatXact* package or the *PITMAN* PC-program by Dallal (1985b). The latter program was applied to the data presented in Table 15.6.

For the comparison of scores before and after the first therapy period the exact p-value for a one-sided test for an increase in competence (because no negative effects are expected overall), using the dependent samples randomization test, is $p=0.001$. Basically the same result is obtained for the exact version of the U-test and the dependent samples t-test with 9 degrees of freedom, which are also carried out by the *PITMAN* program. The p-values for all three test-statistics and all therapy periods are reported in the bottom part of Table 15.6 as well. Very similar to the first B-phase, there is a highly significant increase in performance for the second application of that type of therapy, whereas no significant improvements could be detected for both administrations of the traditional PACE approach.

The study of *differential* improvement is somewhat more involved. For (quasi-)metric data one can compute the difference between post- and pre-test performances for each item taken for the assessment of function A as well as those for the assessment of function B. These two sets of differences can then be compared with a randomization test (or a rank test) for the independent two-samples problem. For the example presented in Table 15.6, the two-sided comparison of difference scores for the first B- and A-phase again using the dependent samples randomization test yields a p-value of $p=0.0195$, indicating superiority of the modified PACE approach. The same holds true for a comparison of the second application of both types of therapy ($p=0.0254$). Moreover, the two B-phases could be compared with each other in order to examine whether the effect of treatment gets smaller or larger in the second instance. Although the mean difference is somewhat smaller, the two-sided p-value of $p=0.1465$ for the dependent samples randomization test is well above the level of 0.05.

If the response measures have only ordinal scale properties the differences of ordinal scores themselves need not be ordinal any more. For example, for an ordinal scale with 7 grade scores 1 to 7, for which the differences between adjacent scores need not be equidistant, it may well be that 7–4=3 represents a smaller change in competence than 3–1=2. The definition of mastery is more complicated as well. If no particular measurement model is assumed, a simple operational definition for graded score totals would require performances to be above some high percentage of the maximum attainable score. For reaction time data an operational definition would be required as well. The individual patient's median reaction time across the set of items should fall below some cut off value possibly chosen as some percentile of the distribution of performances for normal controls if available. Another suggestion would be to require a certain minimum percentage reduction compared to baseline performance.

Conclusions

It has been demonstrated in this chapter that it is possible for the individual aphasia therapist to assess whether specific treatment approaches or methods are effective in reducing certain aphasic symptoms or impairments. Efficacy research of this kind for single-case studies can be carried out quite easily with the aid of a PC. If the control tests are composed of pass/fail items, only two tests for two-way contingency tables, Fisher's exact test or its asymptotic counterpart the chi-square test for two-by-two tables and the exact (or asymptotic) version of the McNemar test, are needed to test all relevant hypotheses of the crossover treatment design, which is well suited to demonstrate modality or task specific treatment effects. It has been pointed out that statistical power considerations should and indeed can be given more attention in designing a single-case study. But proceeding in that way often leads to quite a large number of items being included in a task. Inherent differences in task difficulty pose a definite problem for the interpretation of mastery and the validity of dissociations observed in the data. Although it has been argued repeatedly by cognitive neuropsychologists that the performance of normals is to serve as the adequate point of reference, ubiquitous ceiling effects of normals on many of the tasks appropriate for studying aphasic language performance make this criterion difficult to maintain. If available, data from the general aphasic population can also offer relevant information concerning the gradation of performance on different tasks.

There is evidence that researchers in the field of aphasia therapy are becoming increasingly aware of the methodological problems involved in efficacy studies although the meta-analysis of Schoonen (1991) on the internal validity of aphasia therapy efficacy studies was rather negative about the design quality of published studies. Two recent books edited by Paradis (1993) and Holland and Forbes (1993) and a NIDCD monography (Cooper 1992) devote several chapters to the discussion of general and specific design considerations for therapy studies. The psychometric and statistical considerations in this chapter are intended to help with some of the problems one encounters when inferential statistical procedures are sought for single-subject therapy studies.

References

Behrmann M, Herdan S (1987) The case for cognitive neuropsychological remediation. Die Suid-Afrikaanse Tydskrift vir Kommunikasieafwykings 34:3–9.

Berk RA (Ed) 1980) Criterion-Referenced Measurement: The State of the Art. Baltimore MD: Johns Hopkins University Press.

Blanken G (1988) Anmerkungen zur methodologie der kognitiven neurolinguistik. Neurolinguistik 2:127–47.

Byng S (1988) Sentence processing deficits: theory and therapy. Cognitive Neuropsychology 5:629–76.

Byng S, Coltheart M (1986) Aphasia therapy research: methodological requirements and illustrative results. In Hjelmquist E, Nilsson L-G (Eds) Communication and Handicap: Aspects of Psychological Compensation and Technical Aids. Amsterdam: Elsevier.

Cohen J (1988) Statistical Power Analysis for the Behavioral Sciences (2nd edn) New York: Academic Press.

Coltheart M (1983) Aphasia therapy research: a single-case study approach. In Code C, Muller DJ (Eds) Aphasia Therapy. London: Edward Arnold. (2nd edn 1989).

Connell PJ, Thompson CK (1986) Flexibility of single-subject designs. Part III: using flexibility to design or modify experiments. Journal of Speech and Hearing Disorders 51:214–25.

Cook TD, Campbell DT (1979) Quasi-Experimentation: Design and Analysis Issues for Field Settings. Boston MA: Houghton Mifflin.

Cooper JA (Ed) (1992) Aphasia Treatment: Current Approaches and Research Opportunities. NIDCD Monographs, 2, NIH Publication no. 93–3424.

Dallai GE (1985a) PC-SIZE: a program for sample size determination – version 2.0. Boston MA: USDA Human Nutrition Research Center on Aging, Tufts University.

Dallai GE (1985b) PC-PITMAN: Randomization tests – version 2.0. Boston MA: USDA Human Nutrition Research Center on Aging, Tufts University.

De Gruijter DNM, Vander Kamp LJT (1984) Statistical Methods in Psychological and Educational Testing. Lisse The Netherlands: Swets & Zeitlinger.

Documenta Geigy (1980) Wissenschaftliche Tabellen. Teilband Statistick (8th edn) Basel Switzerland.

Edgington ES (1987) Randomization Tests (2nd edn) New York: Marcel Dekker.

Edgington ES (1992) Nonparametric tests for single case experiments, In Kratochwill TR, Levin JR (Eds) Single-Case Research Design and Analysis. Hillsdale NJ: Erlbaum pp 133–57.

Finney DJ, Latscha R, Bennett BM, Hsu P (1963) Tables for Testing Significance in a 2x2 Contingency Table. Cambridge: Cambridge University Press.

Gulliksen H (1987) Theory of Mental Tests. Hillsdale NJ: Lawrence Erlbaum.

Hambleton RK (1980) Test score validity and standard-setting methods. In Berk RA (Ed) Criterion Referenced Measurement: The State of the Art. Baltimore MD: Johns Hopkins University Press.

Hambleton RK, Novick MR (1973) Toward an integration of theory and method for criterion referenced tests. Journal of Educational Measurement 10:159–70.

Hambleton RK, Swaminathan H, Algina J, Coulson DB (1978) Criterion-referenced testing and measurement: a review of technical issues and developments. Review of Educational Research 48:1–47.

Hasemann JK (1978) Exact sample sizes for use with the Fisher-Irwin test for 2x2 tables. Biometrics 34:106–9.

Hays WL (1963) Measuring progress in aphasia therapy: a multiple baseline study. British Journal of Disorders of Communication 21:47–62.

Holland AL, Forbes MM (Eds) (1993) Aphasia Treatment: World Perspectives. San Diego CA: Singular Publishing Group.

Howard D (1986) Beyond randomized controlled trials: the case for effective case studies of the effects of treatment in aphasia. British Journal of Disorders of Communication 21:89–102.

Howard D, Hatfield FM (1987) Aphasia Therapy: Historical and Contemporary Issues. Hove: Lawrence Erlbaum.

Howard D, Patterson K, Franklin S, Orchard-Lisle V, Morton J (1985) Treatment of word retrieval deficits in aphasia. Brain 108:817–29.

Kay J, Lesser R, Coltheart M (1990) Psycholinguistic Assessment of Language Processing in Aphasia. London: Lawrence Erlbaum.

Kazdin AE (Ed) (1992) Methological Issues and Strategies in Clinical Research. Washington DC: American Psychological Association.

Kearns KP (1992) Methodological issues in aphasia treatment research: a single-subject perspective. In Cooper JA (Ed) Aphasia Treatment: Current Approaches and Research Opportunities. NIDCD Monographs, Vol. 2 NIH Publication no. 93–3424.

Klauer KJ (1987) Kriteriumsorientierte Tests. Göttingen: Hogrefe.

Kratochwill TR, Levin JR (1992) Single-case Research Design and Analysis. Hillsdale NJ: Lawrence Erlbaum.

Lesser R (1987) Cognitive neuropsychological influences on aphasia therapy. Aphasiology 1:189–200.

McReynolds LV, Patel NR (1983) Single-Subject Experimental Designs in Communicative Disorders. Austin TX: Pro-Ed.

Mehta CR, Patel NR (1983) A network algorithm for performing Fisher's exact test in rxc contingency tables. Journal of the American Statistical Association 78:427–34.

Moore DS (1982) The effect of dependence on chi-squared tests of fit. The Annals of Statistics 10:1163–1171.

Paradis M (Ed) 1993) Foundations of Aphasia Rehabilitation. Oxford: Pergamon Press.

Poeck K, Göddenhenrich S (1988) Standardized tests for the detection of dissociations in aphasic language performance Aphasiology 2:375–80.

Pring T (1986) Evaluating the effects of speech therapy in aphasia: developing the single-case methodology. British Journal of Disorders of Communication 21:103–15.

Schoonen R (1991) The internal validity of efficacy studies: design and statistical power in studies of language therapy for aphasics. Brain and Language 41:446–64.

Scott C, Byng S (189) Computer assisted remediation of a homophone comprehension disorder in surface dyslexia. Aphasiology 3:301–20.

Sergent J (1988) Some theoretical and methodological issues in neuropsychological research. In Boller F, Grafman J (Eds) Handbook of Neuropsychology Vol. 1. Amsterdam: Elsevier.

Seron X, Deloche G (1988) Cognitive Approaches to Neuropsychological

Rehabilitation. Hove: Lawrence Erlbaum.

Shallice T (1988) From Neuropsychology to Mental Structure. Cambridge: Cambridge University Press.

Siegel S (1956) Nonparametric Statistics for the Behavioral Sciences. New York: McGraw Hill.

Siegel S, Castellan N, Jr (1988) Nonparametric Statistics for the Behavioral Sciences (2nd Ed) New York: McGraw Hill.

Springer L, Glindemann R, Huber W, Willmes K (1991) How efficacious is PACE-therapy when 'language systematic training' is incorporated? Aphasiology 5:391–9.

StatXact (1989) Statistical Software for Exact Nonparametric Inference. Cambridge, Cytel Software Corporation (Version 2.0, 1991).

Tavaré S, Altham PME (1983) Serial dependence of observations leading to contingency tables and corrections to chi-squared statistics. Biometrika 70:139–44.

Thompson KC (1992) A neurolinguistic approach to sentence production treatment and generalization research in aphasia. In Cooper JA (Ed) Aphasia Treatment: Current Approaches and Research Opportunities. NIDCD Monographs, Vol. 2, NIH Publication no. 93–3424.

Tompkins CA, (1992) Improving aphasia treatment research: some methodological considerations. In Cooper JA (Ed) Aphasia Treatment: Current Approaches and Research Opportunities. NIDCD Monographs, Vol. 2, NIH Publication no. 93–3424.

Wertz RT (1992) A single case for group treatment studies in aphasia. In Cooper JA (Ed) Aphasia Treatment: Current Approaches and Research Opportunities. NIDCD Monographs, Vol. 2, NIH Publication no. 93-3424.

Wertz T (1993) Efficacy of various methods of therapy. In Paradis M (Ed) Foundations of Aphasia Rehabilitation. Oxford: Pergamon Press.

Westermann R and Hager W (1986) Error probabilities in educational and psychological research. Journal of Educational Statistics 11:117-46.

Willmes K (1990) Statistical methods for a single-case study approach to aphasia therapy research. Aphasiology 4:415-36.

Wilson B (1987) Single-case experimental designs in neuropsychological rehabilitation. Journal of Clinical and Experimental Neuropsychology 9:527-44.

Wilson B (1993) Editorial: How do we know that rehabilitation works? Neuropsychological Rehabilitation 3: 1-4.

Chapter 16
Efficacy

ROBERT T. WERTZ

> In an inconsistent and uncertain world, it may be perversely comforting that over the past 80 years doubts, skepticism, and incredulity regarding the efficacy of psychological treatments have been dependably constant and certain. Neither variation in the nature of claimed effects nor apparently authoritative evidence has diminished critics' regular and expectable expressions of mistrust (Parloff, 1986:79).

Every time the issue about the efficacy of treatment for aphasia is raised, we are reminded how unsettled a community aphasiology continues to be. So many of our uncertainties about the kind of discipline we want to be are brought into focus by the efficacy issue - uncertainties about the value of treatment for aphasia, about which treatments are effective and which are not, about how the question of efficacy should be answered. It is not surprising that 23 years after Darley (1972) reviewed the evidence and provided direction for future research, nothing about the issue seems resolved.

Criticism of treatment's efficacy in aphasia ranges from a *Medical World News* article (Anonymous, 1969) that concluded, 'The classic aphasia patient...comes in on a stretcher and isn't talking. When he leaves, he is walking but not talking.' through a *Lancet* Editorial in 1977 that proclaimed, 'assessment of the value of therapy is virtually impossible' to Siegel's (1987) position that asking 'Does therapy work?' is not a proper question for research. More recently, those who would investigate the efficacy of treatment for aphasia cannot agree on how it should be done. Howard (1986) and Caramazza and Badecker (1989), for example, advocate confining efforts to single-case designs. Others (Bates, Applebaum and Allard, 1991; Bates, McDonald, MacWhinney and Applebaum, 1991; Rosenbek, LaPointe and Wertz, 1989; and Zurif, Gardner and Brownell, 1989) believe both single-case and group designs are appropriate methods of inquiry. Thus, the clinician

interested in the efficacy of his or her efforts is told they are not efficacious, it is impossible to determine, or it is not an appropriate question. Those who ignore this counsel will find the means they use –
single-case or group design – rejected by someone.

Nevertheless, aphasic people continue to seek and obtain treatment,
and it seems reasonable to ask whether what they receive helps. The
purposes of the following are to examine the evidence collected to
date in group and single-case designs, to attempt to cull an answer to
the question about whether treatment for aphasia really does any good,
and to speculate where inquiry about the efficacy of treatment may
want to go from here.

Evidence From Group Treatment Studies

Some (Salive, Mayfield and Weissman, 1992; Longstreth, Koepsell and
van Belle, 1987) maintain the most unequivocal method for evaluating
the efficacy of any treatment is a controlled clinical trial. For aphasia,
(Howard, 1986) argues the controlled clinical trial will not produce
useful information about the efficacy of treatment. Regardless of one's
preference for or objection to the controlled clinical trial for evaluating
treatment's efficacy, it has been employed in a variety of designs – some
more controlled than others. The following lists the requirements for
group studies of aphasia treatment, reviews the literature, and provides
some conclusions about what this method has told us about the efficacy of our efforts.

Requirements for Group Treatment Studies

Objections to controlled clinical trials include: patients are too heterogeneous, treatments are too heterogeneous and outcome measures are
inappropriate or insensitive to improvement. One could add the failure
of some group studies to control for time (spontaneous recovery) and
failure to meet statistical requirements essential for inference about
results. All of these objections are appropriate, and an acceptable
group treatment study must answer them. Specifically, attention is
necessary to selection criteria, control for spontaneous recovery, selecting a no-treatment group, outcome measures, the treatment administered, and the statistical requirements of group designs.

Selection Criteria

Aphasic people do differ. They differ in biographical variables – age,
gender, occupation, education, handedness, etc. They also differ in
medical variables – cause of aphasia, time post-onset, severity, type of
aphasia, medical history, etc. These variables are believed to influence
improvement and response to treatment (Darley, 1972; Wertz, 1985). If

these differences are not controlled in a group study, the heterogeneous sample or samples make interpretation of results difficult and application of results impossible. Their control is obtained by establishing rigid selection criteria for patients who are entered in a controlled clinical trial. A review of group treatment studies indicates the selection criteria employed vary from one, aphasic, to numerous.

The problem with selection criteria is that they influence sample size – the more rigid and numerous the criteria, the fewer the potential study patients. Moreover, selection criteria limit application of results to only those patients who would have qualified for entry in the study. Nevertheless, to reduce heterogeneity and sharpen application of results, precise selection criteria are essential. They should include at a minimum: age, time post-onset, etiology, localization of brain damage, neurologic history, medical and psychological status, sensory and motor status, and severity of aphasia. Some of these are discrete, for example, etiology: aphasic subsequent to a first, single, left hemisphere thromboembolic infarct. Others may range, for example, age: 75 years or younger. Those that range may be employed as covariates in the analysis of results. The rule about selection criteria is simple. They are essential. They influence results and the application of results.

Spontaneous Recovery

Demonstrating the efficacy of a treatment requires demonstrating improvement results from the treatment and not from some uncontrolled variable, for example, time. We believe that untreated aphasic people improve, especially during the first few months post-onset. We call this spontaneous recovery (Butfield and Zangwill, 1946), and we believe it results from physiological restitution. Because it occurs, it must be controlled in a treatment study. Otherwise, we do not know how much of the improvement observed results from spontaneous recovery and how much, if any, results from the treatment. The way to control for the influence of spontaneous recovery in group treatment studies is random assignment of study patients who meet selection criteria to treatment and no-treatment groups. This will equate spontaneous recovery between groups. For example, both groups are expected to experience improvement from spontaneous recovery, however, if the treated group displays significantly more improvement than the no-treatment group, the difference can be inferred to result from the treatment.

The rule about controlling for spontaneous recovery is simple. It is essential. Otherwise, it is not possible to infer a treatment effect. And, as every clinician knows, this is the most common question about aphasia treatment's efficacy – 'How do you know they would not have improved if you left them alone?'

Selecting a No-treatment Group

The classical clinical trial evaluates the efficacy of a treatment or treatments by assigning study patients who meet selection criteria randomly to treatment and no-treatment groups. This approach provides control over variables, for example, spontaneous recovery, that may influence improvement. While the design is simple and straight forward, employing it is extremely difficult. Only three aphasia treatment studies (Lincoln, et al., 1984; Katz and Wertz, 1992; Wertz, et al., 1986) have employed a randomly assigned no-treatment group.

The difficulty in utilizing a randomly assigned no-treatment group results from ethical objections. Because aphasia treatment exists, some (Shewan and Kertesz, 1984) believe it is unethical to withhold it. Clinicians believe in what they do, and they are reluctant to refrain from doing it. However, if the efficacy of what they do is to be demonstrated, a randomly assigned no-treatment group is essential.

Some (Vignolo, 1964; Basso, Capitani and Vignolo, 1979; Holland, 1980a; Shewan and Kertesz, 1984) have employed self-selected no-treatment groups for comparison with treated patients. Those who lived too far away to participate in treatment, who could not afford the cost of treatment, who did not want treatment, or who declined to participate in treatment for other reasons became the no-treatment controls. Others (Hagen, 1973) obtained a no-treatment group by establishing a waiting list – the first patients identified were treated, and those who followed were placed on a waiting list for treatment. Both methods are unacceptable because the self-selected no-treatment patients may differ from the treated patients in important characteristics, for example, severity of aphasia (Shewan and Kertesz, 1984). Moreover, one must explain why the self-selected, no-treatment group is probably better than no no-treatment group, but the very nature of being self-selected may influence results.

A potential solution to the ethical objection about withholding treatment is to employ a deferred treatment group (Wertz, et al., 1986). Patients who meet selection criteria are assigned randomly to either immediate treatment or deferred treatment later in the study. The deferred treatment patients do receive treatment, but during their period of deferral, they constitute an acceptable, randomly assigned, no-treatment group for comparison with patients randomly assigned to immediate treatment. Another solution to the ethical objection is to study chronic aphasic patients – those who have been treated and are no longer receiving treatment (Katz and Wertz, 1992). For those patients, nothing is being withheld, because they had already received treatment and were discharged. And, even here, the deferred treatment approach can be employed – chronic aphasic patients are assigned randomly to treatment or no-treatment, and the no-treatment patients are treated later in the treatment trial. The rule about a no-treatment group is simple. To demonstrate efficacy, a no-treatment group is essential, and it must result from random assignment.

Outcome Measures

To demonstrate the efficacy of a treatment, patient performance must be determined pre- and post-treatment. Improvement, if it occurs, is reflected as the difference in performance between these two points in time, pre- and post. Again, this seems to be a simple and straight forward approach. However, problems arise in what constitutes an acceptable outcome measure. Howard (1986) has criticized randomized, controlled treatment trials for employing generalized and insensitive assessment techniques.

Certainly, aphasiologists do not agree on the most appropriate test for aphasia. If they did, we would have only a few. Obviously, we have many. Most would agree that an appropriate outcome measure should be valid – tests what it reports to test; reliable – change reflects improvement or decline and not variability in patient or examiner performance; and sensitive – detects change if it occurs. We diverge on what behaviors should be assessed; whether the tests capture only performance displayed in the testing environment or whether they reveal communicative performance in functional, everyday contexts; and whether they indicate the changes the therapy administered is designed to evoke.

There is ample evidence that most tests for aphasia yield performance that is significantly related (Holland, 1980b; Wertz, Deal and Robinson, 1984). This includes comparison of metalinguistic measures, for example, the *Boston Diagnostic Aphasia Examination* (BDAE) (Goodglass and Kaplan, 1972) and the *Porch Index of Communicative Ability* (PICA) (Porch, 1967), as well as comparisons among metalinguistic measures (BDAE and PICA) and functional measures, for example, Communicative Abilities in Daily Living (CADL) (Holland, 1980b), and the Functional Communication Profile (FCP) (Sarno, 1969). These relationships imply the traditional, metalinguistic measures are capturing a good deal of the information observed with functional measures. Thus, one might argue that any test with a high relationship with other tests is an appropriate outcome measure for aphasia treatment studies.

The question about test sensitivity is more difficult. All aphasia tests do not detect change in aphasia equally. For example, the PICA's 16-point multidimensional scale is extremely sensitive to small changes in behavior, however the PICA's battery of subtests lacks 'top' and may not detect changes in mildly aphasic people. Conversely, the *Western Aphasia Battery* (WAB) (Kertesz, 1982) Aphasia Quotient is over-loaded with oral-expressive language tasks and may not detect changes in other modalities. But, the WAB contains a wide range of task difficulty and is more sensitive to improvement in mildly aphasic people. Neither measure, however, may detect improvement resulting from a very specific treatment.

Some (Wertz, et al., 1981; Wertz, et al., 1986) have employed a battery of measures to capture general language performance (PICA, BDAE); functional communication (FCP, CADL); and performance in specific modalities (Token Test, Word Fluency Measure). The problem with this approach is that a battery of measures takes time and extends the treatment trial. Also, a battery of measures may make interpretation of results difficult, for example, significant group differences on some measures and not on others.

The rule about outcome measures is not so simple. Obviously, the outcome measure employed should have demonstrated validity, reliability, and sensitivity. Beyond these, selection of an outcome measure or measures will be influenced by the specific research question or questions asked. For example, if the question relates to functional communication or the social validity of improvement, a functional communication measure or a means of social validation should be employed. Or, if the treatment is designed to improve a specific aspect of communication, a measure that is extremely sensitive to change in the aspect should be selected. One's selection of an outcome measure or measures may never satisfy all of his or her knowledgeable, professional peers, but every effort should be made to try.

Specifying the Treatment

Selection criteria reduce study patient heterogeneity, but they do not eliminate it. Thus, treatment groups will comprise patients who differ in severity, type of aphasia and the nature of impairment among and within specific language modalities. Even though we lack empirical evidence to support our belief, we assume these differences should be treated differently. This presents a problem in specifying the treatment to be administered in a group treatment study.

Most reports of group treatment studies describe the treatment as traditional, conventional, or stimulus-response. This lack of specificity permits administering a variety of treatments to meet the needs of a variety of study patients. It does not tell the consumer of group treatment research very much about what the treatment was or how the results might be replicated. Most group treatment studies, therefore, have asked the question, 'Is treatment, *in general,* efficacious for aphasia?' This seems reasonable, because aphasia, typically, is treated generally. It does not imply that efforts to fragment the process by asking questions about the patient, therapist, setting, method of therapy, etc., should be shunned.

A group treatment study should be directed by a treatment protocol. That protocol should indicate the type or types of treatment that will be administered, the rationale or theory for the treatment, whether the treatment will be in a single modality or multimodality, criteria for selecting treatment tasks, criteria for moving from one treatment task to another, etc. How and what is treated in each study patient, the amount of time devoted to each task, and the results obtained can be captured in treatment logs. Application of appropriate single-case treatment designs with each study patient can be specified, and the results of each effort should be retained. There is no rule that forbids use of single-case designs within a group design. All of this information, of course, will not be available in a journal report of results because of space limitations. Nevertheless, the information should be collected and available upon request.

Specifying the treatment in a comparison of treatments group design is easier. The research question dictates there will be two or more treatments and that these treatments will differ. Each should be specified in a treatment protocol, and each should be monitored throughout the study. It is not sufficient to demonstrate that treatments differ prior to initiating the study. One must demonstrate that treatments continue to differ throughout the study. A method (Wertz, et al., 1986) for doing this is to record samples of treatment sessions in all groups, periodically, throughout the study and submit them to analysis, for example, with the *Clinical Interaction Analysis System* (Brookshire and Nicholas, 1979).

The rule about specifying the treatment in group treatment studies is simple but difficult to employ. The treatment to be administered must be specified in a general, treatment protocol. A variety of methods is necessary to accommodate differences among study patients and changes within study patients. Use of single-case designs is encouraged, and the results obtained with each design should be retained. When two or more treatments are being compared, the treatments should differ, and they should continue to differ throughout the study.

Statistical Requirements

Schoonen (1991) has criticized studies on the efficacy of language treatment for aphasia for lacking internal validity and statistical power. Many of his criticisms are appropriate. Few group studies have stated the necessary sample size, effect size and statistical power. Some have employed less than appropriate analyses.

A problem that plagues many group studies is inadequate sample size. The number of patients necessary should be determined prior to initiating the investigation. To do this, it is necessary to state an effect size, the desired level of significance, and statistical power. Effect size is the amount of difference between groups, treated and untreated, that is *clinically* significant. It is usually expressed as a difference in the outcome measure, for example, 15 percentile units in PICA Overall performance. To detect small treatment effects, large samples are necessary. To detect large treatment effects, smaller samples will suffice. Efficacy is defined as achieving the desired effect. Thus, the effect size stated should represent what is desired. The typical level of significance employed in aphasia treatment efficacy studies is .05. This seems reasonable. It expresses the probability of making a Type I error, rejecting the null hypothesis when the null hypothesis is true. In an efficacy study, a Type I error would be concluding the treatment was efficacious when it was not. Statistical power influences the probability of a Type II error, accepting the null hypothesis when it is false. In an efficacy study, a Type II error would be concluding the treatment was not efficacious when, in fact, it was (Dronkers and Swain, 1991). The higher the statistical power, the lower the probability of a Type II error. Generally, the larger the sample size, the higher the power. While one can calculate power, there is no precise way of determining exactly what the power should be. At least a power of .80 is desirable. The group study investigator should make an *a priori* statement that includes all of the requirements, for example, 'In order to detect a difference of 15 points in the outcome measure, with a Type I error of .05, and a power of .90, a sample of 35 patients in each group is necessary. This provides the effect size, 15 points in the outcome measure; acceptable statistical significance, p<.05; the power, .90; and the necessary sample size, 35 subjects in each group.

The second problem, less than appropriate analyses, results from using pre- and post-treatment change scores. Randomization will equate groups, but it will not, necessarily, make them identical. Thus, comparison of each group's pre- and post-treatment performance is somewhat cumbersome, because the groups may differ at pretreatment. The preferred analysis to evaluate treatment effects is a repeated measures analysis of covariance in which the pretreatment language score is covaried. Further, other variables that may influence outcome, for example, time post-onset, can also be covaried. An appropriate analysis for comparing groups over time, at different points in the treatment trial, is a repeated measures analysis of covariance that includes the pretreatment, entry, score. If significant group effects emerge, multiple comparisons (Bonferroni method) are appropriate and use an adjusted significance level to provide an overall probability of Type I error of .05.

The rule about statistical requirements is that they are essential. If they are not met, little valid inference about results is possible. Probably the most common problem in most group studies is a lack of statistical power resulting from inadequate sample size. Frieman, et al.'s, (1978) review of 71 treatment trials that reported negative results indicated 67 employed inadequate samples, lacked acceptable power, and ran a high risk of having missed an important treatment effect. Judging from the small samples utilized in aphasia treatment studies, Type II errors are rampant.

Results From Group Treatment Studies

Group studies designed to evaluate the efficacy of aphasia have not been a popular pastime. They are expensive. Nevertheless, several have been conducted. Those that have differ in the number and types of groups investigated. Generally, they can be classified according to the design employed – single treatment group, comparison of treatments, treatment versus no-treatment, and comparison of treatments with no-treatment. None of the group studies has met all of the requirements listed above, thus their results must be interpreted within this limitation.

Single Treatment Group Design

This approach involves selecting a sample of aphasic patients, administering a pretreatment outcome measure, providing a period of treatment, readministering the pretreatment outcome measure, and comparing pre- and post-treatment performance. Some studies (Frazier and Ingham, 1920; Weisenburg and McBride, 1935) report that patients improved. Others (Butfield and Zangwill, 1946; Wepman, 1951; Marks, Taylor and Rusk, 1957; Sands, Sarno and Shankweiler, 1969; Poeck, Huber and Willmes, 1989; and Lesser, et al., 1986) report the per cent of patients that improved. This ranges from 50 to 96 per cent across these studies. One investigation (Aten, Caligiuri and Holland, 1982) administered a specific type of treatment, functional, and reported significant improvement on a functional measure, the CADL, but not on a general, metalinguistic measure, the PICA.

Some (Aten, Caligiuri and Holland, 1982; Broida, 1977) treated patients who were chronic; well beyond six months post-onset. They could argue that improvement resulted from the treatment, because conservative estimates (Culton, 1969; Vignolo, 1964; Lendrem and Lincoln, 1985; Sarno and Levita, 1971) indicate significant spontaneous recovery ends prior to six months post-onset. This, however, is argument and not evidence. Poeck, Huber, and Willmes (1989) employed a similar, but data based, approach. They corrected for spontaneous recovery 'as demonstrated in a previous investigation' and reported improvement in their treated patients that exceeded what could be expected from spontaneous recovery alone. Again, this attempt to control is creative but not convincing. The single treatment group design can indicate aphasia improves, but it will not provide proof that the improvement results from treatment.

Comparison of Treatments Design

This approach involves assigning aphasic patients to different treatments, administering a pretreatment outcome measure, providing the specified treatment to the specified patients, readministering the pretreatment outcome measure post-treatment, and comparing improvement between or among the different treatment groups to determine which resulted in the most improvement. Examples of comparison of treatments studies are comparison of treatment by speech pathologists with treatment by trained nonprofessionals (Meikle, et al., 1979; David, et al., 1982); comparison of individual treatment with group treatment (Wertz, et al., 1981); and comparison of traditional treatment with nondirective counselling (Hartman and Landau, 1987).

Again, comparison among studies is difficult because selection criteria; outcome measures, and the amount, duration, intensity, and, of course, the types of treatment differ. In all studies, patients in all treatment groups made significant improvement. Like the single treatment group studies, none of the comparison of treatments investigations demonstrate the efficacy of treatment for aphasia, because there is no control for time – spontaneous recovery. Therefore, unless one is comparing a treatment with another treatment that has been demonstrated to be efficacious, the comparison of treatments design will only demonstrate whether one treatment is the same as, better than, or worse than the other. It will not demonstrate the efficacy of either treatment.

Hartman and Landau (1987) forgot the comparison of treatments design's inability to test efficacy and interpreted their lack of significant differences between groups as a negative result. This is incorrect. Even though there was no significant difference between their treatment groups, and even though both groups made significant improvement during the treatment trial, Hartman and Landau's design does not permit their results to support or refute the efficacy of treatment. Similarly, the lack of differences between speech pathologist treated patients and trained, nonprofessional volunteer-treated patients (Meikle, et al., 1979; David, et al., 1982) did not demonstrate that either treatment was efficacious even though both groups improved. Moreover, the results certainly do not mean speech pathologists can be replaced by nonprofessionals. Speech pathologists in those studies identified the patients, evaluated them pre- and post-treatment, trained the volunteers, and monitored the treatment.

Wertz, et al., (1981) attempted to make a statement about efficacy in their comparison of individual with group treatment design by utilizing the assumed duration of spontaneous recovery argument. Both groups were treated for 44 weeks. The authors argued that if spontaneous recovery ends by, at the most, six months post-onset, any significant improvement after six months post-onset in either treatment group resulted from the treatment. Both groups made significant improvement between six months post-onset and the end of treatment at 11 months post-onset, but to accept this as an indication of treatment's efficacy, one must also accept the assumption that significant spontaneous recovery is complete by six months post-onset or earlier.

Treatment Versus No-treatment Design

This approach requires two groups – one that is treated and one that is not treated. Patients in both groups are evaluated with an outcome measure pretreatment. The treated group is treated and the no-treatment group is followed untreated. At the end of the treatment trial, the outcome measure is readminstered, and improvement in both groups is compared. If the treated group makes significantly more improvement than the no-treatment group, one can infer the treatment was efficacious. However, this inference must be filtered through the requirements listed earlier for efficacy studies.

Several treatment versus no-treatment studies have been conducted. Three (Vignolo, 1964; Deal and Deal, 1978; Basso, Capitani and Vignolo, 1979) employed self-selected no-treatment patients who, for multiple reasons – patient preference, availability of treatment, geographical location, availability of funding, etc., – did not receive treatment. Vignolo (1964) observed no significant differences in improvement between his treated and untreated patients, however he reported patients who were treated earlier post-onset and received a longer course of treatment made significantly more improvement than patients who did not receive treatment. Deal and Deal (1978) and Basso, Capitani and Vignolo (1979) reported their treated patients made significantly more improvement than their untreated patients. Hagen (1973) compared improvement in treated patients with that in an imposed no-treatment group – the first patients who met selection criteria were treated and subsequent patients were placed on a waiting list. His treated patients made significantly more improvement than his no-treatment patients. Holland (1980a) reported a 'serendipitous' treatment result. A follow-up investigation in the development of the CADL identified some patients who had improved and some patients who had not improved when current performance was compared to previous performance. The search for an explanation revealed that patients who improved had received additional treatment, and patients who did not improve had not received additional treatment. Lincoln, et al., (1984) were the first to compare randomly assigned treated and untreated patients. They observed no significant differences in improvement between groups.

The results of treatment versus no-treatment investigations are mixed. Probably, they should be, because the selection criteria, outcome measures, treatment, and amount, intensity, and duration of treatment were mixed. Five of the six investigations employed self-selected, imposed, or discovered no-treatment and no-treatment groups. Only Lincoln, et al., (1984) used random assignment of patients to treatment and no-treatment. Four of the six investigations report positive results – treatment for aphasia is efficacious. One (Vignolo, 1964) observed an overall, negative result – no difference between treated and untreated patients. However, Vignolo suggested specific selection criteria – time post-onset and duration of treatment – would result in a positive treatment effect. Another investigation (Lincoln, et al., 1984) reported a negative result – no significant difference between treated and untreated patients. While this was the first study that utilized random assignment to groups, the minimal selection criteria, mixing of etiologies, mixing of single and multiple strokes; inclusion of patients with left, right and bilateral brain damage, and failure to provide the amount of treatment prescribed (Wertz, et al., 1986) may explain the negative result.

Comparison of Treatments With No-treatment Design

This approach requires three or more groups – at least two that involve different treatments and one that is not treated. Patients in all groups are evaluated with an outcome measure pretreatment. The treatment groups are treated with the specified treatments, and the no-treatment group is followed untreated. At the end of the treatment trial, the outcome measure is readministered, and improvement among groups is compared. If the treated groups make significantly more improvement than the no-treatment group, one can infer the treatments were efficacious. If one treatment group makes significantly more improvement than the other or others, then one can infer that that treatment was more efficacious. Again, inference is influenced by how adequately the requirements for efficacy studies have been incorporated in the design.

At least five comparison of treatments with no-treatment investigations have been reported. Sarno, Siverman, and Sands (1970) studied severe, chronic aphasic patients. Patients were placed, nonrandomly, in three groups – programmed instruction, nonprogrammed instruction and no-treatment. No significant difference in improvement among groups was observed. Shewan and Kertesz (1984) assigned patients randomly to three treatments – language oriented therapy (LOT) administered by speech pathologists; stimulation therapy (ST) administered by speech pathologists; and stimulation therapy (UNST) administered by trained volunteers, primarily nurses. Improvement was compared among the three treatments, and improvement in each treatment group was compared with a self-selected, no-treatment group. Results indicated that LOT and ST resulted in significantly more improvement than no treatment, UNST did not differ from no treatment, LOT and ST did not differ from UNST, and LOT and ST did not differ. Prins, Schoonen and Vermeulen (1989) assigned patients randomly to two treatments – auditory language comprehension and conventional stimulation. Improvement in both groups was compared with a self-selected, no-treatment group. No significant differences in improvement were observed among the three groups. Wertz, et al., (1986) assigned patients randomly to three groups – traditional treatment administered by speech pathologists (clinic), traditional treatment administered by trained volunteers (home), and deferred treatment (deferred). Clinic and home treatment patients were treated for 12 weeks and then followed for 12 weeks with no treatment. Deferred patients were followed for 12 weeks with no treatment and then treated for 12 weeks. Therefore, during the first 12 weeks, the deferred group constituted a randomly assigned no-treatment group for comparison with the clinic and home patients who were receiving treatment. Results at the end of the first 12 weeks of treatment indicated the clinic group made significantly more improvement than the deferred group, the home group did not differ significantly from the deferred group, and clinic and home groups did not differ significantly. At 24 weeks, after the deferred group had been treated, there were no significant differences in improvement among groups. Katz and Wertz (1992) assigned chronic aphasic patients – one year of more post-onset – randomly to three groups – computerized reading treatment, computer stimulation containing no language stimuli and no-treatment. Results indicated the computerized reading treatment group made significantly more improvement than the computer stimulation and no-treatment groups, and there was no significant difference in improvement between the computer stimulation and no-treatment groups.

Typically, comparison among investigations is difficult because of differences in selection criteria, outcome measures, the treatments administered, and the amount, intensity, and duration of treatment. Two (Sarno, Silverman and Sands, 1970; Prins, Schoonen and Vermeulen, 1989) observed negative results – no significant differences in improvement between treated patients and untreated patients. The other three (Shewan and Kertesz, 1984; Wertz, et al., 1986; Katz and Wertz, 1992) observed treatment administered by speech-language pathologists and computerized reading treatment resulted in significantly more improvement than no treatment. Improvement in patients treated by trained volunteers or computer stimulation in these studies did not differ from improvement in untreated patients. Only two investigations (Wertz, et al., 1986; Katz and Wertz, 1992) employed random assignment to all – treated and untreated – groups.

Discussion

What do the results of group treatment trials tell us about the efficacy of treatment for aphasia? A definitive statement is difficult because of differences among investigations. Few investigations met most of the requirements for group treatment studies. Selection criteria varied widely. Some exercised control for spontaneous recovery by employing a no-treatment group for comparison with a treated group or groups, and only three (Lincoln, et al., 1984; Wertz, et al., 1986; Katz and Wertz 1992) employed a randomly assigned no-treatment group. Outcome measures varied widely among studies, and those that employed the same outcome measures differed too much in other areas – selection criteria, type, amount, duration, and intensity of treatment, etc. – to permit comparison. Similarly, treatments among studies varied widely, and even though some treatments were specified, they were sufficiently general to permit application with study patients who differed in severity and type of aphasia. Finally, the investigations varied in their adherence to statistical requirements. Only three (Wertz, et al., 1981; 1986; Katz and Wertz, 1992) made an *a priori* estimation of sample size, stated a significance level, and calculated statistical power. And, only two of these (Wertz, et al.,1986; Katz and Wertz, 1992) obtained the required sample size to achieve acceptable statistical power. Only four (Shewan and Kertesz, 1984; Prins, Schoonen and Vermeulen, 1989; Wertz, et al., 1981; Wertz, et al., 1986) avoided the use of change scores to evaluate improvement and exercised some statistical control over variables – pretreatment severity, time post-onset, etc. – that may influence results.

Some general observations are possible. First, aphasic people – treated and untreated, generally, improve. Results from all group designs, generally, support this conclusion. The amount of improvement, typically, wanes in aphasic people – treated and untreated – as time post-onset increases. Second, the single treatment group and comparison of treatments designs will not demonstrate the efficacy of treatment for aphasia, because there is no control for time, for example, spontaneous recovery. The comparison of treatments design will indicate whether the results of one treatment is the same as, better than, or worse than another treatment or treatments. Specifically, individual treatment appears to be slightly superior to group treatment (Wertz, et al., 1981). Computerized reading treatment is superior to computer stimulation (Katz and Wertz, 1992). Treatment by speech pathologist does not differ significantly from treatment by trained nonprofessionals (Meikle, et al., 1979; David, et al., 1982; Shewan and Kertesz, 1984; Wertz, et al., 1986). Traditional treatment does not differ from nondirective counselling (Hartman and Landau, 1987); language-oriented treatment and stimulation treatment do not differ significantly (Shewan and Kertesz, 1984); programmed instruction does not differ significantly from nonprogrammed instruction (Sarno, Silverman and Sands, 1970); and auditory comprehension treatment does not differ significantly from general stimulation (Prins, Schoonen and Vermeulen, 1989).

Third, investigations of the efficacy of treatment for aphasia have yielded mixed results. The evidence does not permit an unqualified conclusion that treatment for aphasia is or is not efficacious. Individual investigations must be interpreted according to the selection criteria employed – etiology, localization of brain damage, time post-onset, severity, amount of treatment, etc. This results in some speculations about how much of what may or may not be efficacious for whom. In addition, one must consider sample size, for example, Was there sufficient statistical power to permit adequate control for a Type II error? Finally, the evidence is limited to treatment versus no-treatment and comparison of treatments with no-treatment designs, and these reports must be interpreted further according to the no-treatment group employed – self selected or randomly assigned.

So, what can one conclude? Generally, aphasia treatment does not appear to be efficacious for patients who receive 48 hours of treatment or less and who are aphasic subsequent to single or multiple left, right, or bilateral strokes (Lincoln, et al., 1984). Similarly, severe, chronic aphasic patients who receive a brief course of programmed instruction or nonprogrammed instruction do not improve significantly more than patients who receive no treatment (Sarno, Silverman and Sands, 1970). And, patients who receive two sessions each week for five months of auditory comprehension or conventional stimulation treatment do not improve significantly more than patients who receive no treatment (Prins, Schoonen and Vermeulen, 1989). Conversely, patients who are aphasic subsequent to a left hemisphere infarct improve significantly more than patients who receive no treatment if they receive at least three hours of treatment each week for at least five months (Basso, Capitani and Vignolo, 1979); 18 hours of treatment each week for 12 months (Hagen, 1973); three hours of treatment each week for 12 months (Shewan and Kertesz, 1984); eight to ten hours of treatment each week for 12 weeks (Wertz, *et al.*, 1986); or three to five hours of treatment each week for six months (Katz and Wertz, 1992).

It appears that treatment is efficacious for some aphasic people and not others. Moreover, the efficacy of treatment seems to be influenced by its amount, duration and intensity. Little can be said about the efficacy of specific types of treatment beyond the Katz and Wertz (1992) report that computerized reading treatment resulted in significantly more overall language gains than no treatment. Other group studies that obtained positive results imply that treatment, in general, results in more improvement than no treatment. It seems reasonable to ask and answer the question about overall efficacy before fragmenting the total process. However, subsequent investigations may want to address more specific questions relating to specific types of patients, settings, methods of treatment, etc. The initial work in these areas will be done most economically in single-case designs. Results of these efforts will refine questions and provide direction for subsequent group research.

Single-Case Designs: Contributions to Efficacy

Kent (1985) observed that the clarion call for data on treatment's efficacy has generated 'a flurry of activity loosely grouped under the name of single-subject (or within-subject) designs'. He notes that, 'If these designs are to be the salvation of the scientist practitioner, there is certainly no lack of messiahs.' Kent's prose was prophetic. Howard (1986) heard the call, and suggested, 'A sensible strategy would be to establish whether a particular treatment technique works with one patient, and then investigate whether the same treatment approach applies to other patients with problems of the same type – that is a single-case study with replications.'

Single-case designs, like group designs, have strengths and weaknesses. Certainly, they are economical. One needs only one aphasic person. However, it is difficult to control for sequence and order effects in a single-case design, and there are few statistical procedures for evaluating results or assessing their reliability. Nevertheless, different single-case designs can be employed to answer interesting and important questions: Does a treatment work? Does one treatment work better than another? Are there specific components in a treatment that make it work, and how much treatment is optimal? (Hayes, 1981). Which designs are appropriate for which questions is discussed by Hersen and Barlow (1976), McReynolds and Kearns (1983), and Kent (1985) among others. And, reports by Howard, et al., (1985), Thompson and McReynolds (1986), and Byng (1988) among many others demonstrate how single-case designs can be employed to demonstrate whether a specific treatment was effective for a specific aphasic patient.

Some Single-Case Designs

Clinicians who want to demonstrate that they are accountable and explore the efficacy of their efforts have a variety of single-case designs from which to choose. Like different group designs, different single-case designs will answer different questions. The following provides a brief description of several single-case designs and examples of how they have been employed. General elaboration can be found in McReynolds and Kearns (1983), and specific application in the treatment of aphasia is provided by Rosenbek, LaPointe, and Wertz (1989).

Withdrawal or A-B-A Design.

The components of the A-B-A, or withdrawal, design are: an A phase, pretreatment, where a behavior is evaluated to demonstrate its stability, level, or trend; a B phase where the behavior is treated; and a second A phase, post-treatment, where the behavior is followed untreated to determine its stability. Generally, if performance is stable during the first A phase, untreated, improves during the B phase, treatment, and sags during the second A phase, withdrawal, a treatment effect may be inferred. The problem with this design, like the single treatment group design, is that there is no strong control for time – spontaneous recovery. Further, the requirement that the behavior sag during withdrawals is problematic. This seems more appropriate for some interventions, for example, drug treatment, than for others, such as language treatment for aphasia. A solution to the first problem is to reserve this design for treating chronic patients – those beyond the limits of spontaneous recovery. A solution to the second problem is to acknowledge that aphasic behavior may stabilize at high levels of performance following effective treatment and not sag when that treatment is withdrawn. If performance does sag, the implication is a need for additional treatment.

Bernstein-Ellis, Wertz, and Shubitowski (1987) utilized an A-B-A design to assess treatment for speaking rate reduction in a mildly aphasic patient. Baseline rate, pretreatment, was markedly reduced during treatment with a pacing board. During withdrawal, post-treatment, speaking rate remained at the reduced levels observed during treatment. Moreover, performance generalized to conversation in functional contexts, and the patient's number of content units remained essentially unchanged at the slower speaking rate. One can infer this was a positive treatment result, however, the patient was four months post-onset at the time of treatment, and as indicated earlier, the A-B-A design permits no strong control for the influence of spontaneous recovery.

The A-B-A design can be elaborated with additional treatment or different treatment. For example, Simmons (1980) employed an A-B-B C-B-BC-A design in the treatment of a mildly aphasic blind patient who displayed coexisting apraxia of speech. Treatment was designed to improve sentence formulation, and a modification of the Rosenbek, et al., (1973) eight-step task continuum was employed. The first A phase in the design represented baseline performance, pretreatment, and the B phase represented performance during auditory presentation of treatment. The BC condition combined auditory presentation with braille presentation of treatment, and the second A phase represented follow-up post-treatment. The patient's performance was zero to ten percent correct during the A baseline. This improved to 50 per cent correct during B, auditory alone treatment. During BC, auditory and braille treatment, performance rose to 90 per cent correct. During the second B phase, auditory alone treatment, performance dropped to 50 to 70 per cent correct. When auditory and braille combined were reintroduced during the second BC phase, performance rose to the previous 90 per cent correct level. During A, withdrawal, performance sagged to 75 per cent correct and stabilized.

Simmons' patient was eight-months post-onset when treated. The duration of aphasia and the systematic changes in behavior consequent with systematic changes in the treatment design suggest improvement resulted from the treatment. Further, her single-case design demonstrates a major strength in this approach; its flexibility.

Multiple Baseline Design

This design is similar to the ABA design in that it employs a baseline, pretreatment, A phase; a B treatment phase; and can employ a second A, withdrawal or post-treatment, phase. It differs from the ABA design in that baseline performance is collected on two or more behaviors or sets of stimuli, and then treatment is introduced for one behavior or set of stimuli while the other or others are followed in an untreated baseline or baselines. Improvement on the treated behavior or set of stimuli and less or no improvement on the untreated behavior or set of stimuli permits inference of a treatment effect. Treatment can be withdrawn and introduced systematically across behaviors or sets of stimuli. If improvement occurs only when a behavior or set of stimuli is treated, inference about the efficacy of treatment is strengthened. This design is especially appropriate for assessing treatment's efficacy during the period of spontaneous recovery because of the untreated baseline's efficacy during the period of spontaneous recovery because of the untreated baseline's control for determining the influences of time.

Single-case multiple baseline designs have been very popular in the treatment of aphasia. Examples abound. One is Thompson and Kearns' (1981) use of a cueing hierarchy to improve naming in an anomic aphasic patient. Four sets of stimuli were evaluated in an A, pretreatment baseline. Treatment was systematically introduced, B phase, and withdrawn, A phase, across sets of stimuli. The results indicate performance improved only when a set of stimuli was treated and not when it was followed in the extended, pretreatment, baseline condition. Thompson and Kearns could infer a treatment effect.

A problem in multiple baseline designs is the possibility of generalization – treatment for the treated behavior or set of stimuli generalizes and induces improvement in the untreated behavior or stimuli. Certainly, clinicians seek generalization of treatment effects to untreated stimuli, behaviours and settings. However, if they are too successful in obtaining it, treatment effects are obscured. For example, if a behavior or set of stimuli being followed in an untreated baseline in a multiple baseline design improves as much as the treated behavior, it is difficult to determine whether this results from generalization, spontaneous recovery, or some other uncontrolled variable. Thompson's (1989) review of generalization research in aphasia indicates more effort has been devoted to seeking generalization than differentiating it from unexplained improvement that may not have resulted from the treatment.

Alternating Treatments Design

This design can provide an answer to the relative effectiveness of two or more treatments. Typically, a behavior or set of stimuli is evaluated in a pretreatment baseline. Then, two or more treatments are assigned randomly over a number of treatment sessions. During the treatment phase, the clinician observes improvement resulting from each treatment. If it becomes apparent that more improvement occurs on days when one treatment is administered than on days when another treatment is administered, one has evidence about which is more effective. When this is apparent, some stop the less effective treatment and continue with the more effective treatment in subsequent sessions. Ultimately, treatment can be stopped, and a second A, withdrawal phase can be employed. Like the comparison of treatments group design, the alternating treatments single-case design will not demonstrate efficacy. To permit inference about efficacy, one could combine an alternating treatment design with a multiple baseline design.

Hoodin and Thompson (1983) compared three types of treatment – verbal, gestural and verbal and gestural – for improving verbal labelling in two moderate to severe, nonfluent aphasic patients. Their use of the alternating treatment design indicated verbal and gestural treatment was superior to treatment with either alone. Similarly, Loverso, Prescott and Selinger (1992) employed an alternating treatment design to demonstrate a clinician is more effective and efficient in delivering aphasia treatment than a clinician assisted by a microcomputer. Thompson and McReynolds (1986) demonstrated how creative one can be in combining single-case designs. They utilized an alternating treatment design – auditory-visual stimulation compared with direct-production – and combined it with a multiple baseline design to evaluate the efficacy of each treatment. In addition, they included measures of generalization.

Crossover Design

This approach is similar to a multiple baseline design. In fact, it is sometimes referred to as a multiple baseline, crossover design. Two or more behaviors or sets of stimuli are baselined in a pretreatment condition. Then, one behavior or set of stimuli is treated and the other is followed in an untreated condition. At a specific point in the treatment trial – either predetermined or after criterion performance is reached on the treated behavior or stimuli, the clinician crosses over – stops treatment on the previous behavior or stimuli and begins to treat the previously untreated behavior or stimuli. A treatment effect can be inferred if improvement or more improvement occurs on the treated behavior or stimuli than on the behaviors or stimuli that are untreated. Additional evidence for the efficacy of treatment occurs if the previously untreated behaviors or stimuli improve only after they are treated.

LaPointe (1984) utilized a crossover design to improve naming in an aphasic patient with coexisting apraxia of speech. Split lists – equally difficult stimuli – were employed. One list was treated, and the other was followed in an untreated baseline. The patient's performance improved on the treated list, and there was minimal improvement on the untreated list. When LaPointe crossed over, stopped treatment on the previously treated list, and began to treat the untreated list, performance stabilized on the previously treated list and improved on the list that was now being treated. Thus, Lapointe could infer a treatment effect – improvement occurred only when a list was being treated.

Coltheart's (1983) explanation of the crossover design indicates it need not be limited to sets of different stimuli. He suggests different linguistic functions – different behaviors – can be employed in the design. One is treated, while the other is followed in an untreated baseline. When crossover occurs, the previously treated behavior is placed into extended, untreated follow-up, and the previously untreated behavior is treated.

Changing Criterion Design

This design is appropriate for investigating behaviors that change gradually, that can be shaped through a series of steps, or respond to a hierarchical treatment. Once baseline, pretreatment performance is determined, a criterion to be obtained is set, and treatment is administered to reach that criterion. When criterion performance is reached, the next criterion is set, and treatment is continued. This process continues until the final criterion is met. The treatment may be the same from one criterion to the next, or it may be modified to be more appropriate for the specific stage in the process. Unfortunately, there is no control for time, for example, spontaneous recovery. This can be accomplished by combining the changing criterion design with a multiple baseline design to provide comparison of the treated behavior in the changing criterion design with another behavior that is followed in an untreated baseline.

Rosenbek, LaPointe and Wertz (1989) discuss application of a changing criterion design with a mildly aphasic patient to reduce his verbal intrusions that disrupted his relatively good communication. The number of intrusions produced in response to a specific set of stimuli were determined in pretreatment, baseline sessions. The initial criterion was to reduce these by five. Treatment involved the use of a pacing board in picture description. It had two effects – it slowed, focused and kept the patient's verbal description moving forward, and he hated it. When the initial criterion was met, it was changed to reduce intrusions further by five. This process continued across two additional changes in the criterion. The terminal behavior was five intrusions without the use of the pacing board in describing 40 pictures. This can be compared with 25 intrusions on the same task during pretreatment baseline.

Discussion

Single-case treatment designs have become very popular in the management of aphasia. Not only do they provide some inference about the efficacy of treatment for aphasia, they also provide improved management. Every clinician can utilize single-case designs with his or her patients. Those who conduct group treatment research can utilize single-case designs within the study protocol with each study patient within the groups.

These designs will provide evidence for the efficacy of a specific treatment with a specific aphasic patient. They will not provide everything a group design can, but they can provide some things group designs cannot. For example, they do not require withholding all treatment as is necessary in the classical clinical trial. The pretreatment baseline, A phase, is short, and the post-treatment, withdrawal phase does not preclude treatment on another task, behavior, or set of stimuli. Even in the multiple baseline design, some behavior or stimuli are being treated. Further, single-case designs permit tailoring a specific treatment for a specific patient. They also permit testing a model or utilizing theory-driven treatment. These can be accomplished in group designs, but the process is longer and much more expensive. Most of all, single-case designs are extremely flexible. They permit rapid change in the treatment consequent with change in the patient, thus they need not await the end of a group treatment trial or a specified amount of a specified treatment.

Unfortunately, all single-case designs are somewhat confounded by time. For example, even if a pretreatment baseline appears stable, one must assume that improvement during the treatment phase indicates the results of treatment and not the influence of some unknown or uncontrolled variable. Even in the multiple baseline design, one must assume that the behaviors or stimuli used to control for time in the extended, untreated baseline or baselines have the same probability as the treated behavior or stimuli of improving spontaneously. Further, single-case designs have difficulty in controlling sequence and order effects. For example, A–B–C–A and crossover designs cannot completely explain the influence of the previous treatment on response to the subsequent treatment. Similarly, in the alternating treatments design, one does not know the influence of coexisting treatments on either treatment alone. Finally, analysis of results is problematic. Few statistical measures are available to determine significant improvement. Typically, inference is based on visual interpretation of the data.

Nevertheless, single-case designs provide a powerful, easily applied means to explore the efficacy of aphasia treatment. They are particularly appropriate for answering specific questions about specific patients and providing evidence to skeptics in one's clinical setting. And, over time, through replications with additional patients, treatments can be refined and their efficacy improved or, as importantly, disproved. Ultimately, one can acquire a sizeable amount of data, even within the confines of a single clinic, on the efficacy of treatment for aphasia.

Every Question About Efficacy Has Not Been Answered

While there is a good deal of evidence from single-case and group designs that treatment for aphasia is efficacious for some aphasic people, doubts persist. Moreover, there continue to be questions about efficacy that require answers to improve practice. Little is known about how much treatment is most efficacious; when, post-onset treatment may be efficacious or most efficacious; exactly for whom treatment is efficacious; and what kind of treatment is efficacious. Of course, these questions interact, and the answer clinicians seek is how much, of what, for whom, when?

We might begin our search for these answers by abolishing quarrels about methodology; specifically about the use of single-case *or* group designs. It seems to me (Wertz, 1992) neither design is better *than* the other. They are different *from* each other. The merits of one over the other become apparent depending on the specific research question. It is not necessary for everyone interested in treatment's efficacy to utilized both single-case and group designs. General George Patton observed that when everyone is thinking alike, no one is thinking. It is essential that one utilize a design that is appropriate for his or her research question. More importantly, we should avoid insisting on only one design to the exclusion of the other. Controversy does not demean us. Scientific McCarthyism does.

Kent (1985) proposed several models for intervention research. All models begin with knowledge about existing intervention research – what has been done. The next step in all models is innovation – generation of new intervention procedures and/or new measurement procedures. After this step, the models bifurcate into single-case designs and group designs. These different approaches can interact and influence each other. For example, single-case designs can be replicated to refine research questions and focus research for a subsequent, more expensive group study. Or, the results of a group design may indicate new or persisting questions that are most appropriately answered and refined in a series of single-case designs prior to mounting additional group research. Ultimately, the results of both single-case and group designs permit us to evaluate the efficacy of our efforts. The following utilizes Kent's approach for answering some persisting questions about the efficacy of treatment for aphasia.

Intensity and Duration of Treatment

The optimal amount of aphasia treatment has not been established. Of course, one is prompted to ask, 'The optimal amount of what kind of treatment for which kind of aphasic person at what point in time post-onset?' Nevertheless, waiting for the world to become perfect will be a long wait if those who can move us toward perfection are reluctant to begin, because the questions are too complex.

One might begin to answer the question about intensity and duration with single-case designs and explore the influence of the potential confounding variables – who, what, and when – through replications with different kinds of patients, different kinds of treatment, at different times post-onset. The results of these single-case designs – probably combined A–B–A–B–A multiple baseline designs – could provide selection criteria; specify the treatment; and indicate the amount, intensity and duration of treatment to be employed in a group design. For example, an A–B–A–B–A multiple baseline design will provide a control for time through the extended, untreated stimuli or behaviors, thus permitting inference about efficacy. The alternating As, pretreatment and post-treatment, and Bs, treatment, should indicate when performance requires or responds to more treatment and, ultimately, when it no longer improves with additional treatment. Replications of this approach with similar patients will support or refute the initial observations. Replications with different patients at different times post-onset and with different treatments should indicate the influence of patient, treatment, and time post-onset variables on amount, intensity, and duration of treatment.

When single-case research refines the question – study patient selection criteria, type of treatment, potential amounts, intensities, and durations of treatment, this information can be utilized in a group design that blocks on amount, intensity, and duration, utilizes the appropriate selection criteria and administers the specified treatment. For example, study patients are assigned randomly to different amount, intensity and duration of treatment groups and a no-treatment or deferred treatment group. The results should indicate whether the different amount, intensity and duration of treatment are efficacious – treated groups improve significantly more than the no-treatment or deferred treatment group. Further, comparison between or among the amount, intensity, and duration of treatment groups should indicate which one is most efficacious.

When Treatment Should Occur

The majority of improvement in aphasia appears to occur during the first three months post-onset in patients who are aphasic subsequent to a first, single, left-hemisphere, thromboembolic infarct (Wertz, et al., 1981). For patients who are aphasic subsequent to other causes, few data on when aphasia improves are available. Nevertheless, clinicians need to know when post-onset their efforts are most efficacious. For example, is early intervention most appropriate, because, perhaps, early treatment raises the ceiling for ultimate improvement, i.e., patients treated early attain higher levels of ultimate performance than patients treated later post-onset? Or, should treatment be delayed until it is necessary, i.e., permit spontaneous recovery to exhaust its benefits and focus treatment on the aphasic deficits that persist? We do not know. Basso, et al., (1979) reported patients treated prior to two months post-onset improved more than patients treated after two months post-onset. Wertz, et al., (1986) reported delaying treatment for three months during the first six months post-onset had no significant influence on ultimate outcome after three months of treatment. Again, combining single-case and group treatment designs permit improving our knowledge and, ultimately, improving our practice.

Utilizing single-case designs – probably multiple baseline designs – with a variety of patients who demonstrate different durations of aphasia seems a reasonable place to begin. Through replications, single-case designs will identify variables – patient, type of treatment, duration of aphasia – to be controlled in a group design. When these are apparent, a group design can utilize them in specifying the important selection criteria, type of treatment and duration of aphasia to be investigated. For example, the group design would block on duration of aphasia, i.e., patients one- to three-months post-onset, patients three- to six-months post-onset, etc. All patients would meet all other selection criteria, i.e., cause of aphasia, severity, age, education, etc. Those within the specified time post-onset ranges would be assigned randomly to treatment or no-treatment or deferred treatment. All treatment groups would receive the same type, amount, intensity, and duration of treatment. At the end of the treatment trial, comparison of the treated group with its time post-onset, no treatment cohort would indicate the efficacy of the treatment. Comparison between or among different time post-onset treatment groups would indicate whether early or late treatment resulted in more improvement and influenced the ultimate level attained. A similar group design could investigate one duration post-onset, for example, treatment before six months post-onset. It would assign patients who met the same selection criteria randomly to immediate treatment for six months or to deferred treatment, after six months, and look at amount of improvement at one year post-onset. Comparison of groups at six months post-onset would indicate the efficacy of the treatment – early treatment patients had received treatment during this period, delayed treatment patients had not. Comparison of groups at one year post-onset, after the deferred patients had received six months of treatment, would indicate any advantage in overall improvement or ultimate outcome from early or late treatment.

What Kind of Treatment for Whom

Howard (1986) and Byng (1988) suggest one would not treat all aphasic patients the same. Certainly, clinicians seem to agree, because they do treat aphasic people differently. However, there is no empirical evidence to support or refute this assumption (Wertz, 1993). Single-case and group designs provide means for finding out.

Again, the economical way to begin is with a series of single-case designs to determine patient, treatment, etc., variables that can be applied in group designs. The single-case approach can utilize a specific treatment for a specific type of patient in a multiple baseline design, or it could investigate two treatments in an alternating treatments design with multiple, untreated baselines. The former approach would be replicated with similar and different patients – those whom the specific treatment is predicted to help and those whom the specific treatment is predicted to be ineffective. The latter approach could be employed similarly – one treatment is predicted to be effective and the other is predicted to be ineffective. The alternating treatments design appears particularly appropriate for testing theory-driven or model-based treatment. For example, one treatment is selected because the theory or model predicts it would be effective, and the other treatment is selected, because the theory or model predicts it would be ineffective.

Once again, after the important patient and treatment variables are identified in a series of single-case designs, the information can be utilized in a group design. The appropriate group design would be a comparison of treatments with no-treatment control. Selection criteria can be used in two ways. One is to select only those patients for whom a specific treatment is designed to help. These are assigned randomly to three groups: the appropriate treatment group, an inappropriate treatment group, and a no-treatment group. Comparison among groups at the end of the treatment trial should indicate whether either treatment is efficacious – comparison of the treated groups with the no-treatment group – and whether one treatment is more efficacious than the other – comparison of the treatment groups. The other approach is to employ two sets of selection criteria – one designed to identify patients for whom the treatment is predicted to help and the other designed to identify patients for whom the treatment is predicted to be ineffective. The resultant two groups – appropriate and inappropriate – are assigned randomly to two additional groups – treatment or no-treatment. Thus, we have one treatment administered to two groups, each with its own no-treatment control group. At the end of the treatment trial, comparison among groups should indicate whether the treatment was efficacious for either treated group – both compared with both no-treatment groups – and whether the treatment was efficacious or more efficacious for the appropriate treatment group than the inappropriate treatment group.

Over the Mountains Are Mountains

The above are only a few of the questions about treatment's efficacy that require answers. For example, nothing was mentioned about why treatment is administered beyond the implied 'to improve communication'. Earlier, I defined efficacy as achieving the desired effect. Moreover, I spent some time discussing effect size. We may want to ponder what, specifically, the desired effect is and how large the effect size should be. Statistical demonstration of improvement may be only interesting or curious (Wertz, 1991). It may not warrant the time, effort and expense of treatment. Many seek clinical significance. Fine, but what constitutes clinical significance? And, how is it measured? Answers require attention to the outcome measures employed in aphasia treatment efficacy studies and social validation of the effects and their size that treatment achieves.

Advocating the use of both single-case and group designs may seem cavalier. For most clinicians, only single-case designs are possible within their clinical environments. One should not apologize for this limitation. Kent (1985) observed there is a paucity of reported intervention research, and if we are to have any, it is the clinician who will provide it. Thus, one may want to apologize for not participating. Single-case designs can be employed where and when aphasic person and clinician gather. Group designs will be employed by those who can generate multicenter treatment trials. Sample sizes restricted by rigid selection criteria can only be obtained when several centers provide patients; these group studies should employ single-case designs with the individual patients within the deign's groups.

A Caveat

Parloff's (1986) observation about consistent doubt regarding the efficacy of psychological treatments in an inconsistent and uncertain world need not be troublesome. Efforts to test the efficacy of treatment for aphasia transcend similar efforts in much of Medicine, Neurology, Surgery and Psychiatry (Darley, 1972). We need not apologize for our efforts. However, we should apologize if they are not continued. Probably, the world is not going to become perfect, and, probably, scepticism about the value of treatment for aphasia will continue. Means – single-case and group designs – for reducing that scepticism exist. If clinicians do not employ these means to determine whether what they do for aphasic people does any good, clinicians will be forced to live with answers others make up. That, of course, is unacceptable.

References

Anonymous (1969) Struggling with aphasia. Medical World News 10:37-40.

Aten J, Caligiuri MP, Holland AL (1982) The efficacy of functional communication therapy for chronic aphasic patients. Journal of Speech and Hearing Disorders 47:93-6.

Basso A, Capitani E, Vignolo L (1979) Influence of rehabilitation of language skills in aphasic patients: a controlled study. Archives of Neurology 36:190-6.

Bates E, Applebaum M, Allard L (1991) Statistical constraints on the use of single cases in neuropsychological research. Brain and Language 40:295-329.

Bates E, McDonald J, MacWhinney B, Applebaum M (1991) A maximum likelihood procedure for the analysis of group and individual data in aphasia research. Brain and Language 40:231-65.

Bernstein-Ellis EG, Wertz RT, Shubitowski Y (1987) More pace, less fillers: A verbal strategy for a high-level aphasic patient. In Brookshire RH (Ed) Clinical Aphasiology 17. Minneapolis MN: BRK Publishers. pp 12-22.

Broida H (1977) Language therapy effects in long term aphasia. Archives of Physical

Medicine and Rehabilitation 58:248-53.

Brookshire RH, Nicholas LE (1979) A scale for rating clinician, patient, and session characteristics in aphasia treatment sessions. In Brookshire RH (Ed) Clinical Aphasiology Conference Proceedings. Minneapolis, MN: BRK Publishers. pp 115-23.

Butfield E, Zangwill O (1946) Re-education in aphasia: a review of 70 cases. Journal of Neurology, Neurosurgery, and Psychiatry 9:75-9.

Byng S (1988) Sentence processing deficits: theory and therapy. Cognitive Neuropsychology 5:629-76.

Caramazza A, Badecker W (1989) Patient Classification in neuropsychological research. Brain and Cognition 10:256-95.

Coltheart M (1983) Aphasia therapy research: a single-case study approach. In Code C, Muller DJ (Eds) Aphasia Therapy. London: Edward Arnold. pp 194-202.

Culton GL (1969) Spontaneous recovery from aphasia. Journal of Speech and Hearing Research 12:825-32.

Darley FL (1972) The efficacy of language rehabilitation in aphasia. Journal of Speech and Hearing Disorders 37:3-21.

David RM, Enderby P, Bainton D (1982) Treatment of acquired aphasia: speech therapists and volunteers compared. Journal of Neurology, Neurosurgery, and Psychiatry 45:957-61.

Deal J, Deal LA (1978) Efficacy of aphasia rehabilitation: Preliminary results. In Brookshire RH (Ed) Clinical Aphasiology Conference Proceedings. Minneapolis, MN: BRK Publishers. pp 66-77.

Dronkers NF, Swain BE (1991) Statistical power in aphasia research. In Prescott TE (Ed) Clinical Aphasiology, Volume 19. Austin, TX: Pro-ed. pp 15-19.

Editorial (1977) Prognosis in aphasia. Lancet 2:24.

Frazier CH, Ingham SD (1920) A review of the effects of gunshot wounds of the head: based on the observation of two hundred cases at US General Hospital No. 11, Cape May, NJ Archives of Neurology 3:17-40.

Freiman JA, Chalmers TC, Smith H, Kuebler RR (1978) The importance of beta, the Type-II error and sample size in the design and interpretation of the randomized controlled trial. The New England Journal of Medicine 299:690-4.

Goodglass H, Kaplan E (1972) Boston Diagnostic Examination for Aphasia. Philadelphia, PA: Lea & Febiger.

Hagen C (1973) Communication abilities in hemiplegia: effect of speech therapy. Archives of Physical Medicine and Rehabilitation 54:454-63.

Hartman J, Landau WM (1987) Comparison of formal language therapy with supportive counselling for aphasia due to acute vascular accident. Archives of Neurology 24:646-9.

Hayes SC (1981) Single case experimental design and empirical clinical practice. Journal of consulting and Clinical Psychology 49:193-211.

Hersen M, Barlow DH (1976) Single Case Experimental Designs: Strategies for Studying Behavior Change. New York: Pergamon Press.

Holland AL (1980a) The usefulness of treatment for aphasia: A serendipitous study. In Brookshire RH (Ed) Clinical Aphasiology Conference Proceedings. Minneapolis, MN: BRK Publishers. pp 240-7.

Holland AL (1980b) Communicative Abilities in Daily Living. Baltimore, MD: University Park Press.

Hoodin RB, Thompson CK (1983) Facilitation of verbal labelling in adult aphasia by gestural, verbal, or verbal plus gestural training. In Brookshire RH (Ed) Clinical Aphasiology Conference Proceedings. Minneapolis, MN: BRK Publishers. pp 62-4.

Howard D (1986) Beyond randomised controlled trials: the case for effective case studies of the effects of treatment in aphasia. British Journal of Disorders of Communication 21:89-102.

Howard D, Patterson KE, Franklin S, Orchard-Lisle VM, Morton J (1985) Treatment of word retrieval deficits in aphasia: A comparison of two therapy methods. Brain 108:817-29.

Katz RC, Wertz RT (1992) Computerized hierarchical reading treatment in aphasia. Aphasiology 6:165-77.

Kent RD (1985) Science and the clinician: the practice of science and the science of practice. In Kent RD (Ed) Application of Research to Assessment and Therapy, Seminars in Speech and Language. New York: Thieme-Stratton Inc. pp 1-12.

Kertesz A (1982) Western Aphasia Battery. New York: Grune & Stratton.

LaPointe LL (1984) Sequential treatment of split lists: a case report. In Rosenbek JC, McNeil MR, Aronson AE (Eds) Apraxia of Speech: Physiology, Acoustics, Linguistics, Management. San Diego, CA: College-Hill Press. pp 277-86.

Lendrem W, Lincoln NB (1985) Spontaneous recovery of language in patients with aphasia between 4 and 34 weeks after stroke. Journal of Neurology, Neurosurgery, and Psychiatry 48:743-8.

Lesser R, Bryan K, Anderson J, Hilton R (1986) Involving relatives in aphasia therapy: An application of language enrichment therapy. International Journal of Rehabilitation Research 9:259-67.

Lincoln NB, McGuirk E, Mulley GP, Lendrem W, Jones AC, Mitchell JRA (1984) Effectiveness of speech therapy for aphasic stroke patients: A randomized controlled trial. Lancet 1:1197-200.

Longstreth WT, Koepsell TD, Van Belle G (1987) Clinical neuroepidemiology II. Outcomes. Archives of Neurology 44:1196-202.

Loverso FL, Prescott TE, Selinger M (1992) Microcomputer treatment applications in aphasiology. Aphasiology 6:155-63.

McReynolds LV, Kearns KP (1983) Single-subject Experimental Designs in Communicative Disorders. Baltimore, MD: University Park Press.

Marks M, Taylor M, Rusk HA (1958) Rehabilitation of the aphasic patient: a summary of three years' experience in a rehabilitation setting. Archives of Physical Medicine and Rehabilitation 38:219-26.

Meikle M, Wechsler E, Tupper A, Benenson M, Butler J, Mulhall D, Stern G (1979) Comparative trial of volunteer and professional treatments of dysphasia after stroke. British Medical Journal 2:87-9.

Parloff MB (1986) Placebo controls in psychotherapy research: A sine qua non or a placebo for research problems? Journal of Consulting and Clinical Psychology, 54:79-87.

Poeck K, Huber W, Willmes K (1989) Outcome of intensive language treatment in aphasia. Journal of Speech and Hearing Disorders 54:471-9.

Porch BE (1967) Porch Index of Communicative Ability. Palo Alto, CA: Consulting Psychologists Press.

Prins RS, Schoonen R, Vermeulen J (1989) Efficacy of two different types of speech therapy for aphasic stroke patients. Applied Psycholinguistics 10:85-123.

Rosenbek JC, LaPointe LL, Wertz RT (1989) Aphasia: A Clinical Approach. Austin, TX: Pro-ed

Rosenbek JC, Lemme ML, Ahern MB, Harris EH, Wertz RT (1973) A treatment for apraxia of speech. Journal of Speech and Hearing Disorders 38:462-72.

Salive ME, Mayfield JA, Weissman NW (1992) Patient outcomes research teams and the agency for health care policy and research. AHCPR Program Note, Agency for

Health Care Policy and Research, US Department of Health and Human Services, 697-708.

Sands E, Sarno MT, Shankweiler D (1969) Long-term assessment of language function in aphasia due to stroke. Archives of Physical Medicine and Rehabilitation 50:202-6.

Sarno MT (1969) The Functional Communication Profile: Manual of Directions (Rehabilitation Monograph 42). New York: New York University Medical Center, Institute of Rehabilitation Medicine.

Sarno MT, Levita E (1971) Natural course of recovery in severe aphasia. Archives of Physical Medicine and Rehabilitation 52:175-8.

Sarno MT, Silverman M, Sands E (1970) Speech therapy and language recovery in severe aphasia. Journal of Speech and Hearing Research 13:607-23.

Schoonen R (1991) The internal validity of efficacy studies: design and statistical power in studies of language therapy for aphasics. Brain and Language 41:446-64.

Shewan CM, Kertesz A (1984) Effects of speech and language treatment on recovery from aphasia. Brain and Language 23:272-99.

Siegel GM (1987) The limits of science in communication disorders. Journal of Speech and Hearing Disorders 52:306-12.

Simmons NN (1980) Choice of stimulus modes in treating apraxia of speech: a case study. In Brookshire R H (Ed) Clinical Aphasiology conference Proceedings. Minneapolis, MN: BRK Publishers. pp 302-7.

Thompson CK (1989) Generalization research in aphasia: A review of the literature. In Prescott TE (Ed) Clinical Aphasiology, Volume 18. Boston: College-Hill Press, Little, Brown, and Company. pp 195-222.

Thompson CK, Kearns KP (1981) An experimental analysis of acquisition, generalization, and maintenance of naming behavior in a patient with anomia. In Brookshire RH (Ed) Clinical Aphasiology Conference Proceedings. Minneapolis, MN: BRK Publishers. pp 35-45.

Thompson CK, McReynolds LV (1986). Wh.. interrogative production in agrammatic aphasia: an experimental analysis of auditory-visual stimulation and direct-production treatment. Journal of Speech and Hearing Research 29:193-206.

Vignolo L (1964) Evolution of aphasia and language rehabilitation: a retrospective exploratory study. Cortex 1:344-67.

Weisenberg T, McBride KE (1935) Aphasia: A Clinical and Psychological Study. New York: Communwealth Fund.

Wepman JM (1951) Recovery From Aphasia. New York: Ronald Press.

Wertz RT (1985) Neuropathologies of speech and language: an introduction to patient management. In Johns DF (Ed) Clinical Management of Neurogenic Communicative Disorders, 2nd ed. Boston, MA: Little, Brown, and Company. pp 1-96.

Wertz RT (1991) Predictability: greater than p <.05. In Prescott TE (Ed) Clinical Aphasiology, Volume 19. Austin TX: pro-ed. pp 21-30.

Wertz RT (1992) A single case for group treatment studies in aphasia. In Aphasia Treatment: current approaches and research opportunities. NIDCD Monograph 2:25-36.

Wertz RT (1993) Efficacy of various methods of therapy. In Paradis M (Ed) Foundations of Aphasia Rehabilitation. Oxford: Pergamon Press. pp 61–75.

Wertz RT, Deal J, Robinson AJ (1984) Classifying the aphasias: a comparison of the Boston Diagnostic Aphasia Examination and the Western Aphasia Battery. In Brookshire RH (Ed) Clinical Aphasiology Conference Proceedings. Minneapolis, MN: BRK Publishers. pp 40-7.

Wertz RT, Deal J, Holland AL, Kurtzke JF, Weiss DG (1986) Comments on an uncontrolled no treatment trial. Asha 28:31.

Wertz RT, Collins MJ, Weiss D, Kurtzke JF, Friden T, Brookshire RH, Pierce J, Holtzapple P, Hubbard DJ, Porch BE, West JA, Davis L, Matovitch V, Morley GK, Resurreccion E (1981) Veterans Administration cooperative study on aphasia: a comparison of individual and group treatment. Journal of Speech and Hearing Research 24:580–94.

Wertz RT, Weiss DG, Aden J, Brookshire RH, Garcia-Bunuel L, Holland AL, Kurtzke JF, Lapointe LL, Milianti FJ, Brannegan R, Greenbaum H, Marshall RC, Vogel D, Carter J, Barnes NS, Goodman R (1986) Comparison of clinic, home, and deferred language treatment for aphasia: a Veterans Administration cooperative study. Archives of Neurology 43:653–8.

Zurif EB, Gardner H, Brownell HH (1989) The case against the case against group studies. Brain and Cognition 10:237–55.

Subject Index

Author Index

DEDICATION
To Emily, Lucy and their friends, Hayley, Robert, Vicky, Clare, Emma and Laura.

Studies in Disorders of Communication

General Editors:

Professor David Crystal
Honorary Professor of Linguistics, University College of North Wales, Bangor

Professor Ruth Lesser
University of Newcastle upon Tyne

Professor Margaret Snowling
University of York